CRABS HOLT CO

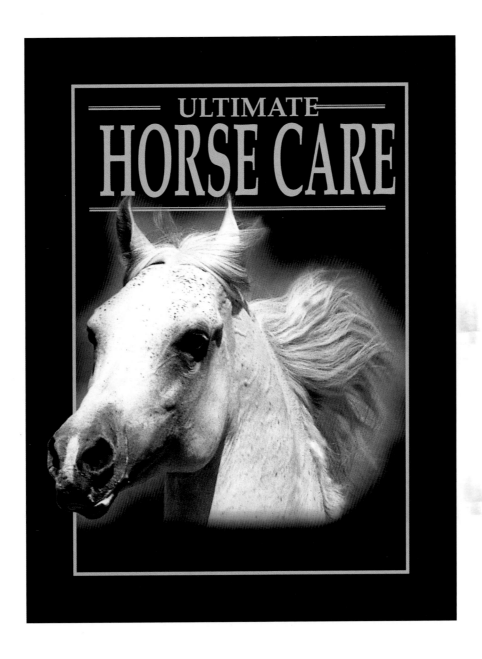

John McEwen BVet, MED, MRCVS

RINGPRESS

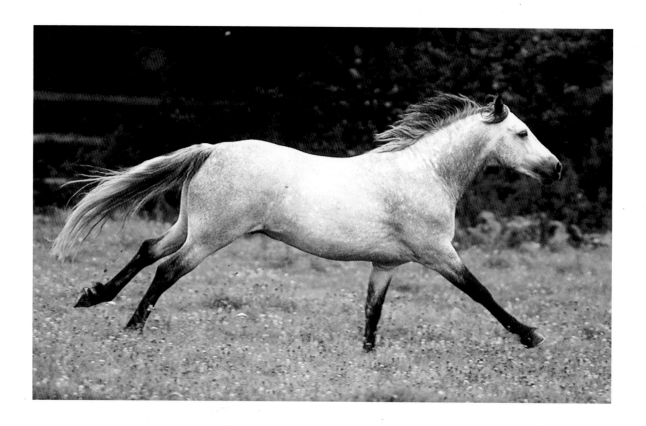

Published by Ringpress Books Ltd,
PO Box 8, Lydney,
Gloucestershire GL15 4YN, United Kingdom.

Project Director: Jackie Budd.
Designed by Rob Benson

The publisher wishes to acknowledge the assistance
of *Your Horse* magazine in the compilation of photographs.

First Published 2000
© 2000 RINGPRESS BOOKS

ISBN 1 86054 186 0

Printed and bound in Singapore through Printworks International Limited

0 9 8 7 6 5 4 3 2 1

CONTENTS

Evolution: The development of the horse. **Nature's horse**: The psychological blueprint. **Implications**: Modern management methods and their impact. **Lifestyles**: Tailoring management to needs. **Communication**: The horse's language.
Practical guides: *Leading • Tying up • Handling the feet • Catching & releasing • Bedding & mucking out • Stable construction • Fencing • Pasture maintenance*

Signs of good health: The grass-kept and stabled horse. **Keeping your horse in good shape**: Feeding; worming; vaccinations; teeth; hoof care. **Causes of disease**: Bacteria; viruses; fungi; parasites. **Signs of ill health**: Indicators to watch for; recognising lameness. **When to call the vet**: Assessing the urgency of a problem. **First aid**: Emergency guidelines; wound care. **Nursing the sick horse**: Priorities for the convalescent.
Practical guides: *Worming • Vaccinations • Teeth care • Grooming • Checking vital signs • Locating the seat of lameness • First aid kit • Giving medication • Methods of restraint • Wound care • Bandaging • Using a poultice • Thrush*

The physiology of digestion: Structure and function of the digestive system. **The horse's nutritional requirements**: Carbohydrates; fats & oils; protein; vitamins & minerals; water. **Types of feedstuffs**: Forage; concentrates; supplements & additives. **Rationing**: Condition scoring; working out a ration. **Practical feeding**: The feeding behaviour of horses.
Common problems of the digestive system
Mouth & teeth: Lampas; parrot mouth; quidding; wolf teeth; infected teeth; step/wave/shear mouth; enamel hooks; eruption cysts. *Digestive disorders*: Dehydration; choke; colic (veterinary examination; immediate care; types of colic; treatments); grass sickness; peritonitis; diarrhoea; poisoning; liver disease. *Urinary disorders*: Renal failure; bladder/kidney stones; cystitis; polynephritis. *Laminitis*: Recognising the signs; causes; feeding the laminitic; shoeing the laminitic.
Practical guides: *The rules of feeding • The rules of watering • Practical feeding: hay • Practical feeding: concentrates • Poisonous plants • Avoiding laminitis*

The physiology of movement: Structure & function of bone; the skeleton; structure & function of joints; the major joints of movement; structure & function of muscle; the major muscle groups; tendons & ligaments. **The horse's foot**: Insensitive & sensitive structures; limb & hoof assessment; the well-shod foot; keeping feet healthy; future trends in farriery. **The dynamics of motion**: Description of movement; the stay apparatus; the reciprocal apparatus; fore-limb and hind-limb movement; gaits.
Common disorders of the locomotive system
Tendonitis (bowed tendons); sweeney; ringbone; locking patella; fibrotic myopathy; osteochondrosis; splints; arthritis; bone spavin; windgalls & bog spavin. *The foot*: Navicular disease; sidebone; pedal ostitis; injury to the coronary band; cracks; corns; infection in the foot.
Practical guides: *Gaits • Interference • Bony & soft tissue enlargements • The hot shoeing process • Routine care – the unshod foot • Routine care – the shod foot*

THE CARDIOVASCULAR SYSTEM
The physiology of circulation: Structure & function of the peripheral cardiovascular system. **The heart**: Structure & functioning of the heart. **How the cardiovascular system works**: The effects of exercise. **Signs of heart disease**: Investigating heart disease; heart problems & pre-purchase examinations; breeding & heart disease. **Blood**: Blood sampling; anaemia.
Conditions of the cardiovascular system
Heart murmurs; regurgitations (leakage from valves); endocarditis; abnormal heart rhythms (arrhythmias).
Lymphatic system
Filled legs/lymphangitis.

THE RESPIRATORY SYSTEM
The physiology of respiration: Structure & function of the respiratory system; respiration during exercise. **Clinical signs of respiratory disease.**

Diseases & disorders of the respiratory system
Infectious diseases: Equine influenza; equine herpes; equine viral arteritis. *Bacterial diseases:* Strangles; Rhodococcus equi pneumonia; pleuropneumonia. *Parasitic diseases:* Lungworm; parascaris equorum infection. *Allergic respiratory diseases:* Chronic obstructive pulmonary disease; summer-associated obstructive pulmonary disease. *Diseases of the nasal cavities & para-nasal sinuses:* Sinusitis; progressive ethmoidal haemotoma. *Diseases of the guttural pouches:* Guttural pouch tympany, empyema/chondroids & mycosis. *Upper airway obstructions:* Recurrent laryngeal neuropathy; dorsal displacement of the soft palate; epiglottic entrapment.
Practical guides: Dust-free management

The nervous system: Structure and function of the nervous system; the spinal cord; reflexes; the peripheral nervous system. **The endocrine system:** Hormones & how they work; the major glands. **The senses:** Sight; hearing; smell; taste; skin and touch. **Learning and memory:** Intelligence, training and memory.

Disorders of the nervous & endocrine systems
Changes in behaviour: Stable 'vices'; head-shaking; self-mutilation; narcolepsy/cataplexy; trauma; hepatic encephalopathy. *Seizures and fits:* Meningitis; epilepsy. *Head and facial abnormalities:* Horner's Syndrome; facial nerve paralysis; trigeminal nerve trauma; vestibular lesions. *Weakness and in-coordination:* Cerebellar hypoplasia/abiotrophy; botulism; spinal cord trauma; vertebral body abscess/osteomyelitis; 'Wobbler' Syndrome; equine degenerative myeloencephalopathy; stringhalt; 'shivering'. *Tumours:* Cushing's Disease. *Paralysis:* Tetanus; radial nerve paralysis; peroneal nerve paralysis; foaling paresis; polyneuritis equi; sacral trauma.

Disorders of the eye
Entropion; eyelid lacerations; conjuncitivitis; corneal abrasions & ulcers; keratitis; uveal disorders; cataracts; retinal disease; optic nerve disease; sarcoids; squamous cell carcinoma; lymphosarcoma; pseuda-tumours.
Practical guides: 'Vice' prevention: lowering stress levels

The skin: Structure and functions of the skin

Disorders of the skin
Pruritis (itching): Insect-bite hypersensitivity/sweet itch; contact dermatitis; louse infestation; chorioptic mange. *Wheals:* Urticaria. *Fungal diseases:* Dermatophytosis/ringworm. *Bacterial diseases:* Dermatophilosis folliculitis & furunculosis/acne.
Photo-sensitisation
Nodules: Collagen granuloma; abscesses; sarcoids; melanoma; papillomatosis/warts; aural plaques; epidermoid cysts.
Practical guides: Prevention & management of sweet itch • Prevention & management of mud fever/greasy heel

Fitting saddlery: Listen to your horse; evaluating new approaches to saddle fit. **Rugs/blankets:** Choosing and fitting horse clothing. **Leg protection:** Fitting and using boots and bandages. **Clipping:** Selecting a suitable clip and the clipping process. **Pulling & trimming:** The right way to a smarter 'look'. **Show preparation:** Bathing, plaiting and final touches. **Travelling:** Methods of transport, travel clothing, hints for trouble-free loading and travelling.
Practical guides: Conventional rules for correct saddle fit (English) • Fitting martingales • Fitting the bridle and bit • Types of rug & rug fitting • Types of boot and their fit • Using exercise bandages • Care of equipment • Clipping • Trimming • Pulling • Bathing • Plaiting the mane • Plaiting the tail • Putting on a tail bandage • Transporting horses

CONTRIBUTORS

EDITOR: JOHN McEWEN BVet, MED, MRCVS has a varied and wide experience in veterinary matters in respect of the competition horse, having been in equine veterinary practice for the last 30 years. Veterinary surgeon to the British show jumping team since 1978 and to the British dressage team since 1984, he also has wide experience of three-day eventing, having assisted at four Olympic Games and major national three-day Championships and has experience in the endurance riding world having been on the jury of appeal for the 1993 and 1997 European Championships (senior and junior). He has been a veterinary surgeon for the Fédération Equestré Internationale (FEI) since the early 1980s.

Senior Veterinary Surgeon to Bath and Chepstow Racecourses, John is also an advisor to the British Equine Veterinary Association, on matters involving equine transportation and EU regulations.

He is Chairman of the International Treating Veterinary Surgeons Association which was created to improve the welfare of the competition horse and to liaise with the FEI veterinary committee on related matters. He has recently been appointed to the FEI veterinary committee.
See Chapter Nine: The Competition Horse.

PROJECT DIRECTOR: JACKIE BUDD is the author of 10 books on horse management and behaviour, including *Reading the Horse's Mind*. She is a regular contributor to *Your Horse*, the UK's best-selling equestrian magazine.
See Practical panels.

DR FRANCIS BURTON PhD has studied horse behaviour for more than 20 years, and has published work on the vomeronasal organ and Flehmen behaviour. In 1990, he received a PhD degree in physiology from Glasgow University, where he currently lectures. Since 1996, he has been Chairman and Scientific Editor of the Equine Behaviour Forum, a unique, voluntary, non-profit-making group which aims to advance the sympathetic management of horses by promoting a better understanding of the horse's mind.
See Chapter Six: The Horse's World (The nervous system and endocrine system; The senses; Learning and memory).

J. MARK CRAIG BVSc, Cert SAD, MRCVS qualified as a veterinary surgeon in 1985. After five

years in general veterinary practice, Mark followed a residency programme in Large Animal Dermatology at the Royal Veterinary College in Hertfordshire where he dealt regularly with referred equine dermatology cases. As well as teaching, he was involved in clinical research projects on the use of evening primrose oil and fish oil in horses with allergies. He obtained his post-graduate certificate in dermatology in 1993. Since finishing the residency programme, Mark has set up his own referral dermatology service in the south of England and the Midlands.
See Chapter Seven: The Skin.

CHRISTOPHER DAY MA, VetMB, MRCVS, VetFFHom is acknowledged as a leading expert on veterinary homoeopathy, giving lectures and holding courses throughout the world. He qualified in Veterinary Medicine from Cambridge University in 1972. He also studied Agricultural Sciences while at Cambridge, useful for his current work on health programmes for organic farms.

He now runs the Alternative Veterinary Medicine Centre in rural south Oxfordshire.

He is a founder member of the British Association for Veterinary Homoeopathy of which he has been Hon. Sec. for approaching twenty years. He gained Membership of the Faculty of Homoeopathy in 1987 and established courses for veterinarians, later becoming Veterinary Dean of the Faculty. In 1991, he was elected Fellow, for his services to homoeopathy.

From 1980, he studied acupuncture, which is now also a major part of his practice along with herbalism and other alternatives. He is External Assessor for the IVAS/ABVA Veterinary Acupuncture courses, which are held at Exeter University. He was the first President of the International Association for Veterinary Homoeopathy and is currently serving a second term of office.
See Chapter Eleven: Alternative Approaches (Introduction; Herbalism; Homoeopathy; Acupuncture).

ROBERT EUSTACE BVSc, Cert EO, Cert EP, FRCVS spent nine years in equine practice in the UK, Eire and Australia before becoming a lecturer in equine studies at Liverpool University. During this period he gained Royal College of Veterinary Surgeons Certificate qualifications in equine practice orthopaedics.

In 1988, he established the Laminitis Clinic as a

referral centre at Bristol University, where he developed a new plastic and steel adjustable shoe for the treatment of laminitis, founder and sinker cases. He published the book *Explaining Laminitis and its Prevention* in 1992. Robert was awarded the Diploma of Fellowship of the Royal College of Veterinary Surgeons for his thesis 'Radiological measurement involved in the prognosis of equine laminitis' in 1993. The Laminitis Clinic moved to purpose-built premises at Dauntsey, Wiltshire, in 1993. In 1997, Robert founded the Laminitis Trust, a registered charity dedicated to supporting laminitis research.
See Chapter Three: Feeding and Nutrition (Laminitis).

TONY GILMORE AMC learnt the value of correct spinal mechanics after receiving treatment, as a child, from John McTimoney, who had developed his human chiropractic technique to encompass vertebrate animals.

Tony was one of the initial batch of students at the McTimoney Chiropractic School (later College). An early Principal of that College, Tony assisted in the development of its animal course and has seen the hard work of the tutors rewarded when the McTimoney Course was awarded the first external validation for a course in animal manipulation. He continues to teach as one of the course's practical tutors.

Tony has worked in all disciplines in equine sport, treating at one time horses for seven separate Olympic teams, and currently has an extremely busy practice treating racehorses.
See Chapter Eleven: Alternative Approaches (Chiropractic).

JANE VM HASTIE (NEE NIXON) MA, VetMB, BSc, MRCVS qualified as a veterinary surgeon at Cambridge University in 1978. She has spent the last 20 years almost solely in equine practice. Jane has a particular interest in the examination of horses for purchase and breeding, and production of the sports horse. She enjoys all aspects of the horse and has owned, produced and ridden internationally top-class working hunters for the last 15 years.
Contributions to Chapter Two: The Horse in Health and Sickness.

TIM MAIR BVSc, PhD, DEIM, MRCVS graduated from the University of Bristol in 1980. After two years in general practice, he returned to the University to undertake research into respiratory disease in the horse. He was awarded a PhD for this work in 1986. He then stayed at Bristol as lecturer in equine internal medicine until 1989 when he returned to specialist equine practice. He obtained the Diploma in Equine Internal Medicine in 1997. He is currently a partner at the Bell Equine Veterinary Clinic in Kent, with particular interests in equine medicine and soft tissue surgery.
See Chapter Five: Life Support Systems (Respiratory system; Disorders of the respiratory system).

SUSAN McBANE has been described by The Equestrian Society book club as "one of Britain's most highly respected equestrian authors". She has been a professional writer and editor for many years, having produced 39 books and having edited two commercial magazines. She is currently editor of Equine Behaviour, the Equine Behaviour Forum's magazine. She has life-long experience of looking after and riding horses in many different disciplines. She teaches classical riding and is a Shiatsu for Horses practitioner.
See Chapter One: Management and Mentality.

JACQUELYN McCANN BVSc, Cert EM (Int med), MRCVS
See Chapter Three: Feeding and Nutrition (Disorders of the digestive system, including colic).

ROBERT OLIVER is one of the country's leading riders and producers of show horses, including hunters, hacks, cobs and riding horses. Robert is a worldwide judge of horses and ponies, and a council member of British Show Hack, Cob and Riding Horse Association and British Light Horse Breeding Society. He is a former master and field master of the Ledbury Foxhounds, and has written several books on showing and stable management.
See Chapter Twelve: Conformation.

DR MARK PATTESON MA, VetMB, PhD, DVC, Cert VR, MRCVS qualified from Cambridge in 1986 and has worked in practice and at the University of Bristol Veterinary School. He holds the Diploma in Veterinary Cardiology, and a PhD for his work in equine cardiology. He is one of only six RCVS Specialists in Veterinary Cardiology. He has written many papers and book chapters on equine cardiology and has spoken at meetings in Britain, continental Europe and the USA.

Mark runs a referral service in cardiology and diagnostic imaging in Berkeley, Gloucestershire, and visits other clinics across the UK and Ireland.
See Chapter Five: Life Support Systems (Circulatory system; Disorders of the circulatory system).

SARAH PILLINER BSc Hons, MSc, BHS Stablemanager is an equine consultant, nutritionist, lecturer, riding instructor and author. She is involved in the development and monitoring of horse care qualifications through her work as an Associate Inspector for the Training Standards Council and as a consultant for the Animal Care and Equine National

Training Organisation. Sarah is Training and Development Officer for the British Horse Trials Association and also tries to find time to ride two event horses.
See Chapter Three: Feeding and Nutrition (The digestive system; Nutritional needs; Planning a diet; Practical feeding).

FIONA POOLE BVSc, MRCVS qualified from Bristol in 1994, and worked at John McEwen's practice for three years while studying for her Equine Certificate. She is currently travelling to expand her knowledge.
Contributions to Chapter Ten: The Next Generation.

JANICE M. POSNIKOFF DVM is a graduate of the Western College of Veterinary Medicine, Saskatoon, Saskatchewan, Canada. She completed her internship at Chino Valley Equine Hospital, Chino, CA, then entered – and is currently practising with Equine Medical Associates, Tustin, CA. Janice is co-author of a monthly column 'Vet on Call' for Horse Illustrated and is co-author of Horses for Dummies.
See Chapter Four: The Horse in Motion (Nature and function of bone and muscle; Joints; The lower limb, tendons and ligaments; Motion; Disorders of the locomotive system).

HAYDN PRICE DWCF has been running a mixed farriery practice for the last 16 years, covering all aspects of farriery, including performance-related equines. A farriery referral unit for specialist areas is linked with the practice.
See Chapter Four: The Horse in Motion (The Horse's Foot).

SIDNEY RICKETTS LVO, BSc, BVSc, DESM, FRCVS is senior consultant to the Royal Stud Farm at Sandringham and was made Lieutenant of the Victorian Order (LVO) in Her Majesty the Queen's Birthday Honours. Sidney is an Honorary Member of BEVA and has developed an international reputation in the field of equine reproductive physiology and clinical pathology.
Contributions to Chapter Ten: The Next Generation.

JO SHARPLES BHSAI is an experienced rider and horse owner who has worked extensively with equine behaviour specialist Richard Maxwell. She worked for several years as a writer for *Your Horse* magazine.
See Chapter Eight: The Horse in Work, Chapter Twelve: Identification and description; (Breeds and types; Colours and marking).

BEN STURGEON MRCVS qualified from the University of Edinburgh, befor spending time as the house physician at the University of Dublin and moving into the Large Animal Practice Teaching Unit at the Easter Bush Veterinary Centre Royal (Dick) School of Veterinary Studies, Edinburgh. He is currently completing a residency in equine medicine. Special interests include vascular and internal medicine.
See Chapter Six: The Horse's World (Disorders of the nervous system).

LESLEY ANN TAYLOR is a qualified stable manager and riding instructor, and has taught in the UK as well as in the US. With an interest in complementary healing, Lesley trained as a massage therapist. Having seen the benefits of massage for both horses and riders, Lesley now promotes an holistic approach to training.
See Chapter Eight: The Horse in Work (Fitting saddlery).

MARY BROMILEY FCSP, SRP, RPT (USA) is a Chartered Physiotherapist. She works with both humans and animals, and pioneered the work of transferring human physiotherapy techniques to animals. She runs weekend and career courses in Equine Sports Massage at the Equine Rehabilitation Unit.
See Chapter Eleven: Alternative Approaches (physiotherapy).

1 MENTALITY AND MANAGEMENT

EVOLUTION

The route horses took through evolution is no secret; the fossil record is clear about it, and this background, combined with knowledge of the types of environment in which horses' ancestors developed, gives us a clear picture of the sort of animals horses are.

OUT OF THE PRIMORDIAL SOUP

By the time the modern horse's most distant direct ancestor, Eohippus or Hyracotherium, had become established about 55 million years ago, it was already a fairly advanced fox-sized mammal, far up its branch of the evolutionary tree from the single-celled organisms which were the roots of all life. It was well able to control its own body chemistry and temperature and reproduced sexually rather than by primitive means. Not only did it eat and drink rather than absorb nutrients through its cell walls, it was actually specialised as a herbivore and already had a strong instinct to stay alive by foraging on leaves, berries and fruits and by avoiding predation.

The earth's environment then was mainly tropical, swampy forest and Hyracotherium was probably striped and/or mottled for camouflage in the dappled forest light. It is difficult to get up any speed in dense forest, so this would not have been a fast animal, but one scuttling and hiding rather than running from danger.

The wariness and alertness still generally prevalent in the horse family stems from its going down the prey-animal route rather than the carnivorous hunter route. Hyracotherium was probably solitary: the modern herd lifestyle had not developed and was not possible in thick forest. Many experts believe that this environment provided the root of the horse's

jumping ability, denying that most horses do not jump naturally (anyone who has seen an untrained youngster jump nonchalantly out of a field or over a ditch or fallen tree must agree). Fallen trees would have formed a daily part of Hyracotherium's life and would be negotiated when scurrying away from predators into the forest's protecting darkness.

THE WONDERS OF WEATHER

Over millions of years, the ubiquitous tropical forests gradually receded as a new phenomenon made its presence felt – changing climate. As the Earth's climate very gradually developed into bands and zones, weather as we know it appeared. Tropical forest eventually settled in a broad belt around the equator, with the climate gradually cooling to north and south until intense cold became established around the poles.

ADAPT OR PERISH

Parts of the Earth also experienced several glaciations, or Ice Ages, leading to the extinction of those species unable to adapt to the cold and the changes it brought in the availability of food and water. Some, though, changed to better fit them to the new conditions and others developed the habit of migrating to friendlier climes.

The land masses were changing through volcanic activity, moving, separating and colliding. This both created new migration routes for the spread of species and cut off others, isolating them to develop in highly specific ways. These millions of years of tremendous upheaval had a great effect on the Earth's flora and fauna, but how did they affect horses? With the changing climate came new environments – deciduous forests, coniferous forests, steppe, tundra, desert, scrub and, the most

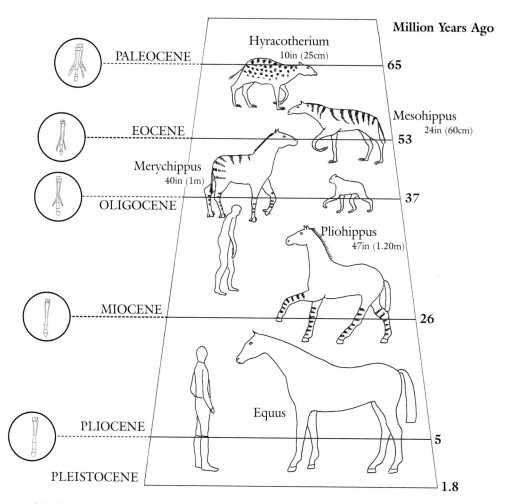

The evolutionary tree of the horse, showing the most important zoological groups and corresponding geological epochs. The insets of the lower foreleg are drawn to a larger scale and illustrate the development of the hoof.

significant for many horse types, open grasslands.

Species adaptation occurs through genetics. Genes can change or mutate, giving a species different mental and physical traits which may, or may not, enable them to exist in a new environment. Hyracotherium was followed by many successors which mutated in this way, enabling them exist and thrive in their new environment.

As surroundings became open, predators could see their targets easily. The prey animals had to develop speed to run away rather than rely on hiding, and the predators had to develop the traits of creeping up on them and the speed to run and catch them. The evolving horse types developed elongated, more powerful, longer-striding legs and the number of toes gradually reduced to one – an ultimate specialisation for speed.

Hyracotherium's teeth had been fairly small and

weak – all it needed to chew its fairly soft food – with a correspondingly small head and short neck. It browsed at all levels and was small. But grass is tough and grows on the ground, so the head and neck had to lengthen so that the animals could reach down from above their longer legs, and the teeth had to become big and strong.

Another change was in the body and digestive system of the evolving horse. Grass is less nutritious than the berries, fruits and young leaves available all year round in the formerly season-less tropical forests. The horse's ancestors had to eat more and more grass to obtain enough nourishment. This called for a capacious digestive system geared to processing large amounts of bulky fibre passing through it constantly. A larger abdomen was needed which was much heavier (due to its content of gut and grass), necessitating a stronger, longer spine to support the gut which is suspended from it. The whole body had to be balanced and developed to support its own weight, to digest grass almost constantly and to be able to instantly get up high speed to escape predators.

The trait of alertness developed in the horse, working in conjunction with very acute senses for detecting predators: eyes high up on the head to see above the grass and almost radar-like ears with which to pick up the smallest sound from long distances in any direction. Another phenomenon developed in horses – that of living in herds. They learned that predators usually killed only one animal per hunt, whose carcass lasted them for days. By living among others of your kind, the likelihood of that individual being you was greatly reduced.

WHAT ARE WE LEFT WITH?
This unimaginably slow evolutionary process has created, in the horse, one of the most specialised animals in the world. One so specialised that, had it not possessed, in Man's eyes, more useful and attractive physical and psychological qualities than any other animal, it would by now almost certainly be extinct. This is not an unreasonable claim, given how Man's extreme fecundity and, hence, his propensity not only for farming every square metre of the planet he possibly can but also for hunting to excess every creature which takes his fancy, has already ensured that there are no truly wild horses left. The legacy of evolution has left us with an animal we generally find physically beautiful, spiritually appealing, fast, strong, 'trainable', sociable and, above all, adaptable.

NATURE'S HORSE – THE PSYCHOLOGICAL BLUEPRINT

Nature's aim is the survival of entire species, not the welfare or survival of individuals. This may seem strange, because unless the individual members of a species survive, the species itself will not. In practice, however, the natural system works admirably.

When horses lived naturally, the loss of individuals was commonplace, as it is within remaining free-living equine species such as zebra. The carnivores responsible for most of these losses survive by means of mental cunning and physical prowess: they have to be wily enough to stalk their prey, fast and agile enough to catch it (as in the case of the cat family) or with the endurance to wear it down (the way of the dog family), and strong or clever enough to

bring it down, solely or with help, and to kill it.

The prey animals have to be alert to every rustle in the grass and every shadow in a bush. They must be mentally able to read the predators' body language and intelligent enough to assess whether they are in hunting mode or merely passing through. In the final analysis, they must be not only wary enough not to let a hunter get too close but also physically strong and fast enough to be able to keep out of its reach during the ultimate chase.

The horse's mentality, that of a typical herbivorous prey animal, became formed during millions of years of this lifestyle. Like any animal, its main drives are survival and reproduction which together achieve Nature's overall aim – the survival of the species.

SURVIVAL
To survive, wild and feral equidae need six things:-

1. *Food*, usually found all around, growing on the ground. Horses developed migratory habits, where possible moving on from a grazed-down area to fresh pastures sometimes many miles or kilometres away. However, their food supply is subject to seasonal growth and it is natural for feral horses and other wild equidae to lose weight in winter. The 'autumn flush' of carbohydrate-rich grass helps, but this is an individual survival test: those not able to store and metabolise their body-fat to best effect will have starved by the time the spring flush comes, so will be unable to breed and perpetuate their weakness. Their bodies provide food for others. It is Nature's way.

2. *Water*, often not so readily available, but within reasonable trekking distance. Some feral horses or ponies, depending on their locations, are observed regularly to drink only once a day, usually in the evening. Zebras have been seen to drink only every few days when their preferred grazing grounds are many kilometres from the water holes. Watering points are dangerous places where predators, knowing the food must come eventually, lie in wait.

3. *Shelter* from the elements, or an effective skin and coat. Horses developed thick or thin skins, and coarse, wiry hair coats or finer ones, according to the type of protection needed in the climate where they and their ancestors developed. Some horses live in totally exposed areas, others in regions where there is ample shelter from cliffs, hills and woods. Feral horses are not, however, prone to sheltering in caves, which attract predators.

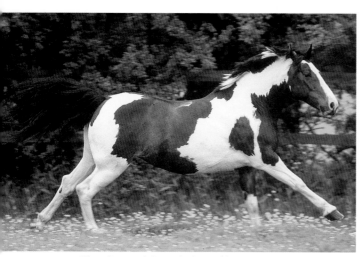

The winner of the evolutionary lottery was Equus, a wary plains-dweller specialised for speed.

4. The safety of numbers in the herd. *Company* is crucial to a feeling of security for most horses, certainly feral ones. Lone horses are at great risk, although they do exist, if not by choice. When colts reach puberty the herd stallion usually banishes them from the herd (and this can happen with fillies, too). Until these individuals can find other rejects to join in a bachelor band, or are able to take over a herd or gather some mares or fillies of their own, they wander alone, surely bewildered and frightened. Solitude is an unnatural state for horses.

5. *Space* all around them to survey their surroundings and to run away when necessary. Horses as a species seem, understandably, to be claustrophobic. Given a choice, they choose the

highest ground on which to rest as this offers the best vantage point and view of danger for many miles around. Feral horses grazing on low ground or in valleys are known to post lookouts on higher ground, and to take their turn on watch. Domestic horses instinctively do the same, if their surroundings permit.

6. Finally, to survive in Nature (and, indirectly, in domesticity, too), horses need physical strength and agility, translated in domestic horses as *athleticism* due to the work we demand of many of them. Horses are big animals weighing around 500kg or about half a ton. They spend little time lying down, particularly flat-out asleep, as they are at their most vulnerable like this, when vital seconds lost getting up can mean the difference between being caught by a predator or escaping. Even so, most will lie down sometimes but must be able to get to their feet and accelerate to their top speed in less than four or five seconds. Sheer speed is needed, with an element of endurance to keep going once a horse realises it is him or her that the hunter is after.

REPRODUCTION

Reproduction is one of the horse's strongest instincts (it even stops them eating sometimes!). Survival of the species being paramount in Nature's scheme of things, it is not surprising that during spring, summer and early autumn, feral horses (and those of their domestic counterparts free to do so) are greatly preoccupied with giving birth to the results of last year's activities and with courting and mating and nurturing foals until they are able to cope on their

Freedom, food, space, society: herd living on the open grasslands provided all that was needed for the survival of Nature's horse.

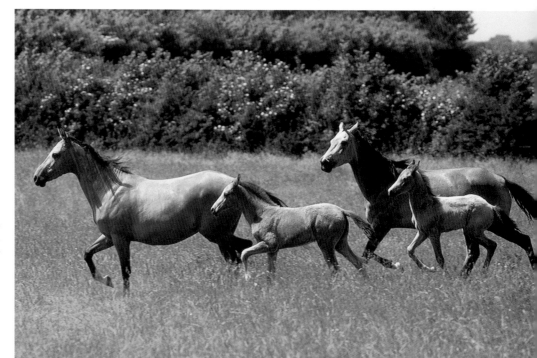

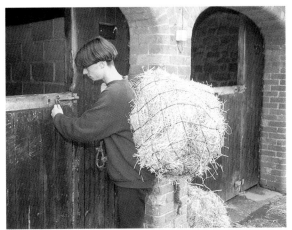 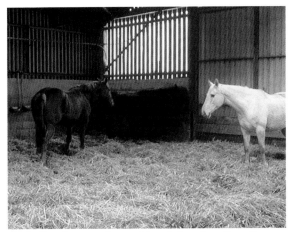

Occupying the digestive system by the increased use of low-energy, high-fibre forage and organising shelter that allows for some natural exercise with company, are two ways of adapting domestication to suit the horse's natural lifestyle.

own. Mares come into season mainly due to lengthening daylight hours but also to climatic temperature and availability of food. Mating can occur repeatedly for a few days till the stallion's chosen mare-of-the-moment goes out of season.

Besides impregnating his mares, the herd stallion will take a great interest in his own foals (although he may kill a previous stallion's foals). Although it is the dam-foal unit which is the most important in ensuring the survival of the next generation, the stallion will play a role in socialising them.

IMPLICATIONS

We have discussed the qualities horses possess which make them so attractive to us – their strength, speed and spirit, their sociability, adaptability and relative ease of training. We know very well what kind of animal Nature created – a fast-running, almost constantly grazing and moving animal which feels safest living in close (tactile) contact with its own kind and in open spaces where it can scan the horizon for trouble.

That being so, why do we persist in so often managing horses in a way which is completely alien to the lifestyle described? Sometimes isolated, often unable to touch and communicate properly with others, frequently confined most of the time to small (expensive) cells in which they can barely walk, if at all, let alone gallop, and which are usually closed in above and on three sides allowing the horse only one outlook? The answer is simple: for our convenience.

Another question: that being so, why is it that so many generations of domesticated horses have not only survived but appear to have thrived under this

totally inappropriate management? Answer: because the horse is so extremely adaptable. This single, overall quality of adaptability is the main reason for the horse's continuing existence on Earth. By adapting to Man's changing requirements, the horse has ensured his survival.

One final question: if horses are doing so well, our management of them cannot be so very wrong, can it? The answer to this requires some explanation.

WHAT WENT WRONG?
Some types of horse, usually the quieter or more stolid types, and particularly those given several (not just one or two) hours of work or exercise a day, do seem content, physically healthy and secure in their routine. Most horses in the westernised world, however, are privately owned leisure mounts used for sport or casual pleasure riding. For the most part, these individuals are under-exercised, over-confined, very short of social contact and mental occupation and inappropriately fed.

Research suggests that well over three-quarters of horses kept in traditional westernised (note the small 'w') management systems, where they are individually stabled with insufficient fibrous food and exercise, show behavioural abnormalities of some kind. These are not merely formal stable vices, but other abnormal actions such as head twisting and tossing, mouthing, regular aggression, leaning/rocking on the stable structure, chewing wood or stable equipment, door-banging, wall-kicking, pawing, 'sulking', lethargy and depression, being unduly temperamental or highly strung or showing generally 'difficult' behaviour. Physical ill-health (mainly respiratory) and injuries also occur due to poor housing and inappropriate exercising.

It is clear, then, that horses do not in fact adapt to our management methods as well as we might think.

A BETTER WAY

Taking the six survival elements detailed in the Nature's Horse section of this chapter, let us see how these can be applied to domestic horses to create a more appropriate lifestyle for them.

1. *Food:* Nowadays, plenty of high-nutrient fibrous feeds are available, such as short-chopped forage feeds (often based on alfalfa) and haylage (hay that is cut and sealed before the drying process is complete), commercially or farm-produced. This can replace moderate hay and much cereal-based concentrate such as oats, barley and maize or corn, large quantities of which do not suit the horse's fibre-geared digestive system. Such fibrous feeds produce excellent work results without favouring metabolic disorders such as colic, azoturia, laminitis, filled legs and so on.

The horse can spend much longer periods of time eating, as he evolved to, remaining occupied and satisfied. The old idea of drastically reducing the horse's fibre (hay) to a third of the diet in hard-working horses has also now been scotched: the ratio of fibre to concentrates should never be less than 50:50 for even the hardest-working horses.

2. *Water:* Most domestic horses have water constantly available and this is the safest way to manage them. It is now known to be dangerous to take away a performance horse's water more than an hour before work. Water passes through the system quickly, and depriving a horse of the chance to drink can make him uncomfortable, interfere with his metabolism and favour dehydration. In very cold climates, water heaters may be needed.

3. *Shelter:* Even the toughest equines appreciate shelter sometimes, but in domesticity they should all, from sensitive Thoroughbreds to hardy natives, have much more choice as to when to use it. Housing, or a paddock shelter, from which the horses can come and go as they need, is not difficult to arrange, with a little imagination. The result is animals who are far more contented than those condemned to either imprisonment or exposure.

4. *Company:* Most horses have a deep need of other equine companionship and, in its absence, latch on to other species as being better than nothing. If horses must be individually stabled, they should be turned loose (not necessarily in a field) with a friend or

friends for several hours a day to meet this need. Stable walls which are solid up to the roof should be abandoned (they do not help prevent the spread of disease) in favour of bars or grilles from back-height upwards, so that compatible neighbours can touch and smell each other. Choose companions carefully, to avoid fighting, stall-kicking and injury.

5. *Space:* Horses should have more than one outlook from stables or covered yards to satisfy their instinctive need to see all around them. Studies in the USA have shown, by monitoring blood pressure, heart rate and skin tension, that domestic horses were calmer and more content with an all-round view. Closed-in stable yards should be opened up where possible so that the occupants can see the surrounding locality.

6. *Exercise:* Physical strength and agility is improved by allowing the horses to exercise at slow, steady gaits, ideally at liberty, as much as possible. The equine body does not thrive optimally on 22 hours of confinement with only one or two hours of abrupt work, despite proper warming up and cooling down. Liberty, horse-walkers, being led from other horses in safe surroundings and long-reining or in-hand walks around the lanes are all recommended. Lungeing should be restricted, as constant circles are physically stressful and mentally boring.

LIFESTYLES

Horses and ponies specialised to survive in different environments. Types evolving in hot climates have differing features from those evolving in cold ones and will need differing management. We classify horses and ponies as hot-bloods or cold-bloods with warm-bloods, obviously, coming in between. Note that these terms refer to the animals' physical and temperamental characteristics, not their body temperatures.

HOT-BLOODS

Commonly called 'blood' horses, these types evolved in hot regions. Needing to lose body heat easily, they have fine coats and thin skins with blood vessels near the surface to allow heat to radiate out through the skin. The fine coat and mane and tail hair assist this. Even the winter coats of such animals are not long and heavy. The head of the hot-blood type is short and relatively narrow with large nostrils, allowing hot air to be breathed out. The ears, which hold plenty of

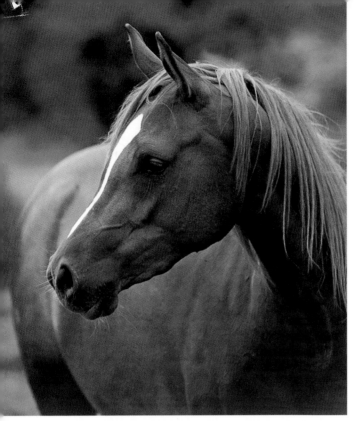

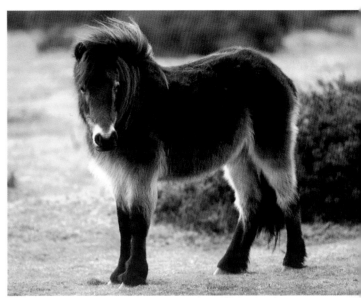

The hot-blood's specialist adaptations to life in a hot, dry climate were physical and psychological. They produced a fine-skinned, narrow-bodied horse that is sensitive and quick to react.

Survival in the harshest of conditions created the cleverness and toughness of the world's native pony breeds and the strength and dependability of its cold-blood draft horses.

blood, are large to dissipate heat, and their necks and bodies are often long and oval-shaped, again to facilitate heat loss in comparison to a more rounded body.

Long legs and a tail held away from the body again assist air circulation and heat loss. Such horses sweat freely as a way of evaporating away heat.

Although some hot-bloods need increased amounts of food to keep weight on, not all do, and Arabs, particularly, are normally 'good doers' or 'easy keepers'.

COLD-BLOODS

These comprise British native ponies and cobs and heavy horse breeds. The main concern of the cold-blood types is retaining heat, so these have larger heads with longer air passages to warm cold air which could otherwise chill lungs and heart, and the nostrils are smaller and narrower. The ears are small and neck short and thick, with a rounded body and short legs. Their tails lie close to the body and the skin sweats less freely. Coats are thicker and longer, creating a greater overlap to retain an insulating warm-air layer next to the skin, and the mane and tail hair is long, thick and wiry for added protection.

Most cold-bloods have super-efficient metabolisms and retain condition with relatively little food (at least, very little concentrate food, much of which is not good for them).

WARM-BLOODS

Cross-breeding between hot-bloods and cold-bloods has produced a huge variety of 'warm-blooded' breeds world-wide. These vary in type depending on their precise ancestry, but breeders have long aimed to combine the class and athleticism of the Thoroughbred and Arab with the toughness and dependability of draft and pony types. They range from the agile and workmanlike American Quarter Horse to performance-bred continental sports horses such as the Trakehner, Holstein and French Selle Francais.

TEMPERAMENT

When deciding on appropriate management, an individual horse's temperament and inclinations are as important as his physical features. Most hot-bloods have alert temperaments, which make them more active than cold-bloods. Some are highly-strung and full of nervous energy, not taking well to a life of confinement. Racing stables (full of young, confined Thoroughbreds) seem to have more than their normal share of stereotypies or stable 'vices', possibly as a direct result of this.

In contrast, most cold-bloods are placid: saving energy conserves heat and insulating body fat, so galloping it off is inadvisable in cold climes.

Naturally there are exceptions to every rule. Some cold-bloods or native types have quite sharp, reactive temperaments and some Thoroughbreds are as placid as old dogs. Thoroughbreds and similar types can also be deceptive as they may stew things up inside, letting out their frustrations in abnormal behaviour in the stable rather than hotting up under saddle.

Many Arabian horses have very gentle if sensitive temperaments – although, due, it seems, to changing fashions in the show ring, this is not so much the case as formerly, in some families.

THE HORSE FOR YOU

Many equestrians have a penchant for a particular breed or type of horse. This is fine, provided that they can provide the facilities and the lifestyle that animal needs. In the UK, problems occur mainly with native ponies and cobs and similar types being kept on over-rich, improved agricultural grassland (quite opposite to their ancestral keep) which causes serious physical problems, particularly laminitis. These types need poor or restricted grazing plus good exercise and yarding with moderate-nutrient hay or forage feeds.

Working owners with restricted turnout facilities and exercise time, conversely, should not take on responsibility for a hot-blood which needs to be on the go much of the time. It is down to every prospective horse owner or carer to be both realistic and responsible. You either have to be able to fit your facilities and time budget to your horse, or buy the type of animal which will be well and content on what you can provide.

DAILY NEEDS

Every horse needs food, water and exercise daily. Those living out may provide for themselves, given facilities, but stabled horses must be waited on 'hand and foot'. The most practical system for most owners and horses, given normal facilities in the UK where yarding is still unusual, is the combined system, in which the horse spends some time stabled and some at grass. Yarded horses live communally and can be kept in together or allowed access to a surfaced pen or to pasture.

Stabled horses need checking early morning, their clothing adjusting, haying up, feeding and watering, with exercise later, followed by grooming. Working owners may quarter (give a brief tidy-up) and exercise first thing, leaving the horse with his breakfast and an ample hay and water supply. Mucking out needs doing early. If someone can check the horse mid-day, he can be hayed-up and watered again, perhaps fed, droppings skipped out (removed) and clothing adjusted, if worn. A walk out would be desirable. In the evening, more exercise should be given and the horse fed, hayed, watered, groomed and mucked out. Quite a day for the working owner!

Using the combined system (depending on the season), the horse can be in during the day (in summer away from flies and sun) or at night (on cold winter nights). When in, he must be provided with ample hay and water, possibly feeding, mucking out and light grooming. 'Man-made' exercise is not essential unless he needs to be fit. Otherwise, treat as grass-kept.

Grass-kept animals must be checked twice daily. A great deal can go wrong in twelve hours! Their water supply must be clean and ample, the fencing and gates checked and their shelter facilities and surrounding ground kept in good shape. To keep

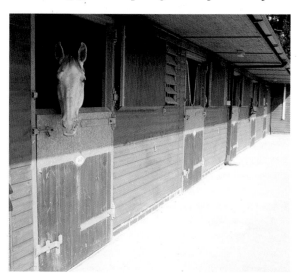

A system where the horse is stabled by night during the winter but turned out by day combines the best of both worlds. Solely grass-kept animals will still require daily supervision.

Stabled horses rely on human help for every need, entailing a heavy commitment in time and expense. Adequate exercise is essential.

LEADING

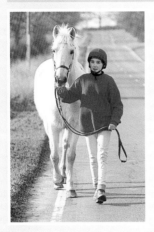

◀ *Horses should be used to being led from both sides to prevent 'one-sidedness' and because they must be led on the public highways with the handler between horse and traffic. Any other practice is highly dangerous. When being led on the highway, a horse should be wearing a bridle. For safety, handlers should wear strong boots and, ideally, gloves and a hard hat.*

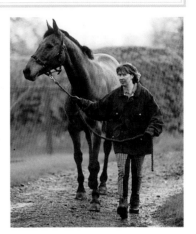

Walk level with the horse's head and neck so ▶ you will not be trodden on should he skip sideways, but far enough in front so he does not catch your heels. Tie a knot on the end of your rope to help prevent its being pulled through your hand. Never wrap it round your hand and always hold up the spare end.

TYING UP

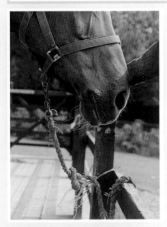

◀ *Horses should only be tied to a wall, fixed fence or other immovable object. Always use a quick-release knot.*

It is often recommended that horses are tied to a string ring (not binder twine which is too strong) which will snap and free the horse should he pull back. However, once a horse has learned that he can break away when tied up, this is likely to become a habit. Short of being re-trained to the halter, such horses should only be tied in enclosed areas where they cannot reach danger, such as a yard with closed gates, and should never be left alone, or they should be held by an assistant. If alone, use a longer rope and learn to work holding it in one hand with your tools.

HANDLING THE FEET

Despite the trust that this involves from a flight animal, horses learn to allow their feet to be picked up relatively easily. It helps if the feet are always done in the same order. Position the horse so his first foot is not bearing much weight, then ask for the hind foot on the same side and work around the horse from there. Stand close alongside the horse, facing the tail.

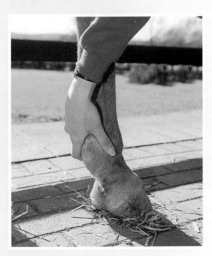

◀ *Get your farrier or vet to show you the spot just above the fetlock where a quick pinch of a nerve will result in a reluctant horse lifting a 'fixed' foot.*

If you need to do a two-handed ▶ job on a foot, learn to hold the foot between your thighs, like a farrier, and if he really plays up just open your knees to free it. Teach your horse that "Stand" means stand, in any position, until you say otherwise.

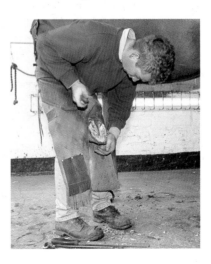

CATCHING AND RELEASING

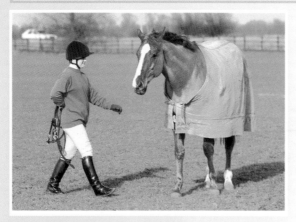

◀ *Approach a loose horse in a relaxed but confident way, avoiding any sudden movements. Hold the headcollar/halter down by your side and walk at an angle towards the horse's shoulder, speaking to warn him of your approach.*

A void taking a bucket into a field where there is more than one horse. A titbit can be kept in the pocket to reward your horse for being caught. Stand alongside and put the lead rope around the neck, then carefully put on the headcollar.

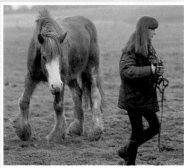

◀ *Reluctant horses usually come if left until last, fearing being alone. If a horse goes away from you, move him on steadily until he becomes fed up and curious. Then walk away as if you do not want him after all, and he is likely to follow. Learn your horse's psychology, as different ones react to different ruses.*

Never let horses charge away from you ▶ when turning loose as it can ultimately break your fingers or leave you vulnerable to a kick. Turn towards the gate, making the horse stand and wait. Remove the headcollar whilst holding the mane at the poll, then release very subtly, stepping back out of harm's way.

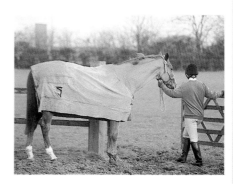

BEDDING AND MUCKING OUT

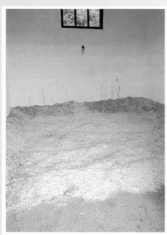

T he whole point of mucking out is to remove droppings and wet bedding! If you would not be happy to spend a night on your horse's bed, then don't expect him to either. Thin, mean beds get dirtier quicker, offer no protection and are cold, and therefore are in no way money-saving.

Banking around the sides helps reduce draughts ▶ and reduces the risk of the horse becoming 'cast'.

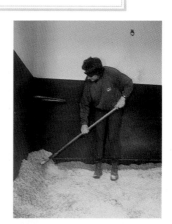

◀ *Even if your horse has no respiratory problems, dust-free bedding is worth the extra cost in cleaner air, horse and clothing (human and equine) and improved health and comfort.*

Wood shavings

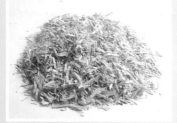

Aubiose (hemp)

Hygiene is all-important. ▶ Deep litter beds, where droppings only are removed and fresh bedding added on top, should be completely cleared at least every 12 weeks. Never put any horse on a former occupant's bedding. Wash and disinfect the box (with horse-safe disinfectant) and put in all fresh bedding.

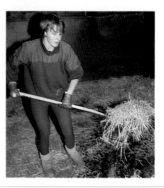

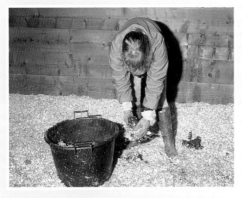

◄ Skipping out regularly helps keep the bed clean.

The muck-heap ▶ should be kept tidy and be situated well away from the stable area.

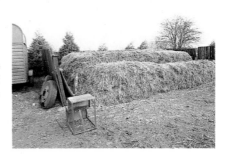

STABLE CONSTRUCTION

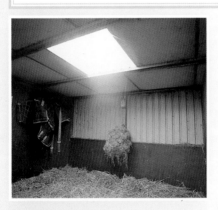

◄ Latest research indicates that, to feel secure, individually-stabled horses need boxes equal to their 'personal space', i.e. 15 ft square minimum. Two settled friends can, however, live in one box of that size.

Good ventilation should be ▶ ensured by windows and ridge-roof ventilators (ideally open-ridge roofs protected by full-length cowling).

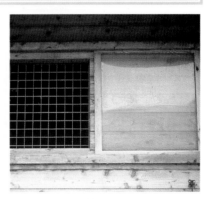

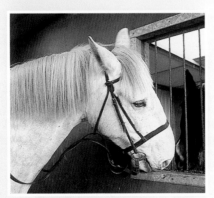

◄ Viewpoints on all sides add to the horses' feeling of security, with closure facilities should strong winds blow right in. 'Talk holes' between boxes in rows give the occupants the reassurance of seeing and sniffing their neighbours.

Most stables are too low for ▶ safety or health. Ceilings should be high enough for a horse to rear (even if he never does) without hitting his head. Doorways must also have the height and width to allow easy access and avoid knocks.

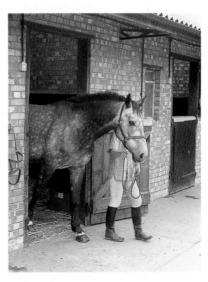

Good repair is essential. Projections within the stable should be avoided and fittings kept to a minimum. Tie rings should be at the horse's head height and hay nets always be well-secured to reach no lower than shoulder level even when empty.

FENCING

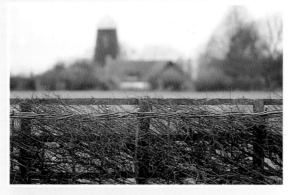

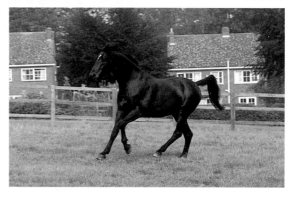

Thick, high, prickly hedges make the best fencing and windbreaks. Whatever other materials you use (wooden posts and rails; flexible synthetics; smooth, taut wire; diamond mesh, etc.), fencing should be very strong, with well-sunk and secure posts, be non-toxic and easily maintained.

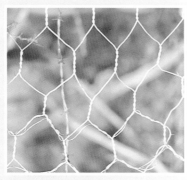

◀ Imagine what injuries your horses could sustain on any particular type of fence – because if you can think of it, they can do it. Barbed wire, square mesh, chicken wire, metal railings (especially with spiked tops) and wooden palings, are all dangerous or too weak.

Gates must be sturdy snd safe, and ▶ be easy to open. For security, try to have all gates opening onto private roads or property, safely blocking off those on public highways.

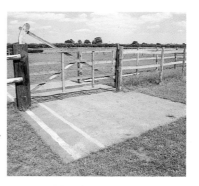

PASTURE MAINTENANCE

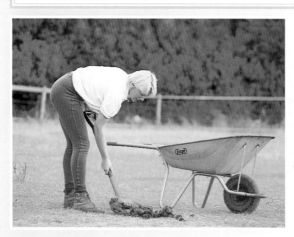

◀ Horse droppings contaminate land with their smell if not removed within 30 minutes! Gradually, lavatory areas spread as horses dung on the edges, cutting down the area they will graze. Spreading land with cattle manure before its annual rest disguises the smell, but check with your vet the implications of hormones or chemicals it may contain.

Picking up droppings is the single most valuable element in preventing parasite infestation. Monitor the pasture regularly for poisonous weeds whose toxins can cause neurological or liver damage.

Cutting or 'topping' any long, rank areas as they ▶ appear will encourage even grazing, as will keeping other livestock such as sheep or cattle, and harrowing (right).

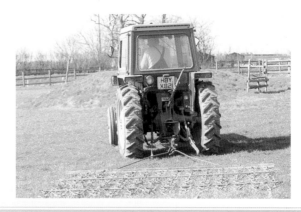

down parasite infestation, droppings must be removed from the field every three days at the longest, more often in warm, moist weather when worms breed most frequently. Rugs (blankets), if worn in winter, must be removed twice daily and changed to dry off, if necessary.

Careful watch must be kept for lice infestation in long coats, and for mud fever on the legs and rain rash on the back. In summer, sore eyes are a sign that your shelter is inadequate. Heavy-cotton fly fringes on breakable headcollars help.

COMMUNICATION

One of the most significant changes for the better in human/horse relationships in recent years, and one which was well overdue, is our increasing interest in and understanding of how horses communicate between themselves and with other animals, including humans.

Only a human generation ago or less, the attitude was very much: "The horse must know who's boss; what he thinks is insignificant; he has to do as he's told and you have to make him or he'll walk all over you." Now, most equestrian magazines feature regular major articles on the horse's point of view of his life and work, improving horse/human relationships, creating a partnership with your horse and so on.

None of this is possible, though, if we do not understand what the horse is saying.

To achieve a harmonious relationship with discipline and mutual respect, as in nature, it is essential for each species to understand the other. Horses learn quickly to associate particular words (which are simply sounds to them) with actions desired. Being minutely perceptive, visually-orientated animals, horses also quickly learn human body language and signals. However, once a person can understand, 'speak' and, ideally, think, in what American horseman and trainer Monty Roberts has called 'equus' (the horse's body language), he or she is able to communicate instantly and surely – back and forth – with any horse. This is the language that horses everywhere understand naturally. As Roberts has pointed out, horses from different lands do not need interpreters.

Conversely, relying upon a strange horse understanding vocal commands can lead to trouble, because the horse may not have been taught the same commands that the handler or rider habitually uses. This can create uncertainty, insecurity, frustration and even anger – and all horse-people know where that can lead.

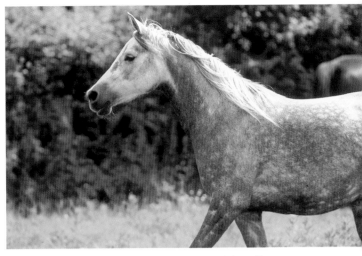

Subtle nuances of posture and muscle tone involving all parts of the body combine to create an overall impression of mood. A healthy and happy horse gives off all the 'vibes' of well-being and satisfaction with life.

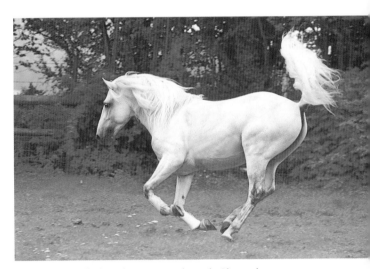

Outline gives the best clue to general mood. Alarmed or aroused, everything is 'up', demanding attention.

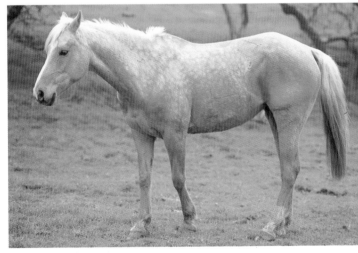

The relaxed horse has a softer, more low-key outline, whereas the dull or uncomfortable animal is noticeably 'down' or 'tucked up'.

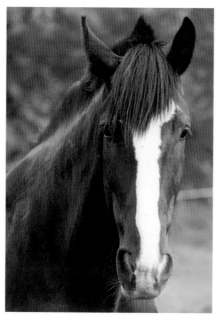

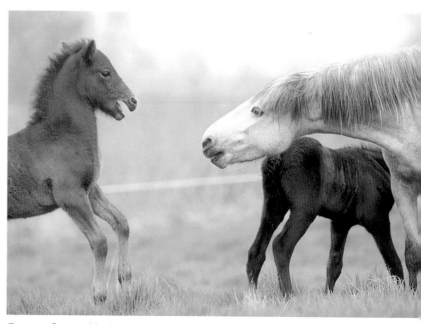

Facial expressions are remarkably varied and expressive. Eyes, muzzle and ears can all convey a range of feeling or intent, from pain, submission or fatigue to interest, alarm or aggression. With their 180 degree rotation ability, ears can operate individually or in tandem to focus on the source of intriguing sounds.

Ears are flattened back out of danger when threatening, or in a fast gallop. Here a foal displays the typical submissive 'mouthing' gesture, signalling to the dominant older horse that he means no harm.

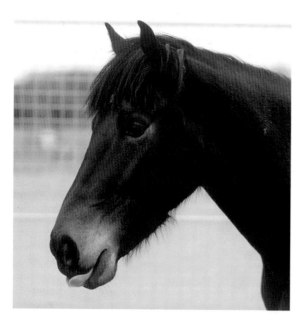

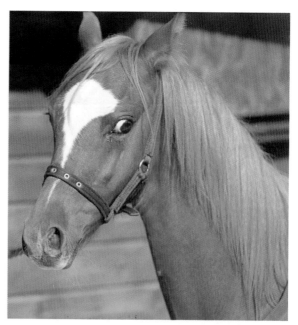

'Licking and chewing' is another sign of submission.

Under stress or in anger, the nostrils and muzzle will tighten in tension and the eyes widen or roll to attempt a better all-round viewpoint.

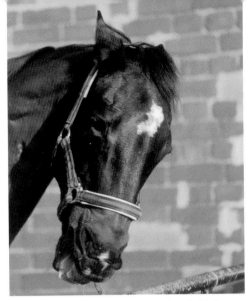

Disgust or discomfort shows in this wrinkled muzzle, lips and eyes.

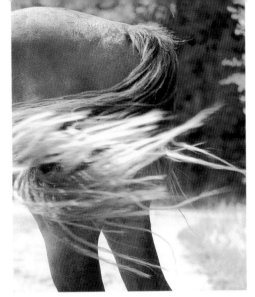

Expression is not confined to the head and neck. A swishing tail demonstrates irritation or anger.

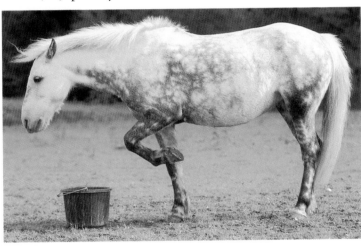

Legs can be used to indicate impatience, as here, or threat behaviour.

A NEW VOCABULARY

So, then, the answer is to learn to understand, speak and think Equus. You can always teach the horse Human as well!

Horses do make vocal sounds and use them regularly. However, their main means of communication is not vocal but visual – a system known as body language. Horses detect and instantaneously translate the slightest nuance of a sign shown by another animal or human. This is essential to their understanding not only herd-mates but also the intentions of predators.

Their general posture and 'air' give the first impression of mood. We can often sense, in horses we know well, how they are feeling simply by 'vibes' and aura, or whatever you want to call it. We just 'know'. Even when other body signs seem to be absent, this can often alert us to slight illness, pain, sadness or discontent. Another day, we know just as surely that, although not particularly active, the horse is feeling fine. This is a sense that grows the more we tune in to horses; it is very noticeable that those with no real feel for them never acquire it.

MORE SPECIFIC SIGNS

The head and neck often give the next impression of mood. Ears pricked forward mean alertness, interest or sometimes alarm. Flopped to the sides they may indicate doziness, relaxation or not feeling well: if to the sides but not relaxed, the horse is listening intently to something he cannot see. Ears pointed back can mean aggression, dislike, fear or simply maximum effort. To decide which, you often have to combine them with the expression in the eyes and, to some, this can be difficult to decipher. It can only be said that a soft or bright, interested light in the eyes means 'good', a hard, sharp one says 'danger' or 'determination' and a dull, glazed or sunken look signifies not feeling good.

Some horses use their muzzles to indicate to humans, for example an empty feed or water tub, an itch that needs scratching or a painful place. They also often bite at their flanks if suffering colic or foaling pains. The nostrils are very expressive: if pulled up, narrowed and wrinkled at the top, this shows aggression, dislike or pain; soft, relaxed nostrils are self-explanatory and rounded, firm (flared) nostrils show great excitement, fear, sometimes distress or, obviously, that the horse is breathing hard after work.

The head and neck held low, with eating motions from the mouth and a submissive or questioning expression, usually indicate submission. However, ears and nostrils hard back and the muzzle outstretched means aggression, and a snaking, side-to-side movement of head and neck is used, not only by stallions, for assertively herding or moving other horses.

A leg stamped usually signifies irritation, often from an insect, or possibly impatience or pain. The horse may turn to look at the place, snap at it or just turn his eyes and ears in its direction.

The tail also indicates mood and will thrash firmly in anger (as opposed to the relaxed swishing at a fly), rise into an arch when excited or interested, clamp between the buttocks if cold or frightened, or just hang relaxed and loose.

GETTING THROUGH

Learning these signs tells you what your horse is thinking, but you can use body postures to inform and even control him.

• A straight-on, square-shouldered, high-headed posture with a confident or even aggressive stare (like a dominant horse) will stop most horses in their tracks and may even send them away from you. To emphasise this, raise your arms and stretch your fingers: all but the most dominant horse will then try to get well out of your reach.

• You can show a friendly intent by slightly drooping your head and shoulders, not looking hard at the horse and standing or walking at an angle to him, as friendly horses do to each other.

• Rubbing a horse on the forehead (even though horses do not do this to each other) and/or withers (which, conversely, is a main spot for mutual communication or grooming) shows him you are friendly and indicates trust if he allows himself to be touched.

Even though our bodies are not the same shape as theirs, horses instantly recognise these postures and actions in humans. By using them automatically, you can understand and communicate clearly with any horse of whatever mood or status – and increase his learning by teaching him your own language, too.

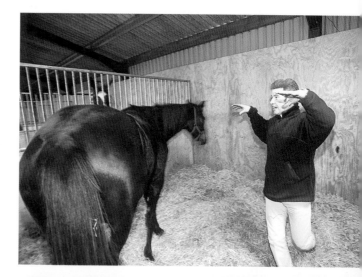

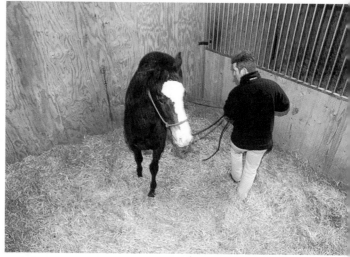

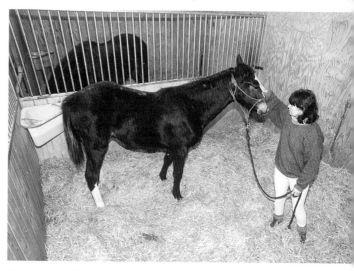

Despite the differing body shape, horses respond to our use of body language signals that correspond to their own.
Top: A dominant posture will cause the horse to back off and move away.
Centre: A rounded, 'low' body shape is unthreatening and invites friendship.
Bottom: Desirable behaviour is rewarded with satisfying contact, through a friendly rub between the eyes.

2 THE HEALTHY HORSE

EARS: *Alert and active. No over-sensitivity on handling. No head-shaking.*

NECK & MANE: *No ridge of fat on the crest. No signs of rubbing or itching.*

BACK: *Well-muscled. No sores or over-sensitivity. Spine easy to feel but not protruding or hidden by layer of fat.*

MUSCLES: *No tension, tightness or spasm.*

HINDQUARTERS: *Rounded and well-muscled, without being fat.*

EYES: *Clear and bright with no discharge. Salmon-pink membranes (eyelids).*

EXPRESSION: *Alert and content.*

TAIL: *No signs of rubbing or itchiness.*

NOSTRILS & MOUTH: *Mucous membranes pink in colour. No nasal discharge.*

ABDOMEN: *Evenly-rounded barrel without any 'pot-belly' (a sign of worms). The ribs can be felt but not seen. No 'poverty lines'.*

TEETH: *In good condition with no sharp edges to the molars.*

BODY CONDITION: *Well-covered, without being fat.*

RESPIRATION: *Breathing not strained when at rest.*

COAT: *Shiny, with no patches of hair loss or sores.*

PASTERNS: *Should be on a straight axis, at a correct angle to the foot.*

HOCKS: *No swellings, lumps or bony enlargements.*

LOWER LEG: *No scars, bony or fibrous enlargements. No signs of thickening of the tendons.*

KNEES: *No puffiness, lumps or scarring.*

CHEST: *The ribs are just covered, so they can be felt but not seen.*

SKIN: *Elastic; able to spring back to smoothness within 2-3 seconds of being pinched.*

HOOVES: *Strong, good quality horn. Correctly trimmed and shaped to balance the foot. Well-shod, with foot neither too long with heels too low, nor too short and 'boxy'. Healthy sole and frog. A matching pair.*

THE HEALTHY HORSE: *Signs to look for*

25

SIGNS OF GOOD HEALTH

Familiarity with the horses in his care under their normal circumstances and their normal environment, is a feature more important than any other in a good horse-master. Knowing each individual's peculiarities and being able to assess anything which appears to vary from the normal is crucial to maintaining horses' well-being.

It takes approximately one year to become really familiar with any horse. The carer needs to have a good working relationship with that horse through all four seasons and during the various types of work which the horse has to undertake.

THE GRASS-KEPT HORSE

The majority of horses spend a percentage of their life out in the field – their most natural environment.

As discussed in the previous chapter, it should always be remembered that the horse is a social animal with a pronounced herd instinct. Horses prefer to be with their own kind and any group will establish its own peer structure. The good horse-master must be aware of the normal relationship between horses in the group and note any signs which vary in their usual behaviour.

A healthy horse will follow a similar pattern during a 24-hour time-span when out in the field. He will usually graze and/or lie down for the same periods, in roughly similar positions in the field, depending on the other conditions at the time. It is,

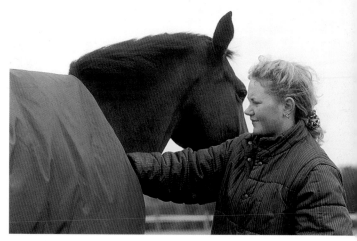

Warmth must be checked at every visit. Feel underneath the rug at the shoulder – the skin should be warm but not clammy to the touch.

of course, usual for a horse to shelter in the shade or in very warm, bright weather. In very wet or windy weather, the horse will usually stand 'tail into the wind'; he is quite likely to ignore light rain, snow and frost, and stand in whichever part of the field he requires for grazing in these weathers.

On first looking at the horse in the morning, check that he is standing in his normal manner. Although alternate hind legs may be rested, the body weight would not normally be taken off a front leg.

A healthy horse should be alert: when called from the gate he should follow his usual behaviour. This may range from being focused, head up, ears forward and looking at the person coming towards him, to, in some cases, showing signs of anxiety or simply mischievous behaviour – e.g. disappearing in the opposite direction!

Once the horse is caught then there are a number of signs which are always the same in a healthy animal. The expression should be bright, with eyes sparkling in the sunlight and always clear. The sclera or white part of the eye should be truly white and the membranes of the eyelids a salmon-pink colour. There should be no discharge from the eyes and any discharge from the nose should be slight and of watery content. The coat should be of good texture and if not covered in mud, should be shiny and healthy with a firm, pliable skin tone. The horse should be neither too plump nor too thin (see Assessing condition, page 64).

When looking at the field, note whether the faeces are normal (or at least normal for that particular horse), whether he has eaten all his food (either hay or concentrate food which has been left for him

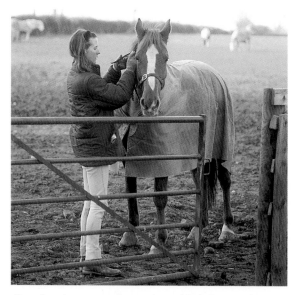

Grass-kept horses must be caught and looked over twice daily. A brief glance from the gate could easily miss signs of injury or ill-health.

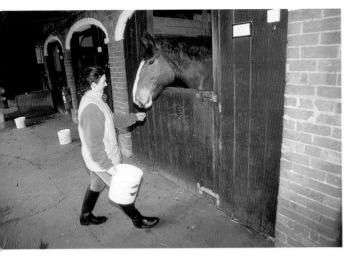

Appetite is a good indicator of well-being. As a rule, horses love their food!

since the previous visit), and whether there are any signs of abnormal behaviour in the field, such as skid marks, hair on the fences, broken rails, etc.

Check to see that water has been drunk since you last visited, and if there is a water trough that it is clean and fresh. The horse should follow you quite happily from his field to stable, with no signs of reluctance when led, and walk with an even and well-balanced stride usual for that particular animal.

THE STABLED HORSE

In a stable the same criteria apply, but look particularly for the character of the horse's faeces and that he has eaten all his food and licked the bowl clean. It is easier to determine if the stabled horse has been in any distress overnight as his rug may have slipped, or he may have been cast, as indicated by hoof marks against the wall or disturbed bedding.

Next assess whether the horse is keen and looking for his next feed. Whether he is out in the field or in the stable, he should eat his breakfast with relish or at least in the manner in which he normally progresses through his food.

Behaviour after the first meal is significant. Does the horse move back intp the stable to rest, and is the manner in which he stands normal? Does he stand looking over the stable door with interest? Or lie down for a rest? The key factor is to know how your horse normally behaves.

EXERCISE

Preparing the horse for exercise, note whether he shows his usual behaviour when tied up, whilst being brushed off, having his feet picked out, being tacked up and led out to the mounting block. The horse should be mounted with ease without showing any unusual behaviour when the rider sits in the saddle, or when first asked to walk forward.

At our veterinary practice every horse which is able to trot up is trotted up at 9am every morning in a straight line on a hard, flat, level surface to assess their demeanour and gait. This is a very well worthwhile exercise to detect any early signs of lameness and any characteristics which the horse is showing which are out of the ordinary.

THE MOST IMPORTANT SIGNS OF HEALTH

- General demeanour
- Brightness of eye
- Whether he has eaten his food
- Character of the faeces
- Whether the limbs are normal in shape, feel and degree of warmth.

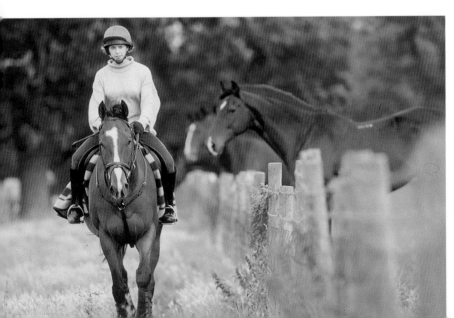

Be aware during exercise of any indications that the horse is not 'right'.

Be aware of any variance from your horse's normal performance during the ride. After exercise when the horse is tied up and his tack removed, his behaviour should also be noted.

When a horse is put loose in his box or out in the field he will invariably firstly drink if thirsty, then eat, snatch a mouthful of straw or hay or grass and then often roll. A healthy horse will usually roll right over two or three times, then shake when it gets up.

The horse should be visited at regular intervals after exercise to note whether he is showing his usual post-exercise behaviour, i.e. no signs of abdominal discomfort and eating his food in the normal manner. Faeces and urine should be constantly monitored.

KEEPING YOUR HORSE IN GOOD SHAPE

There are various essential features of horse-mastership involved in maintaining the horse's well-being. These all involve keeping at the back of your mind, at all times, the fact that the horse is a free-ranging, herd animal. In his natural state he will be with a number of other horses, walking for many hours a day to search for food. He will be a trickle feeder, i.e. eating little and often.

FEEDING
The horse's alimentary tract has become adapted to this method of living over many hundreds of thousands of years. Always bear this in mind when trying to produce the best performance from a domesticated horse.

No horse should ever be without food for more than six hours. A suggested feeding regime to set up such a situation for the stabled horse would involve feeding that individual's daily concentrate (hard feed) ration split between four feeds a day, preferably given at 6.30am, 12 noon, 4pm, and 10pm. He should be given sufficient hay or haylage to enable him to continue eating until after midnight. Perhaps the best way to ensure trickle feeding is achieved is to see that the horse has enough hay for a little to be left in his net or rack each morning.

Oat or barley straw as bedding has the advantage that if the horse eats a little this will boost the fibre content of his diet and enable the trickle feeding process to continue. Some horses, of course, are true gluttons and this would not be satisfactory for them.

Other features of management to ensure the horse

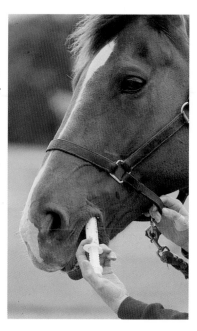

All horses will carry a quantity of internal parasites. By following a strict worming programme, this burden can be kept to an absolute minimum.

is well maintained are that he should always have a constant clean water supply and that his feeding and watering utensils should be cleaned out every day. For more on feeding, see Chapter Three.

ROUTINE HEALTHCARE
The other programmes which should be attended to on a regular basis include worming, vaccination, teeth care and hoof maintenance.

Worming
Worming is a vital part of responsible horse care. The amount and frequency of treatment depends on the intensity of grazing and pasture management. Ideally, horses should be wormed every six to eight weeks, especially when pasture is intensively grazed. (However, the interval between dosings is dependent on the age of the horse and the type of wormer used.) The removal of faeces is a crucial element in parasite control, as it not only prevents the horse becoming re-infected with worms but also helps with fly control, and maintains good-quality pasture. Horses will not eat the rank grass which develops in the 'toilet' areas of the field, and grass dies under fresh manure.

Worming treatment must be carried out on a very regular basis. If in doubt, follow the instructions of one of the larger manufacturers of horse wormers (anthelmintics) and stick to this, or ask your vet for advice with regard to worming in your particular situation.

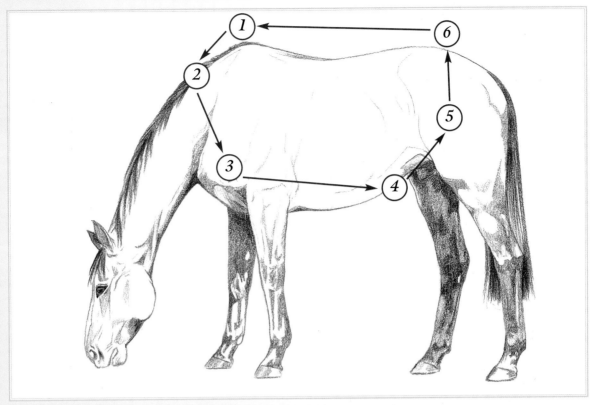

LIFE CYCLE OF LARGE REDWORM

1. *Grazing horse eats worm eggs present on grass.*
2. *Larvae hatch in intestines and burrow through gut wall.*
3. *Around 12 days later, worms migrate into liver.*
4. *In 6-7 weeks, worms move to kidneys, pancreas and spleen, maturing about 17 weeks after infestation.*
5. *Mature worms burrow back through bowel wall, causing bleeding and ulceration.*
6. *After mating, females lay eggs which are passed out in droppings.*

All horses carry internal parasites and all pasture is infected to a varying degree. It is when the level of the parasitic 'burden' increases that extensive damage can be caused to the gut and internal organs. Control is based on breaking the life-cycle through a regular worming programme and good pasture management.

INTERNAL PARASITES AFFECTING HORSES

REDWORMS: Most common equine parasite in UK and Ireland. Small (around 1cm) or large (up to 5cm) varieties are both coloured red from blood sucked from the gut.

ROUNDWORMS: Long white worms that can reach up to 40cm. Mainly affect youngsters up to four years old – very common in North America.

PIN OR SEATWORMS: Thin worms up to 8cm long. Yellow eggs laid under the tail can cause itching.

THREAD OR HAIRWORMS: Vary in colour from brown to red. Often less than 1cm in length.

TAPEWORMS: Flat, white worms of up to 10cm in length and 1cm width. Shed egg-filled sections (like melon seeds) in the droppings.

LUNGWORMS: Live in the respiratory system, where they can cause a chronic, debilitating cough. Thrive in donkeys, who are rarely affected by them but readily pass them on to less-tolerant horses grazing the same pasture.

BOTS: Fly larvae that infest the gut after eggs laid on the horse's coat are ingested.

SIGNS OF HEAVY WORM BURDEN

- Intermittent colic
- Loss of condition
- Pot belly
- Staring coat
- Diarrhoea
- Also itching around rectum, respiratory problems, urinary problems.

CONTROLLING WORMS

Keeping the pasture clean is the cheapest and most effective parasite control measure. Removing droppings at least twice a week will reduce infestation to a minimum. In particular where pasture cannot be cleaned this frequently, a strategic worming programme is essential. Wormers are available in paste or granule form from saddlers and agricultural suppliers or the veterinary surgery. No single type of wormer controls all parasites. All brands contain one of three basic 'active ingredients' – pyrantel, ivermectin and fenbendazole or benzimidazole. Each is aimed at control of particular varieties of parasite.

Resistance to medication occurs more quickly when wormer type is changed too often. Working on a three-yearly cycle, choose one type of active ingredient to use regularly every six to eight weeks throughout the year (autumn>autumn or spring>spring), changing to another type for the next year and the third for the following year.

'One-off' doses are required at these times each year to tackle specific worms:

Late summer:	Pyrantel at double dosage	Tapeworm
Mid-winter & mid-summer:	Ivermectin	Bots
Autumn:	Fenbendazole daily for five days	Migrating large redworm & encysted small redworm

Ideally, all horses sharing a field or yard should be wormed at the same time using the same product. Stabling for 48 hours after treatment reduces the level of re-infestation. New arrivals should be treated before being turned out. Give sufficient dosage for the body-weight of the animal.
- Stabled horses are not free from the risk of infestation. Worm eggs are present on stable floors and dirty utensils.
- An averagely-infested horse passes over 30 million worm eggs every day. Over-grazed or 'horse-sick' pasture carries the heaviest worm burden. Allow at least one acre per horse, and rest pasture for a minimum of six weeks three times a year.
- Dose foals from six weeks of age.

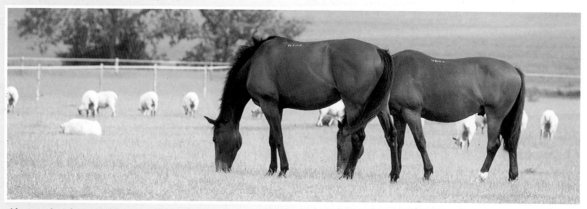

Alternating horses with other livestock helps reduce the worm burden. The vet can monitor your worming programme by regularly analysing dung samples.

Vaccinations are available to provide protection against tetanus, equine influenza, equine herpes virus (EHV, or rhinopneumonitis), equine viral arteritis (EVA) and encephalitis – all potentially serious or fatal diseases. Horses should be routinely immunised against those diseases from which they are most at risk in the region where they live. Tetanus protection is essential for all horses of all types. In the UK, this is frequently given in the same injection as vaccine against equine flu, with additional EHV and EVA immunisation given to breeding stock as appropriate. Full, certified vaccination against flu is a compulsory requirement for competition under the rules of racing, BHTA horse trials or when attending any event held on a racecourse in the UK.

In North America, the flu vaccination is generally combined with one for EHV, which must be repeated every three months to maintain immunity. Here encephalitis, frequently spread by biting insects, is a serious problem, and immunisation against this is also advised usually within an annual tetanus booster.

Guidelines for vaccination against tetanus & flu in the UK

	Initial course	First booster	Subsequent boosters
TETANUS	two vaccinations six weeks apart	one year later	every other year
EQUINE FLU	two vaccinations (21-92 days apart)	150-215 days after second vaccination	every year (no more than 365 days after previous booster)

VACCINATION
Tetanus: Vaccination against tetanus is absolutely essential. A horse owner who does not have his horse vaccinated against tetanus in this day and age, in my opinion, is negligent and not a fit person to care for a horse. Tetanus is a most serious and distressing condition, both in terms of suffering and loss of use of the horse. Foals can be vaccinated from the age of twelve weeks. Whatever the age, the primary vaccination is followed by a second vaccination six weeks later, then a further booster one year later and biannually thereafter. All horses should be vaccinated (see Tetanus, Chapter Six).

Equine influenza: The effectiveness of equine influenza inoculation is continually improving and there are a number of different brands of vaccine available on the market. The purpose of this vaccination is to decrease the load of flu virus in a population of horses and hence reduce the risk of outbreaks in the competitive horse, particularly the racehorse and sports horse when they mix at competition level. In order for horses to compete in the UK both under the rules of racing and under the majority of the various sports horse disciplines, competing horses are obliged to be vaccinated against equine influenza. This must be certified by the vet who has administered the vaccine and the information contained in the horse's passport.

Equine herpes virus (EHV) also known as **Rhinopneumonitis:** This viral disease will cause both abortion in the pregnant mare and respiratory tract signs in all horses. Some individuals also suffer in-coordination and paralysis. At present it is not obligatory for any type of horse to be vaccinated against EHV but it is highly recommended in the Codes of Practice for horse breeding, to attempt to prevent the spread of this disease amongst breeding stock. Pregnant mares should be vaccinated at 5, 7 and 9 months' gestation (see EHV, Chapters Five and Ten).

TEETH
The horse has evolved as a grazing animal and his teeth are adapted for that purpose. Teeth start to appear soon after birth and continue to erupt from the gum for most of the horse's life, so problems can occur at any stage but are often not recognised for some time. Correcting dental problems is likely to improve the horse's ability to eat, his general condition, and comfort with the bit.

Signs that a horse has teeth problems include the inability to eat properly, quidding (dropping food whilst eating), foul-smelling breath, weight loss, dribbling, head-tilting, head-tossing, and fighting or chewing the bit.

Horses should have their teeth checked properly every six months. Without looking carefully inside the mouth many tooth problems will not be

As the horse's lower jaw is narrower than the upper jaw, the side-ways grinding action causes uneven wear on the outer edges of the molar teeth. This results in sharp edges, which if left unattended can lead to severe discomfort and problems with eating, digestion and ridden work.

These sharp edges need filing ('rasping' or 'floating') by a vet or specialist horse dentist every six months or a year. Only veterinary surgeons are legally allowed, in the UK, to perform more complex procedures such as extraction and orthodontic work.

SIGNS OF MOUTH/TEETH PROBLEMS:

- Excessive dropping of food from the mouth ('quidding')
- Foul-smelling breath
- Loss of condition
- Head-shyness
- Reluctance to be bridled
- Evasion of the bit, unsteadiness of the head, snatching the reins, 'yawing', bucking

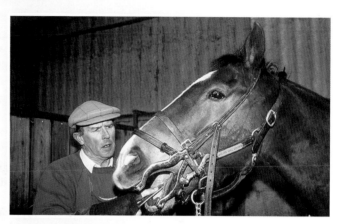

The grinding action of the teeth creates sharp edges on the outside of the molars that must be routinely rasped, or filed away, to avoid soreness and bitting problems.

detected and if ignored they will become worse. In the UK, at present it is only legal for veterinary surgeons to carry out dental treatment, i.e. extraction and orthodontic procedures. However, there is a widespread prevalence of non-qualified people who have been rasping ('floating') horse's teeth for many years. Currently, the Royal College of Veterinary Surgeons is suggesting the formation of a group of equine dental technicians who are taught in equine dental anatomy, physiology and appropriate techniques of dental manipulation. These people would have to pass an approved exam and become registered, after which they would then be permitted to perform a number of techniques, notably dental rasping, without supervision.

More complex procedures such as removing dental hooks or loose teeth would still need to be carried out under direct veterinary supervision, and all other forms of treatment such as teeth repulsion and filling tooth roots, could only be carried out by vets. Unregistered persons carrying out dental procedures could then be prosecuted, and this would help prevent the occasional suffering which undoubtedly occurs in horses throughout the UK at present with unqualified people attempting to treat horses' teeth.

HOOF CARE

Regular hoof care by a registered farrier is absolutely crucial to the well-being of your horse and to maintain his performance. Horses require farriery attention between every three and six weeks depending on the rate of growth of the hoof wall and type of work the horse is performing (see Chapter Four).

It is essential that the farrier is not only trained in the correct fitting of the shoe to the hoof, but also trained to balance the horse's foot to its conformation, so preventing abnormal wear of the hoof capsule that causes lameness, e.g. corns.

A list of UK-registered farriers, including those with higher qualifications enabling them to perform more complicated forms of orthopaedic trimming

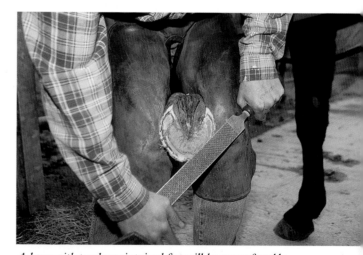

A horse with poorly-maintained feet will be uncomfortable and never reliably sound. Proper foot-care is essential, and a regular expense that the responsible owner must be prepared to budget for.

GROOMING

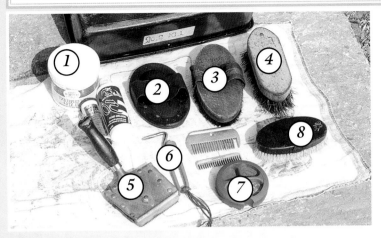

Besides smartening the appearance, grooming is important to help keep the skin and coat healthy, particularly in the stabled horse. A regular grooming session is also an opportunity to spend time with your horse, keep an eye on his general condition and check him over for minor injuries.

1. hoof preparations 2. rubber curry comb 3. body brush 4. dandy brush 5. metal curry comb 6. hoof pick 7. mane combs 8. water brush

THE FIELD-KEPT HORSE

Mud must always be removed when dry, using the fingers, the dandy brush or rubber curry comb. Brushing wet hair is likely to scratch and chafe the skin.

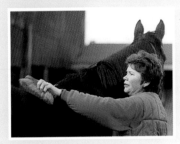

◀ *A field-kept horse will appreciate being allowed to keep a reasonable amount of natural grease in his coat. Avoid over-enthusiastic use of the body brush. As a regular grooming routine, concentrate on making the horse comfortable and tidy. Sponge the eyes, nostrils and dock daily, pick out the feet and remove dried mud from the coat, particularly on areas where the tack will go.*

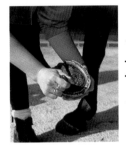

◀ *Pick out the feet, working from heel to toe, and wash any mud off the outside.*

THE STABLED HORSE

Grooming every day is necessary to clean the skin of a stabled horse and improve circulation and muscle tone. The horse can be made tidy before a ride (known as 'quartering') but thorough grooming is best done after exercise when the pores are open. Most horses have ticklish areas and some are sensitive-skinned all over. Tackle these areas with tact!

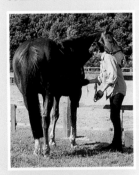

◀ *Tie the horse up securely for grooming, preferably in an enclosed or sheltered place. In cold weather or with clipped horses, leave a rug or blanket on, folding it back in sections as you go.*

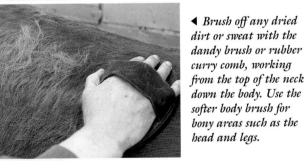

◀ *Brush off any dried dirt or sweat with the dandy brush or rubber curry comb, working from the top of the neck down the body. Use the softer body brush for bony areas such as the head and legs.*

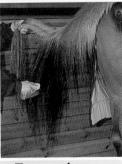

▲ *Tease out the mane and tail hairs with the fingers, then work through it with the body brush.*

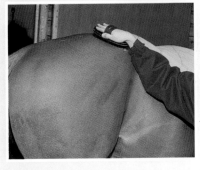

◀ *Starting at the top of the neck, body brush using long, firm, circular strokes in the direction of the hair. Hold the brush in the hand nearest the head.*

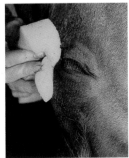

▲ *Sponge the eyes, nose and dock, using a separate sponge for each.*

and surgical shoeing, is available from the Farriers Registration Council.

This kind of attention to detail in your horse's routine care will undoubtedly help maintain his health and, consequently, his performance. It is a sensible idea, whenever the horse is wormed, vaccinated, has his teeth rasped or is shod, to carry forward in your diary the next time that the procedure will need to be carried out. In this way these essential parts of horse maintenance are less easily overlooked.

CAUSES OF DISEASE

BACTERIA

The most commonly encountered effect of bacteria is to cause contamination of wounds. Any wound on any part of the body may be contaminated by bacteria which are always present in the environment but most often will affect the horse in dirty conditions such as mud, water courses, dirty stables and, in particular, low-lying wet conditions. The tetanus organism is an example of a bacterium that can cause death once it has entered the blood stream.

Bacteria are always passed into wounds by touch, in other words, either from contamination of the surrounding area or by human touch. Contaminated wounds are first noticed by four important signs, namely the presence of heat, pain, redness and swelling of the affected area. All or any of these signs may indicate bacterial infection.

Bacteria may also enter the bloodstream through being ingested or inhaled, and then affect a major organ, i.e. the heart, the lungs, the intestines, the liver, the kidney, the ovaries, the uterus or the brain, or indeed the lining of any body cavity such as the thorax or the abdomen, causing pleurisy or peritonitis respectively.

VIRUSES

A virus is spread by aerosol droplet, generally not over a distance greater than 20 metres. Viruses may cause anything from marginally poor performance to severe disease, and death – in the case of rabies, for example, which is transmitted by biting or blood contamination.

The common viruses simply cause poor performance, but may also cause equine influenza, abortion, ataxia and lack of coordination.

FUNGI

Fungi are spread by touch. The most common fungal infection in the horse is ringworm (see Chapter Seven). Ringworm may affect any part of the horse's skin and is usually observed as small circles about the size of a small coin producing raised lesions where the hair drops off and new hair then develops underneath. However, ringworm may be exhibited as any shape and size on the horse's skin – in fact there is no such thing as a 'normal' ringworm lesion. Ringworm is passed from horse to horse by touch or quite commonly from cattle to horses by touch. Ringworm spores and hyphae can live in woodwork for longer than ten years. This is another common cause of an outbreak of ringworm, from post and rail fences and, more particularly, from wooden cowsheds, etc.

PARASITES

Two forms of parasites commonly affect horses. **Intestinal parasites** may be controlled by a suitable worming programme, as described on page 30. Signs of intestinal parasites include ill thrift, a poor, dull coat, staring coat, enlarged abdomen, weight loss along the topline, dullness and lethargy, intermittent or profuse diarrhoea, and colic.

The other type of parasite is the **ectoparasite** family – those which live in the skin, such as lice and mange. Lice generally affect the 'hairier' horse in the UK during the winter months and are commonly seen by areas of hair loss and scratching behind the ear, down the front of the face, the underside of the neck, along the flanks and at the top of the tail.

Mange is usually seen in the heavier horse with unclipped legs, principally with irritative scaly areas of the skin, the back of the knees, down the tendons and back of the fetlocks of all four feet.

Whatever the type, control is based on interrupting the life-cycle of the parasite involved, requiring regular cyclical treatment as will be advised by your vet.

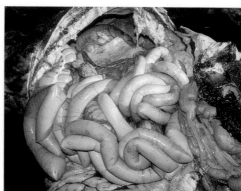

Only a post-mortem will reveal the extent of worm damage.

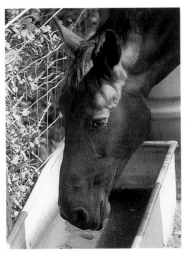

Keeping an eye on the amount your horse is drinking is more difficult for a grass-kept animal. However, normal drinking and urination patterns are important indicators of health.

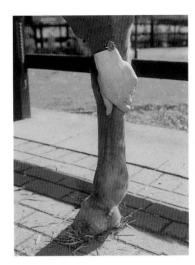

Feel each limb both before and after exercise to check for injury, heat or swelling. To detect problems, it is important to be familiar with the normal shape and feel of an individual's legs.

SIGNS OF ILL HEALTH

The observant carer will immediately be aware of any sign which varies from what is normal for his horse, and will immediately wonder if the horse is showing any sign of ill-health as a result. Any alteration from normal behaviour should be carefully observed and followed up, whether this is noticed in the field or stable.

Ten-stage check for signs of ill-health

1. Change from normal behaviour. Lying down or standing away from the other horses in the field, lying down in the stable when he would generally be standing, not coming for his food or eating it up when he is generally a greedy horse – these are the first things to notice. As you enter the stable, does the horse move away from you as he normally would and move over when asked, or is he reluctant?
2. Change in the amount which the horse drinks, i.e. more or less than normal.
3. Change in the faeces. Are they firmer than usual, looser than usual, more or less frequent? Does he show any signs of faecal contamin - ation of the walls of his stable, of his tail or hind legs that are not normally present?
4. Look more carefully at the horse. Are his ears forward and his eyes bright, or are his ears cold, damp at the base and backward? Is he showing signs of malaise? Are his eyes anything other than clear: are they cloudy, is there any form of discharge? Are the mucous

membranes a brighter red or paler than the normal salmon-pink colour? The gums, the mucous membranes of the eyes and, in the mare, the lining of the vulva, should all be this salmon-pink. Note and observe any variation.
5. Signs of discharge. Any one-sided discharge, thick mucus, mucoid discharge or any smell from the nose is abnormal.
6. Check the horse's coat. See if there is change from the night before. Is it shiny or dull, is he sweating or cold?
7. Take the temperature, pulse and respiration. A pulse greater than 50 beats per minute, a respiration greater than 20 breaths per minute and a temperature greater than 102F or 40C may be a sign of ill-health.
8. Palpate the horse's limbs. Do they all feel the same as usual in terms of temperature and any soft-tissue swelling? Pay particular attention to contour and firmness. The horse should be standing squarely on his front feet, only resting alternate hind limbs. Pointing or lifting of one fore-foot is abnormal.
9. Urination. Notice whether the horse is urinating normally, that the urine is a cloudy yellow as it should be, and whether there is the usual smell in the stable.
10. Abnormal swellings. Moving back to the horse himself, take a look to check there is no swelling between his jaws or in the angle of the jaw which might indicate that either his lymph nodes or his salivary glands are swollen. Next, look closely in his axilla and, particularly, up inside his hind legs to see if any of the lymph channels are swollen and painful.

CHECKING VITAL SIGNS

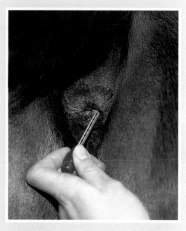

TEMPERATURE
- Wait for at least 15 minutes after exercise before taking a temperature reading. Do not take it immediately after the horse has passed droppings.
- Shake the thermometer so that it reads less than 35 C (95 F). Grease the end with Vaseline.
- Standing to one side, lift the tail and insert the thermometer into the rectum with a gentle, rotating movement. Hold there for at least one minute, then remove and read immediately.
- Sterilise after use.

Normal range: 38 – 38.5 C (100 – 101.5 F).

Temperature varies between individuals. Find out what a horse's 'normal' is when well, for comparison. Higher temperature readings suggest infection or fever. Low temperature is typical of shock or hypothermia. Foals normally have a slightly higher temperature – up to 102F.

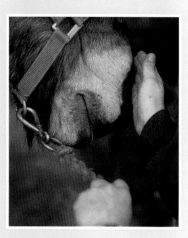

RESPIRATORY RATE
- Breathing should be even, regular and barely noticeable. Rapid, laboured, irregular, shallow or painful breathing is abnormal.
- First watch the breathing from a distance of 2 metres (6 – 7 ft) by observing the movement of the flanks, abdomen or ribs. Each rise and fall is counted as one breath.
- Additionally, watch the nostril movement or gently place one hand over a nostril and feel the air movement in and out.

Normal range: 8 – 16 breaths per minute.

The normal pulse:respiration ratio is 3:1 (even during strenuous exercise). Rates over 20 breaths per minute are abnormal in the UK, although in less temperate regions can rise as far as 32 on a hot day. Very obvious or strained breathing efforts suggest respiratory problems or disease.

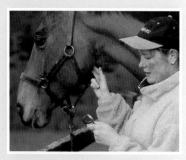

PULSE
- The pulse is the pressure from the heartbeat. The rate (number of beats/time frame) will increase with stress and excitement. For an accurate reading, the horse must be calm and at rest.
- Place a finger (not a thumb) on an artery close to the skin surface, for example:
  the facial artery passing under the lower jaw
  the median artery on the inside of the fore-leg
  the digital artery on the outside of the fetlock joint
- Count the beats for 20 seconds and then multiply by three. To check the heartbeat itself, feel with the palm of the hand, or place a stethoscope behind the point of the left elbow, with the fore-leg slightly forwards.

Normal range: 35 – 42 beats per minute at rest
            (up to 45 bpm in foals, young horses, small ponies).

Normal rates vary with breed, age and bodyweight. Establish what is normal for your horse. Heartbeats over 60 bpm at rest are cause for concern. In colic cases, the pulse rate is a good pain monitor.

If your horse appears to simply be a little dull and out of sorts and you can make no headway in pinpointing the cause, take him out of the stable, remove all his clothing and trot him up on a hard, level surface, looking for any signs of stiffness or lameness. Run your hand over his body, including over every site where the tack will touch, most particularly the saddle and girth area and where the rider's weight would be over his lumbar muscles. Are there any signs of pain there from the rider's weight or from rubbing of the tack?

Any of the signs above may indicate that the horse is in ill health. Consider carefully as to whether the horse should continue with his normal feeding and exercise, whether these need to be adjusted, and whether the vet should be consulted.

RECOGNISING LAMENESS

Many lamenesses can be detected before the horse ever comes out of his box. More severe lameness will often show itself through some of the more general signs of ill health already discussed. A sound horse will stand with his two front feet together and bear an equal amount of weight on each foot. The horse may alternately rest one hind foot and then the other, but the resting or 'pointing' of a fore-foot is not normal. The fore-leg cannons should be vertical, and the pelvis level and symmetrical when viewed from behind. Be wary if the horse is standing unusually still.

Lameness can be most easily detected by the horse trotting straight out of his stable in the morning, as any variation from normal can be noted. We all know that some older horses which have done more work will be a little stiff. By becoming familiar with the stiffness in each particular horse, the variation from normal can be detected at an early stage and, by reducing work or giving appropriate treatment, a worsening of the situation may be prevented.

Often lameness can show only as slight unlevelness and the source (known as the 'seat') is not obvious. Various tests can be carried out to help determine the exact location of the problem.

TROTTING UP

The horse should be trotted up in a straight line, as described in the panel overleaf.

A horse's head is very heavy. When a leg is painful, the horse tries to keep weight off it by moving the head up as the lame leg comes down – resulting in the 'bob' of the head that accompanies the action of a lame horse. This bob, or nod, is most commonly seen in front-limb lameness, though it can occur in severe hind-limb lameness too. If a fore-limb is lame, it may

be difficult to detect whilst watching the horse trot away from you, but as he comes towards you the head can be seen to nod down as the sound leg hits the ground. Where lameness is in a hind leg, the horse will generally nod when the lame leg hits the ground – this is in an attempt to shift weight forwards, off his lame leg. More importantly with regard to hind-limb lameness, when the horse is trotting away from you, the oscillation (swing) of the point of the hip will be greater in the lame than the sound limb.

It is only possible to detect subtle lamenesses on a hard, flat, level surface. The handler must fix his eye on an object from the observer, so the horse is trotted in a perfectly straight line. No pressure must be put on the head of the horse, which must be encouraged to trot with his spine straight along the line the observer is watching. Some horses will always turn their heads towards the handler, in which case ask the handler to go on the opposite side, or use a person on both sides to keep the head straight. With his head turned towards the handler, to the less-experienced eye a horse can appear lame in the fore-limb on that side.

Detection of hind-leg lameness can often be aided by placing a large sticky-tape cross at symmetrical points on the horse's hindquarters, i.e. the tubersacrale. This helps to reveal which side shows the greater rise, and hence impression of lameness.

Other tests that may be performed include turning the horse in a tight circle before trotting it towards the observer. Turning a horse is useful for determining many lamenesses, in particular subtle ones. Corns are an example, as discomfort from these will be exacerbated as the horse twists his foot on the ground as he turns.

In addition, some lamenesses, for example splints and foot problems such as bruising or heel pain, are made worse by trotting on hard surfaces and better on soft going. Other conditions, such as soft tissue problems (e.g. tendon or ligament injuries and joint problems) are worse on softer footing.

FLEXION TESTS

Flexion tests can help determine which part of the leg is causing the greater degree of pain. Here the limb is held in a certain position for a short period of time and the horse trotted away. Most horses do show slight unlevelness for a few strides, but the unsound horse will show very lame. If the flexed position has exacerbated the lameness it is likely that the site of lameness is within the arc of flexion. Flexion tests on the knee or fetlock are best interpreted by your vet.

Systematic evaluation, beginning with careful observation of the horse at rest, will often reveal the location of lameness.

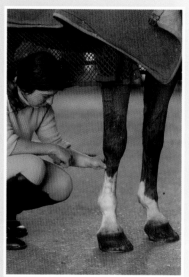

◀ *Examine the limbs for any signs of heat, pain or swelling. Pick up each foot and check the sole for a foreign body, bruising or puncture wound. If warmth is felt, compare this to the other legs.*

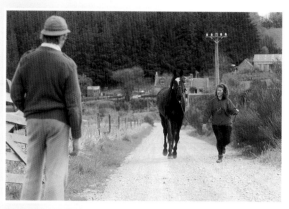

▲ *Have the horse trotted up in a straight line on a hard, non-slippery, level surface. The handler should be positioned midway along the neck and allow enough slack in the rope or reins to give freedom of movement. The horse must be turned away from the handler, giving a continuous view to the observer. Begin by walking away from the observer, turn, then walk back and past. Repeat this in trot. Aim for a gentle, steady pace.*

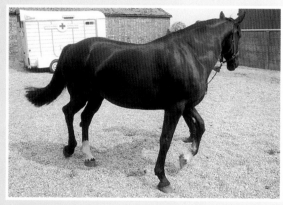

▲ *Lameness frequently becomes more obvious on a circle. Standing by the girth area, turn the horse in small circles in both directions. Larger circles, on the lunge, are particularly useful for showing up fore-leg lameness. Ridden exercise may exaggerate hind-limb lameness.*

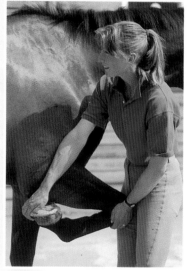

◀ *Flexion can indicate whether lameness is located in a joint. To test for hock lameness, hold up the hind leg for $2^1/_2$ minutes, flexing all joints well. Put the leg down and trot the horse away immediately. Most horses show slight unlevelness for a few strides. Unsound horses show very lame. Flexion tests on the knee/fetlock should be interpreted by your vet.*

TROTTING UP: OBSERVER'S CHECKLIST

- Shut the eyes and listen to the rhythm of the footfalls. The sound horse places its footfalls evenly and regularly. Listen for irregular beat or loudness/quietness.
- Open the eyes and watch one part of the horse at a time.
- As the horse trots away, watch for any sinking of the hindquarters, indicating hind-limb lameness.
- As the horse trots towards you, look for any nodding of the head.
- When a dip is detected, determine which leg is hitting the ground at that time. In fore-limb lameness the sinking or nodding occurs as the horse places weight on its sound side; it is lame on the opposite fore-leg.
- As the horse trots past watch for shortening of the stride. Assess the swing of the limbs and flexion of the joints and how the feet are placed on the ground.
- Now re-examine the suspect limb.

Emergency – essential to contact vet immediately:

- Road traffic accidents involving any damage to horse or rider.
- Haemorrhage: Particularly wounds involving large areas of skin and muscle and arterial bleeding, as judged by bright red blood which escapes from the horse's body in spurts. Haemorrhage may also occur underneath skin, appearing as a rapidly-developing pocket of fluid. Hypovolemic shock is a risk.
- Foalings: Where either the mare has produced any marked straining or any part of the foal or the after-birth appears and nothing further has happened within 15 minutes.
- Fractures or suspected fractures: The horse should not be moved.
- Colic: All cases of suspected colic should be discussed with a vet and not left for a period to see if they will recover on their own.
- Azoturia: As with colic, the case should always be discussed with the veterinarian.
- Endotoxic shock and colitis-X: If the horse shows increased pulse and profuse diarrhoea, for however short a period, a vet should always be made aware of the situation.
- Lymphangitis: An acute and painful condition causing severe swelling of a leg and lameness. If suspected, advise your vet.
- Wounds: Particularly those related to dangerous sites which include joints, tendon sheaths and bursae. Any indication of heat, pain, swelling and redness is a sign of infection and inflammation.
- Temperature, pulse and respiration variations: Notify the vet if your horse's temperature is greater than 40C or 101.5F, the pulse is greater than 50 bpm or respiration rate over 20 breaths per minute.

Do not delay calling vet if:

- Your horse has not passed faeces for longer than 12 hours, if he has not eaten or drunk for more than 6 hours, has showed lameness for more than 36 hours and if there is no improvement or if this is unusual for the horse.
- There are signs of a respiratory infection, particularly those involving swelling of the lymph nodes between the jaws. A one-sided nasal discharge may indicate a sinus infection.
- Your horse has any unusual skin lesions.

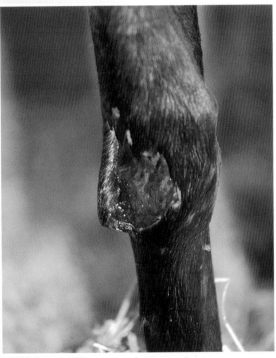

Wounds that are deep, over one inch long, or situated on or close to the joint will need immediate veterinary attention.

FIRST AID

The most essential feature of all first-aid is to do no harm. In an emergency situation, stand back and take a few seconds to assess:
- Firstly, is there any human involvement and any human being at risk? If so, how can that risk be reduced?
- Secondly, is the problem life-threatening to the horse? If so, what steps should be taken to remedy the situation?

Let us deal with first-aid incidents you may encounter, in order of importance.

ROAD TRAFFIC ACCIDENTS
Whenever a horse is involved in a road traffic accident, the Police should be informed. Make sure

A simple first-aid kit should be kept in both the lorry and the yard, and any items that are used replaced immediately. Use a clean, covered container clearly marked First-Aid, containing:

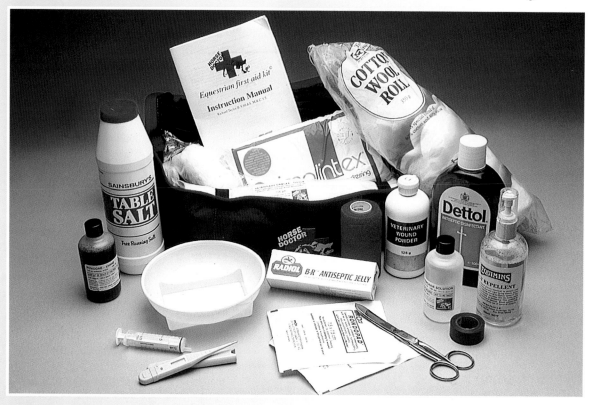

Sterile saline solution or diluted disinfectant: To clean wounds.

Antiseptic scrubs/swabs: Swabs enable cleaning of wounds where there is no water supply. Washes to be used at very dilute concentration (i.e. 1 tsp:1 pint).

Wound powder/ointment: Prevent new infections entering wound. Do not use on horse yet to be seen by vet. Creams and ointments are more easily absorbed. Powders avoid need to touch skin, but are only absorbed where skin is broken.

Antibiotic aerosol: Helps prevent infection without damaging tissue. Spray gently from correct distance.

Dressings: To cover and protect wounds without sticking and to promote healing.

Bandages: 1) 10-15cm wide stretchy crepe for use over padding; 2) elastic adhesive bandages; 3) long, non-stretch stable bandages.

Gamgee: Padding that can be cut to size for use under bandages, as pressure pad, for swabbing, or as emergency splint. Synthetic types available.

Cotton wool: For cleaning wounds, mopping up, or dabbing on powders. Not suitable for direct application to moist wounds or as bandage padding.

Poultice: Particularly effective for puncture wounds (see p.48)

Cold pack: Cooling action aims to reduce inflammation and ease strains.

Scissors: Must be sharp and have blunted ends.

Thermometer: An ordinary household one will do.

Disposable hand gloves: Help prevent infection entering an open wound.

Tweezers/forceps: To remove splinters, etc.

Vaseline/petroleum jelly: To help insert thermometer. Also protects soft tissues from soreness or chafing.

Stockholm Tar: Traditional mildly-disinfectant vegetable tar hoof dressing that helps seal cracks.

- A first-aid kit must be kept where it may be needed. Put together three kits, for the yard, for travelling and for hacking.
- Lock all medicines out of reach of children.
- Write vet's phone number prominently on kit.
- First-aid kits are intended for immediate, emergency action only, not to deal with major incidents, illnesses or replace the attention of a vet.

there is no human being at risk and always deal with this problem first. The horse, if possible, should be removed from the main highway or at least to the roadside, before trying to prevent the incident becoming more serious by alerting on-coming traffic, in both directions, of a problem.

SEVERE HAEMORRHAGE

In the horse it is unlikely that wounds to the limbs will prove fatal, and in any case, stemming haemorrhage of these areas is relatively easy. However, stemming haemorrhage to major vessels in the axilla, the groin, the jugular vein or carotid artery or stake wounds to the abdomen are more difficult to deal with. The best method is to use a clean bed sheet, pushing this into the affected area and holding it tightly in place until the vet arrives. If a sheet is not available, any clean clothing material is satisfactory. Cleanliness is essential, but to quell the haemorrhage it may be necessary to use whatever is available.

Haemorrhage to wounds on the limbs is controlled by using a tourniquet between the wound and the heart. Either a hunting stock, hunting tie, tail bandage or Vetwrap can be placed between the wound and heart and tightened firmly for four minutes, then released for 10 seconds. This should be continued until veterinary help arrives.

With all forms of haemorrhage it is essential to try to keep the horse still and, if possible, warm. Remove anything from the immediate environment which might startle the horse.

FOALING

A sensible and practical rule of thumb with regard to foaling emergencies is that if a mare has produced any large strains or any part of the after-birth or foal has appeared, yet nothing further occurs for 15 minutes, or if the placenta seperates first, then call the vet. Do not attempt to manipulate the foal yourself.

If the foal's nose is showing, make sure that the nose and mouth are cleared from after-birth so that the foal is able to breathe.

FRACTURES

Any horse that is suspected of having sustained a fractured limb or back, should not be moved, other than to clear it from the direct line of road traffic. The saddle and accompanying tack should be taken away and the horse kept warm, but it is best to keep a bridle on so that the horse can be properly held. If he should show an interest in eating he should be allowed to, as this will often encourage the horse to keep still.

A horse that is lying down with a suspected fracture must not try to rise. By placing a knee just behind the horse's ear, facing the horse's front leg (i.e. the handler's face facing the horse's feet), the horse should be encouraged to lie still, flat on his side. This will prevent both the handler from being hurt and the horse from rising.

Do not try to apply any form of first-aid to a limb which is suspected of being fractured.

COLIC (see also Chapter Three)

If you decide that your horse has colic, whilst waiting for the vet the horse should be kept warm and be allowed to lie down if he will lie quietly and not hurt himself by rolling. Putting a bridle on and walking the horse gently around the yard is advisable if there is any risk he might endanger himself by rolling, but only if there is a real risk of this.

Check that there are no sharp objects in the stable that the horse can hurt himself upon, such as salt-lick containers, loose buckets, or any projecting nails or wood. Make sure that the bedding is deep and well stacked against the walls. Try to prevent the horse from banging his head on the floor, particularly around his eyes. *Do not* give him anything to eat or drink and try to keep him warm, preferably with a light 'breathable' rug or blanket over straw that will maintain warmth but allow any sweat to evaporate.

AZOTURIA

Azoturia or rhabdomylisis is commonly mistaken for colic and vice-versa. Azoturia can be brought about by a number of different factors (see Chapter Four).

An episode of azoturia can range from the mild, which may only result in poor performance, to the more severe, where the horse exhibits some muscular stiffness and mild discomfort such as pawing the ground, an occasional looking at his flanks, slight breaking out with sweat and some stiffness over his loins.

Where the horse is in severe distress, it is unable to walk around his box, may urinate bright red urine and shows marked discomfort as with colic.

In the most extreme cases, the horse lies down and is unable to rise due to the severity of muscle cramp which may occur in any of the large muscle masses of his body.

The important first aid factor is that if you believe that the horse has any form of muscle cramp he should not be moved on further – in reality the muscle tissue is being destroyed. All movement must stop. Make the horse warm with rugs, and get transport to take him back to his stable. Once home, warmth and calm are an essential part of the treatment. A heat lamp, rugs with straw underneath and leg bandages are all important. Watch the horse carefully to see if he drinks. Inform a vet about anything other than the very mildest azoturia, giving the vital information as to whether and how much the horse has drunk and, in particular, the colour of the urine. If the horse's urine is brown or red in colour, this is a real emergency and the vet should be contacted without delay. Treatment with fluids, steroids, anti-inflammatories and vasodilators must begin immediately.

No advice can be given with regard to diet at this stage until the vet has seen your horse. Do not attempt to treat the horse yourself by altering his diet as it is impossible to estimate the cause of the dietary problem without laboratory analysis. It is better to give the horse hay or haylage and a proprietary convalescent diet until advised otherwise by your vet.

RESPIRATORY DISEASE (see Chapter Five)
Good nursing is the key to the treatment of respiratory disease. The horse should be placed in a well-ventilated but warm and draught-free stable. He should be bedded on paper or dust-extracted straw or wood shavings. All food should be fed at ground level. He must be kept warm and be encouraged to eat little and often. Feeding and drinking utensils should be regularly cleaned so that no nasal discharge contaminates these and puts the horse off his food and water.

SHOCK & COLITIS-X
A horse will become shocked if he experiences a trauma that he is totally unused to, e.g. a road traffic accident, a fall whilst undergoing an athletic activity, or from disease.

Recognisable signs of shock include the horse becoming dull, a rapidly-rising pulse, cold ears and clammy skin, increasing respiration, paling colour and some lack of coordination.

Under all these circumstances the horse should be placed in a warm, airy, environment and kept warm as described above, including leg bandages, tail bandages and hood. He should be encouraged to drink warm water but should not be given anything to eat whilst his pulse is raised. Should the pulse rise above 60 beats per minute, a vet should be contacted immediately.

The development of diarrhoea creates a crisis when combined with a rising pulse as the horse may develop the condition known as colitis-X, where severe shock rapidly develops and may cause death. This is a more common syndrome in practice than is generally recognised and it is important that horse-keepers are aware of this potential problem. To repeat, any horse which has a rapidly rising pulse, shows all or some of the signs of shock and has diarrhoea (in particular, profuse diarrhoea) should be considered an emergency case. Veterinary attention should be sought immediately.

WOUNDS (see panel page 46)
Wherever a wound occurs, control of haemorrhage is of paramount importance. Next most important is the necessity to do no harm, that is, not to introduce infection into a wound which previously is not infected.

If the wound occurs whilst the horse is at exercise and a vital structure may potentially be penetrated, the horse should be transported home rather than being asked to go under his own steam and so allowing dirt to be sucked into the affected area.

The common sites for serious infection are:
• joints
• tendon sheaths
• tendons
• bursae, including the navicular bursa in the foot.

Good first aid is essential and can make all the difference in a successful treatment and recovery. If possible, take the horse into a clean, well-lit box. Thoroughly groom the horse whilst keeping the wound covered with a light dressing, so that dirt from the rest of the body does not later contaminate the site of the wound.

Next, cold-hose the wound for five minutes to remove any surplus debris and reduce pain and inflammation. Clip any long hair from around the wound so that its extent can be seen, taking care not to let any hair or dirt enter. Do not investigate the wound yourself with either your finger or any form of probe. This must be done under as sterile conditions as possible.

Once the wound has been assessed and hosed, the site can be gently flushed with saline, but do not be tempted to apply any powder, spray or ointment. Simply cover the area with a light, sterile, bandage until the vet arrives.

GIVING MEDICATION

- Powders or liquids can be given in dampened feed. Give the feed at the horse's usual meal-time, masking the smell if necessary using molasses, treacle, honey or apple juice. Watch to make sure the ration is eaten. Do not leave any unfinished food with the horse. If the feed is refused, powder can be made into a paste using icing sugar and given in a syringe, smeared on to the back of the tongue or hidden in a cored apple or carrot. Avoid giving drugs in liquid form by mouth.
- Syringes of paste provide a more direct method especially useful for horses that are off their feed or very sensitive to anything added to the feed. Check if the dose has to be pre-set before pressing plunger on syringe. Squirt paste carefully into the corner of the mouth in the bit space, on top of the tongue and pointing down the throat. Press the plunger in one go. Hold up the horse's nose until he has swallowed.
- Pills and tablets are best placed inside a cored apple, carrot or ripe pear. Small tablets, such as homoeopathic remedies, can be slipped in between the inside of the lips and the gums.
- Injections may be intravenous (into a vein), intramuscular (into a muscle), subcutaneous (under the skin) or intra-articular (into a joint – very specialised). Intramuscular injections are usually given into alternate sides of the neck or quarters. Intramuscular injections only can sometimes be given by the owner, under instruction from the vet.
- Give the whole course of any treatment, until finished.
- Check drug, dose and patient carefully before administering.
- Follow the vet's instructions.
- Tell your vet immediately if the horse is not getting his medication. It may need to be given in a different form – by injection or, where appropriate, by stomach tubing.
- If competing soon after course of treatment, check drugs are permitted.

NURSING THE SICK HORSE

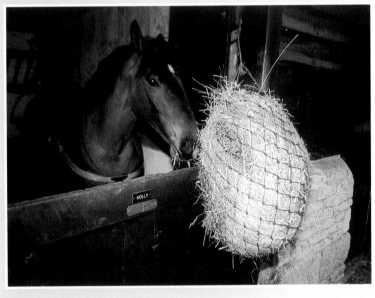

◀ *Correct nursing will aid recovery.*

- Make the horse feel as comfortable and relaxed as possible. Provide a clean bed in a well-ventilated stable. Keep the horse warm but not over-hot. Use layers of lightweight rugs or blankets.
- Monitor horse carefully, recording vital signs regularly. Follow any instructions given by vet. Give plenty of attention, but avoid over-fussing.
- Groom lightly, but pick out feet and sponge eyes, nose and dock twice a day. Clean the sheath area weekly.
- Massage the legs of horses on box rest twice-daily then apply stable bandages. Avoid a deep bed for a lame horse.
- Reduce or cut out concentrate feeds and replace with quality hay. Feed little and often. Feed should be palatable, laxative, easily-digested and low in protein and carbohydrates. Add succulents (e.g. carrots, apples) as appetisers. Warm bran mash or 'invalid' mixes are suitable. Fresh water should be constantly available (preferably from a bucket, to allow for easy monitoring).
- Take steps to prevent boredom.
- Infectious horses should be isolated (ideally 400m downwind for highly-infectious diseases). Tend to sick animal last, using separate overalls, utensils and kit. Wash hands and rinse off boots afterwards. Disinfect stable and gear thoroughly after recovery.

Sick or injured horses are often anxious and unpredictable. For safety's sake and to allow treatment to be carried out properly, the horse must be effectively but sympathetically controlled. The degree and type of restraint depends on the horse's level of education, maturity, character and the type of injury or disease.

When giving first aid or medical treatment:
- wear sensible clothing, including strong footwear, gloves, hard hat
- enlist knowledgeable help if needed
- choose a safe, enclosed area
- handlers should always stand on same side as the person dealing with the horse
- begin with minimum restraint, only increasing it if necessary.

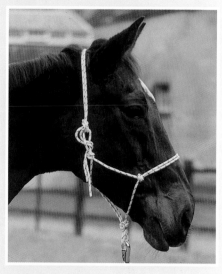

◄ CONTROLLING THE HEAD

Control of the body and limbs is almost impossible without control of the head. Wrapping the lead rope or stud chain once around the nose gives some extra control, but a bridle is far more effective than any normal headcollar or halter. A pressure halter (shown left) can be used with care, or a Chifney bit. Avoid hanging on to the head. Talk quietly to the horse to calm and distract him. Gently rub or scratch the neck or crest.

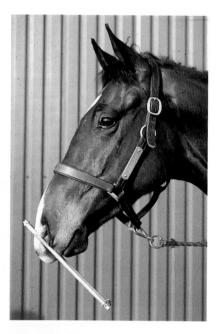

TWITCHING ►

The twitch is thought to work by stimulating production of the body's natural sedatives, endorphins. A proper humane twitch is preferable to an improvised broom handle with loop of twine. Use a twitch on the top lip only, never on the lower lip or ear. The assistant stands to one side. If a loop twitch is used, gather as much upper lip as possible into the loop and twist slowly until the pressure is firm. Knot the lead rope to the twitch handle to prevent it swinging if handler loses grip. The loop can be tightened or loosened slightly if horse gets restless. Reassure horse and rub neck. Clamp-type humane twitches can be applied then fastened to the headcollar to leave one hand free. Relax twitch pressure at regular intervals. If horse continues to resist, have another assistant grip the neck skin.

HOLDING UP A FORE-LEG
Useful with well-handled horses. Keeps horse still and prevents cow-kicking. Position horse four-square with weight evenly distributed. Have fore-leg held up on same side as procedure (use opposite leg if a fore-leg is being treated). Do not allow the horse to lean on the assistant.

GRIPPING SKIN OF NECK
Good for head-shy horses, but only works for short procedures, e.g. bandaging. Grip and squeeze a handful of loose skin on the side of the neck, near the base.

FOALS
Foals and weanlings panic easily, often rearing and rushing backwards if restrained by the head.

Handle foals close to the mare. Approach calmly. Cup one arm under and round the neck and the other round the rump, so the body is cradled between the two.

Weanlings can be backed against a wall or safe fence with the tail held firmly near the base to prevent flipping backwards or sitting down. An assistant works a hand gradually up the neck, cups the ear and squeezes firmly but gently to restrain the head.

HOLDING DOWN
Use to prevent injury when horse is flat-out but struggling intermittently to get up, without success. Put a headcollar and lead rope on horse. With your full weight, kneel on the extended neck and put a hand on the head.

OTHER FIRST-AID GUIDELINES
• Keep the horse clean, warm and dry.
• Remove anything in his stable or surrounds that may injure him further.
• Prevent the horse injuring himself further either by biting, kicking or rubbing the affected part.
• Prepare for the vet's arrival by having a clean, well-lit box with a hard, dry, standing. Ensure that there are at least two clean buckets of warm water available for the vet and a good handler with whom the horse is familiar.
• Keep the horse as calm as possible. This may involve calming down nearby humans, barking dogs etc.

NURSING THE SICK HORSE

Throughout the convalescence of a sick horse it is essential to maintain good movement of the horse's gut. Horses are designed to have a small amount of food making its way through their digestive system at all times and to take in food by moving slowly around their environment; they also are animals with a marked herd instinct – all features to be kept in mind when reducing stress in the sick horse.

GUT MOVEMENT
A horse should be fed little and often with food that is appetising and easily digestible. Make small amounts of hay or haylage available at frequent intervals, in an amount that will maintain a good body weight.

If haynets are used to supply the hay or haylage, tie these up high enough so that the horse cannot get his feet into the net when they are empty. The site of feeding of forage will depend on the nature of the injury. Avoid feeds dropping into wounds, sore eyes, etc. when forage is placed too high. Equally, it is important that the horse, whatever his injury, can easily reach the hay without too great an effort. Never leave the horse without food for longer than six hours.

Many horses normally unaffected by dust will develop a stable cough if they have to remain inside for a continuous period, and it may be necessary to feed some form of haylage under these circumstances.

CONCENTRATE FEED/GRAIN
This must be markedly reduced in line with the amount of work which the horse is getting. If he is on continual box rest, the use of some form of convalescent diet which is palatable and which is easily digested and will encourage gut movement is strongly recommended. The horse should be fed at least four times a day and if the meal is not eaten immediately, any remaining should be removed and discarded. Stale food is likely to put the horse off any other food. The inclusion of diced carrot and apple will be appreciated.

WATER
Clean water should be readily available at all times. If electrolytes are used, it is sensible to have one bucket of electrolytes and one bucket of ordinary water should the horse not care to drink the electrolytes. Using water buckets rather than automatic drinkers is advisable during nursing, allowing the carer to assess how much water has been drunk during each 24-hour period.

Nothing puts a horse off more from eating and drinking than dirty feed and water containers.

WARMTH
The next essential is to keep the horse warm. This may involve using light 'cooler' sheets with light-weight woollen rugs or blankets, woollen leg bandages and possibly the use of a hood. Also, plenty of deep bedding, well-stacked around the edges and right up to the door so that when the horse stands with his head over the door his front feet are on a soft surface. The only exception to this is in the case of severe leg problems where a deep bed may hamper movement.

PEACE AND QUIET
For complete rest, quietness is essential. Whilst remembering that a horse will gain comfort and security from the presence of at least one friendly companion, if possible he should be placed in quiet area of the yard, away from the 'hubbub' of everyday life.

VENTILATION
The sick box must be well ventilated, away from draughts but with a good upward ventilation either through a large vent in the roof or vents at the eaves of the stable. Make sure that the eaves and rafters are not dusty and dirty and that there is nothing projecting in the stable that the horse may hurt himself on.

CLEANLINESS

Cleanliness is crucial when nursing, both in terms of feedstuffs and of the bed. Picking up droppings and clean out the bed regularly, particularly if the horse is suffering from a wound, so that all faeces and urine are kept away. Should the horse have a nasal discharge it is sensible to feed and water with the utensils on the floor to allow gravity to encourage drainage. Utensils should be regularly cleaned and the water should be regularly changed.

If the horse has diarrhoea then plait and tie up his tail. As there should be nothing tight for any length of time around the skin of the dock, the tail should be plaited and turned up and stitched on to itself below the end of the dock (see Chapter Eight) otherwise a pressure necrosis may develop. Any diarrhoea or discharge from the urino-genital system should be regularly removed with clean, warm water.

Similarly, the horse's sheath should be cleaned regularly, as, when the horse is stabled constantly, this will soon become dirty. The job is best done with a very dilute soft-soap solution and using a pair of kitchen gloves, rinsing afterwards with warm water. It is common for such discharge from the sheath to mark and stain the inside of both hind-legs and this also should be removed regularly.

Pick out feet at least twice daily to avoid thrush (see panel page 48). If the horse is to be stabled for a long period, consider removing the shoes and remember to pay attention to hoof trimming to prevent problems associated with over-long feet.

BANDAGING OF WOUNDS

Generally speaking, cold hosing is the best method of cleaning wounds. Maximum constriction of the veins and capillaries occurs after four minutes cold hosing, but hosing can be continued for 20 minutes to help reduce heat in the tissue from inflammation and stimulate the circulation, and so healing. The wound and surrounding hair should then be dried using paper towels, working from the centre outwards so as never to contaminate it with debris from the surrounding tissues.

Any bandages that are applied should always be relatively loose, only firm enough to stay in place (see panel).

Bandages should always be clean and dry; wet bandages should never be applied to horse's limbs. When wounds require the use of cleaning agents, wear rubber gloves to prevent contamination, and clean from the centre outwards using cotton wool and clean warm water plus the recommended cleanser. Discard the cotton wool afterwards and take a separate piece for working outwards again. Never put a soiled piece of cotton wool back into the clean water or cleaning agent or use it more than once.

EXERCISE

Exercise will generally stimulate gut movement but may not be possible, depending on the nature of the condition being treated. Take advice regarding exercise from the vet attending the horse.

WOUND CARE

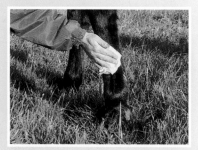

▲ *With any wound, the priority is to stop the bleeding. The simplest way to do this is by applying pressure. Press a pad (e.g. gamgee, or any clean cloth) firmly against the wound. Hold in place for at least five minutes, bandaged if appropriate.*

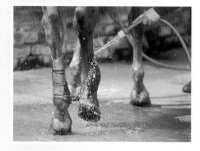

▲ *Once bleeding has stopped, clean the wound. Avoid causing more damage or introducing infection. Hose gently with fresh cold water or wipe (from the centre towards the outside) carefully with cotton wool and clean water or antiseptic wash, or an antiseptic swab. Do not apply ointment, powder or spray if a vet's attention is needed.*

Where a foreign body is stuck in a wound, leave it in place if possible. In the case of foot penetration, note the position, angle and depth of the object. Do not break off nails etc. in the sole, or attempt to move a horse with a nail in its foot.

Wounds on the horse's body area are generally best left unbandaged. On the legs, bandaging helps keep a wound clean, holding the edges together and providing protection to the site. A bandage can consist of up to four layers: a sterile dressing, a layer of padding (cotton wool or gamgee), a layer of crepe (brown gauze) bandage to hold the padding in place, and a protective outer layer. Antibiotic ointment or spray alone is usually sufficient for small scrapes.

THE LOWER LEG

- Use moderate pressure – a finger should fit down easily inside.
- Check often for slippage or rubbing, particularly at pressure points such as the bulbs of the heel, fetlock and back of the knee.
- Replace bandages regularly or at least every 24 hours.

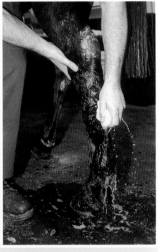

▲ *Step one: Clean the wound thoroughly using clean water or a diluted antiseptic wash. Apply a sterile dressing, but avoid swamping the site in powders or ointments. Wrap plenty of padding around the dressing.*

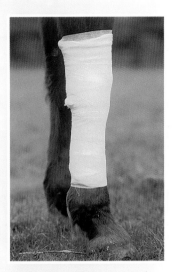

▲ *Step two: Using a stretch crepe bandage, begin at the top and work down to the coronary band and up again, to finish halfway up the leg. Wrap evenly but not too tightly. Secure by snipping and splitting the free end, wrapping around the leg in different directions and tying at the front of the leg.*

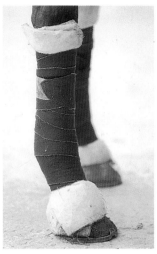

▲ *Step three: Self-adhesive bandage or a stretch-fabric stable bandage provides a final protective layer over gamgee. Bandage firmly and avoid bunching – each layer should come about halfway up the previous one. Secure well, but using no tighter pressure than the bandage itself.*

THE KNEE AND HOCK

The back of the knee is left unbandaged to avoid pressure on the accessory carpal and to make it easy for the horse to move around. The same technique is used for bandaging the hock (as shown).

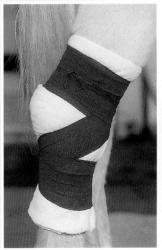

◀ *Cut dressing and padding to required size and apply to affected area. Using stretch crepe bandage, wrap around the leg above the joint, taking in the top of the dressing. Take the bandage diagonally down and wind around the leg below the joint. Bring the bandage diagonally back up across the joint, forming a figure of eight. Finish by winding around the leg above the joint again and securing.*

USING A POULTICE

A dressing can be used to alter the temperature of an injured or infected area. Applying warmth will stimulate the local blood supply and so promote healing of a sprain or injury. The application of a cold dressing works to reduce inflammation.

Traditional bran and Kaolin have now almost universally given way to medicated dressings such as Animalintex. These have a wide range of applications and can be used wet or dry, cold or hot. The minerals and salts impregnated in the dressing draw fluid or pus from a site and will encourage an abscess to rupture.

NB: In North America, an unmedicated hot or cold dressing would be termed a compress, whereas in the UK, the term 'poultice' is used more generally.

Cut the poultice to the size needed to cover the injury site. Pour on boiled water that has cooled to about 100 F (no hotter than your hand can stand easily). Squeeze to remove excess water. Do not put extremely hot or cold poultices in contact with the horse's skin.

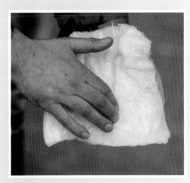

◀ Place on site of injury, polythene backing outwards. A layer of foil can then help retain warmth and prolong the activity of the poultice.

Secure in place using gamgee and ▶ bandaging. For a foot infection, cover whole foot with sacking and secure, or protect using a waterproof poultice boot or Equiboot.

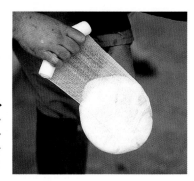

O nce a hot poultice has cooled, it has no effect. After no more than eight hours, remove, wash area and replace. If necessary, keep the old poultice to show vet what has been extracted. Discuss with vet if no real improvement after 48 hours.

Poultice for as short a period as possible. Continue for 36 hours after any pus has appeared on the poultice, but no longer. Repeated poulticing will waterlog the skin and make any wound slow to heal. Poultices are helpful for puncture wounds, especially to the foot, but are often counter-productive in more open types of wound.

PREVENTION AND TREATMENT OF THRUSH

Convalescing horses are particularly at risk from thrush, an unpleasant condition involving decay of the frog, which can affect any horse kept in damp or dirty conditions.

Thrush is caused by the anaerobic bacteria **Sphaerophus necrophorus**. Infection creates a foul-smelling, black, tarry discharge and, if the sensitive tissues become involved, will lead to lameness.

- Keep bedding scrupulously clean and dry
- Clean out feet twice daily, paying particular attention to the cleft of the frog and the grooves alongside it (paracuneal grooves)
- If signs of thrush are seen, any infected tissue must be pared away by the farrier or veterinary surgeon. The frog and sole must be treated daily with anti-bacterial wash provided by the vet, or a 4% iodine or 10% formalin solution, until the condition has completely cleared. Antibiotics may be needed – and a tetanus booster if the horse has not been properly immunised.

3 FEEDING AND NUTRITION

The horse evolved to eat grass. Its natural feeding pattern involves endless and varied grazing, eating small amounts often – indeed, horses will spend up to 60% of the day grazing if allowed to do so. This type of feeding pattern is known as 'trickle' feeding and the horse's digestive tract is ideally suited it.

A natural equine diet consists of grasses and vegetation containing large amounts of fibre. Today's horse, however, leads a completely different lifestyle to that of his ancestors. He is enclosed in stables and paddocks, no longer able to roam freely. In addition we add to his diet concentrate cereals, which reduce both the amount of time he spends eating and the quantity of fibre he takes in. As a result, our horses are prone to illnesses such as colic, azoturia and laminitis and to suffering temperament problems. The aim of the horse owner should be to feed the horse in as natural a way as possible, keeping him both happy and healthy.

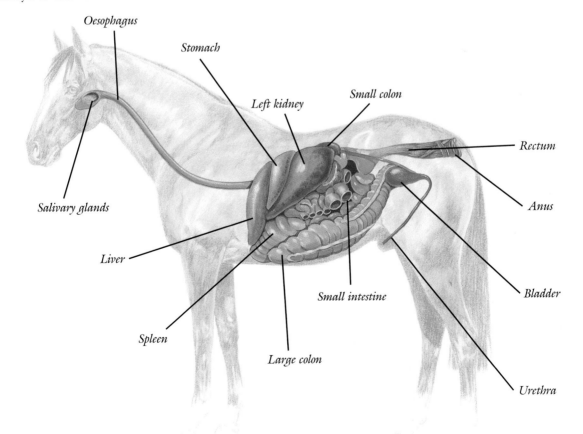

Oesophagus
Stomach
Left kidney
Small colon
Rectum
Salivary glands
Anus
Liver
Bladder
Small intestine
Spleen
Large colon
Urethra

THE DIGESTIVE SYSTEM

A basic understanding of how the equine gut works will help an owner to design a feeding programme to suit the horse's natural lifestyle. The function of the digestive system of the horse is to take in food, break it down and remove nutrients from it.

The digestive system can be divided into seven parts:

Fore gut
mouth
oesophagus (or gullet)
stomach
small intestine

Hind gut
large intestine
rectum
anus.

As a whole, the gut is about 100 feet (30m) long and it takes about 65-75 hours for food to pass through it. It is looped and coiled to fit into the abdominal space and there are several changes in diameter and direction.

MOUTH

The horse grazes by carefully selecting food with its highly mobile lips and then cropping it with the incisor teeth. The food is passed to the back of the mouth by the tongue, where the grinding molar teeth chew the material. Equine teeth differ from human teeth in that they grow continually throughout the life of the horse. This growth compensates for the wearing down of the molars caused by this constant grinding action. The horse's teeth should be regularly checked and rasped if necessary to remove any sharp edges (see Chapter Two, Teeth Care). As the horse chews it produces saliva which wets and lubricates the food before it is swallowed via the **pharynx** and passed into the **oesophagus** on its way to the stomach. Occasionally, food becomes lodged in the oesophagus and this is known as choke (see page 72).

STOMACH

The **stomach** of the horse is small compared to that of other animals. Holding about 7-13 litres (2-3 gallons), the empty stomach is roughly the same size as a rugby ball. If too much feed is given at one time it will be pushed out of the stomach before it has

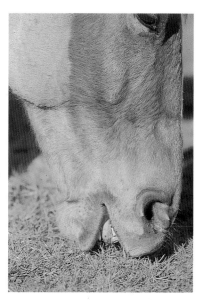

The horse's mobile lips, sharp incisors and elongated jaw packed with heavy-duty molars evolved to bite off and grind a diet of tough grasses.

time to mix thoroughly with the gastric secretions which help to begin digestion, and this can lead to colic. The horse should therefore be fed little and often to avoid digestive upsets.

Feed breakdown begins in the stomach. However, food material is only in the stomach for about 45 minutes and this limits the amount of digestion which can take place. Once food has passed into the stomach it cannot be regurgitated back, so unlike humans, the horse is unable to vomit.

SMALL INTESTINE

Food passes from the stomach to the **small intestine.** The small intestine is where most of the breakdown and absorption of the concentrate part of the horse's diet takes place. Digestion of food in the small intestine is similar to that which occurs in simple-stomached animals such as humans and pigs. Its total length is about 21m (70ft) with a capacity of 55-70 litres (12-16 gallons). Material takes about 60 minutes to travel along this length to the large intestine.

LARGE INTESTINE

From the small intestine, any undigested food and fibre enter the large intestine, which is made up of the **caecum, large colon, small colon** and the **rectum,** and is approximately 8 metres (25 feet) long. The partially digested food reaches the caecum approximately two hours after a meal and remains in the large intestine for 36-48 hours. It is here, in the horse's hind gut, that the fibre found in plant cell walls is broken down.

Fibre refers to complex substances such as cellulose

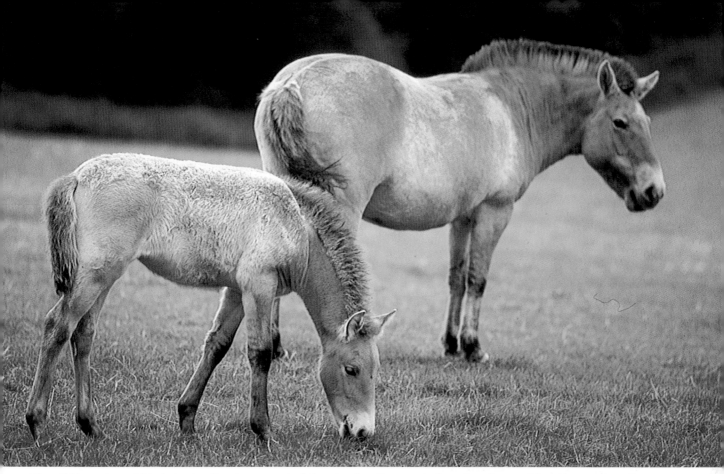

The wild horse is a trickle feeder, its digestive system is designed to handle a steady flow of small quantities of low-quality, fibrous food.

and hemi-cellulose which are resistant to digestion by enzymes in the small intestine. Micro-organisms, bacteria or 'bugs' in the horse's large intestine are able to break down digestible fibre by a process called fermentation, allowing the horse to thrive on its natural fibrous diet. These bugs also synthesise B-vitamins for use by the horse.

The population of bugs will vary according to the nature of the diet – horses fed on grass have a different bacterial population to those on a high concentrate diet. If a diet is suddenly changed, the digestive process is disrupted and the horse may suffer from colic, constipation or diarrhoea. In order to avoid such problems, changes to the diet should be made slowly over a period of time. This allows time for the bacteria to adapt to a different diet.

The quantity of micro-organisms in the digestive tract of the horse is huge, numbering more than ten times all the tissue cells in the body. More than half the dry weight of faeces produced by the horse consists of bacteria. Water is absorbed as food passes through the large intestine.

THE PHYSIOLOGY OF DIGESTION

The digestive processes that take place in the horse are different from those in other grass-eaters such as the cow, which is a ruminant. In the horse, easily-digested food material is first broken down by digestive enzymes in the small intestine. Only insoluble material reaches the large intestine for bacterial fermentation. This insoluble material is mainly cellulose.

The digestion of fibre is entirely reliant on micro-organisms, which ferment cellulose, releasing energy-producing substances known as volatile fatty acids (VFAs). These are absorbed into the bloodstream and converted to energy.

In the wild, the horse is a trickle feeder, eating a mainly fibrous diet. This is very efficient: in an all-hay diet, over 70% of the horse's energy is derived from hind-gut digestion. In contrast, stabled horses are given high-starch concentrates which pass rapidly through the gut. There is often insufficient time for them to be completely digested by the enzymes in the small intestine. Remaining feed passes into the caecum, which is not only wasteful but can also cause severe digestive upset and temperament problems. It is this inadequate processing which results in cereal feeds having what is known as a 'heating' effect. We can help this situation by feeding fibre in the form of chaff with the concentrate feed and giving the horse probiotics in times of stress.

51

THE RULES OF FEEDING

Over the years, certain 'rules' of feeding have developed to help feed horses more safely and efficiently. Not only have the majority of these guidelines stood the test of time, but our knowledge of the anatomy and physiology of the horse's gut now shows that many are indeed based on sound scientific principles.

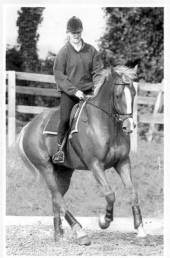

◀ *Feed each horse according to individual needs.*

Feed good-quality feed. ▶

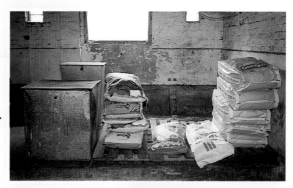

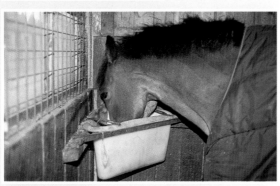

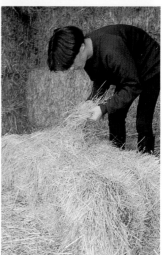

Feed sufficient ▶ *bulk food.*

◀ *Feed little and often, from clean containers.*

- **Feed according to age, size, type, temperament, condition and work being done.**
- **Feed little and often.**
  Several small feeds throughout the day suit the horse's natural lifestyle. A horse has a relatively small stomach and will obtain less benefit from one large feed per day.
- **Do not make sudden changes to the diet.**
  Make sure all changes are introduced gradually, as a sudden change in diet may upset the microbial population in the hind gut.
- **Allow the horse time to digest its food before exercise.**
  Once a horse is working it will stop digesting its food, so plenty of time should be allowed between feeding and exercise.

- **Keep all feeding utensils clean.**
  A horse will be put off its food by dirty equipment and mangers.
- **Feed only good-quality feed.**
  It is false economy to feed second-rate food as this can lead to respiratory and digestive disorders.
- **Ensure a constant supply of fresh, clean water.**
  Colic can be caused by the horse drinking a lot of water after a large feed.
- **Feed a balanced diet.**
- **Feed sufficient bulk food/forage.**
  Horses need bulk and natural fibre in their diet in order to digest their food properly. Even a horse in hard, fast work will require at least 50 per cent of its ration as bulk.

NUTRITIONAL REQUIREMENTS

Feeding is one of the most critical factors in preparing a horse for growth, work or competition and is a combination of science and experience built up over a number of years.

A well-balanced diet contains the correct levels of minerals, vitamins, energy, protein and water. The nutrients required for a balanced diet fall into the following categories:-

- carbohydrates
- water
- fats and oils
- minerals
- protein
- vitamins
- fibre.

CARBOHYDRATES

Carbohydrates are the horse's major source of energy and include such substances as sugar, starch and fibre. Carbohydrates provide the energy needed for all body processes such as breathing, the beating of the heart and muscle contraction. Carbohydrates may be roughly divided into two groups:

- Soluble carbohydrates – starch, sugars (spring grass, cereals)
- Insoluble carbohydrates – cellulose, hemi-cellulose (fibre).

Soluble carbohydrates, such as sugars and starches, are built up from units of glucose formed into long chains. During digestion these are broken down to glucose and absorbed into the blood. Any glucose surplus to immediate requirements is stored as glycogen. Once the glycogen stores are full, any further glucose will be converted to fat and deposited in fat stores around the horse's body. In other words, feeding too much energy-giving food will make the horse fat.

Insoluble carbohydrate makes up a large proportion of the natural diet of the horse – it is the cellulose and fibre found in grass and hay. Fibre is not broken down to any great extent in the small intestine but passes to the large intestine, where it is acted on by the gut bacteria and other micro-organisms to provide an energy source for the horse. The energy from the breakdown and fermentation of fibre is released more slowly and this steady supply

of 'slow-release energy' is much more natural for the horse. Remember, the horse is designed to eat fibre, not starch. Keeping starch levels down will result in a happier horse.

Remembering the rule of good feeding 'feed plenty of bulk', the fibre level in the ration should never fall bellow 50 per cent. An adequate level of fibre is essential to maintain the flow of food through the gut. Fibre also tends to open out the digestive mixture, allowing the digestive juices to act on the feed more efficiently. Additionally, fibre helps to retain water and electrolytes in the large intestine, acting as a reservoir of fluid for the working, sweating horse.

Cereals such as oats, barley and maize contain high amounts of starch and are therefore known as 'concentrates'. Hay contains more fibre and is known as a 'forage'. Good-quality forages are an excellent source of energy for horses and should not be considered as merely 'fillers'.

CALORIE-COUNTING FOR HORSES

We are all familiar with the concept of counting the calories in food when dieting. High-calorie foods are fattening: they contain more energy than we burn up and the excess is laid down as fat. High-calorie foods include sugar, starch (carbohydrates) and fat.

When we are looking at the energy value of feeds for horses, we use the metric version of the calorie, the joule (J). To make the figures easier, the term 'megajoules' of digestible energy per kilogram is used (MJ DE/kg). Thus a high-energy food like oats

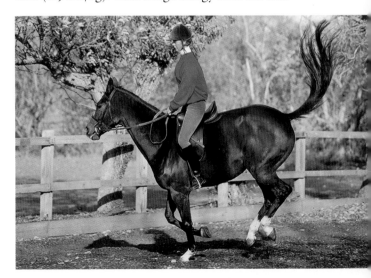

Excess energy created by a diet too high in calories for the horse's workload is the cause of many behavioural problems.

may contain up to 14 MJ DE/kg, while a low-energy grass hay may only contain 7 MJ DE/kg – half as much as oats.

If the horse is fed too much energy, there will be serious consequences:

• Receiving too much energy can make the horse hyperactive.
• Excess energy is stored as fat; horses are less athletic if they are over-weight, and working fat horses strains muscles, tendons and joints.
• Most seriously, too much carbohydrate can affect the horse's metabolism – for example, a carbohydrate overload from rich spring grass or stealing from the feed bin can lead to laminitis (see page 82).

FATS & OILS

Fat contains 2.25 times more energy than carbohydrate and can be stored in the body and used as a source of energy when it is required. Fat has been used for some time to supplement the diets of endurance horses and other performance horses with much success. Just as excess glucose can be converted to fat, fat can be converted to glucose and used for muscle contraction. The addition of 300 ml (1 cup) of sunflower or soya oil to each of three feeds supplies as much energy as 1 kg (2.2 lbs) of oats. High-fat compound feeds are now available from some horse feed manufacturers.

PROTEIN

Protein is required for growth and to rebuild and replace body tissue lost through wear and natural wastage. The need for protein is greatest in the young, growing horse. Once maturity is reached, the protein requirement is reduced and only enough is required to replace worn body tissues and support the slow growth of tissues such as skin, hoof and hair. The horse's dietary requirement for protein is not greatly increased by work – in fact, feeding excess protein to working horses can be detrimental. It is highly unlikely that a mature horse will be deficient in protein, particularly if it has access to good grazing.

Proteins are made up of simple units called amino acids. The most important essential amino acids are lysine, methionine and tryptophan. Some proteins contain more of the essential amino acids and these are referred to as high-quality proteins. Lysine is most likely to be deficient in the horse's diet, particularly when a cereal or 'straight' ration is being fed and the horse has limited grazing.

VITAMINS

Vitamins are a complex group of organic substances that are essential, in small quantities, for the normal metabolism of the body. A deficiency in the diet will result in dysfunctional metabolism and eventually clinical disease.

Vitamins occur naturally in certain foods, but some can be made by the horse from materials in the diet. There are approximately 15 vitamins which are known to be essential to equine health. Actual vitamin requirements will, however, depend upon several factors, such as pregnancy, growth, age and level of work.

Vitamins can be divided into two groups;
• fat-soluble vitamins – A, D, E and K
• water-soluble vitamins – C and B-complex.

VITAMINS REQUIRED IN THE HORSE'S DIET

WATER-SOLUBLE VITAMINS	FAT-SOLUBLE VITAMINS
C – ascorbic acid	A – beta-carotene
B1 – thiamin	D – cholecalciferol ("sunshine vitamin")
B2 – riboflavin or lactoflavin	E – tocopherol
B3 – niacin	K – phylloquinone
B5 – pantothenic acid	
B6 – pyridoxine	
B12 – cyanocobalamin	
B15 – pangamic acid	
folic acid	
choline	
inositol	
biotin (Vitamin H)	

Fat-soluble vitamins can be stored in the body, particularly the liver. Most of these are plentiful in fresh green herbage and the horse can store sufficient over the summer months for later use during the winter. Most of the **water-soluble vitamins** are manufactured by the micro-organisms in the hind gut and therefore are unlikely to be deficient unless the horse has received antibiotic therapy or is highly stressed or ill.

MINERALS

Wild horses are able to meet their mineral needs by selectively grazing and roaming over huge areas of land with different soil types. The modern domesticated horse relies upon good feeding and pasture to supply its mineral requirements.

Minerals are inorganic substances found throughout the horse's body and are crucial for health and development. At least 21 minerals are known to be essential to the equine. Some are required in larger amounts and are known as macro-minerals or major minerals; those required in small amounts are known as trace elements or trace minerals.

MAJOR MINERALS	TRACE MINERALS
Calcium (Ca)	Copper (Cu)
Phosphorus (P)	Zinc (Zn)
Magnesium (Mg)	Manganese (Mn)
Potassium (K)	Iron (Fe)
Sodium (Na)	Iodine (I)
Chloride (Cl)	Selenium (Se)
	Cobalt (Co)
	Molybdenum (Mo)

WATER

Approximately 70 per cent of the body weight of the horse is made up of water. The supply of water is very important and thirst will cause death in a much shorter time than hunger. A loss of barely 8 per cent of body water causes illness and loss of 15 per cent can result in serious dehydration. Horses require an average of between 8 and 12 gallons of water per day; the quantity varies according to the animal, the work, the weather and the diet.

Water is required for many different life functions such as:
• temperature regulation, i.e. sweating
• saliva

• replace liquid lost in breathing
• maintaining blood volume
• enabling nutrients to pass through the gut wall in solution
• urine, which is necessary to get rid of the waste products of the various body functions
• milk production.

TYPES OF FEEDSTUFFS

Feeds for horses fall into two main categories:
• Forage – grass, hay, haylage, alfalfa, dried grass, grass cubes and commercially-produced chaffs
• Concentrates – straights, compound feeds.

FORAGE

Forage is the most natural feed for horses and is a vital source of fibre, essential for normal gut function and all-round health. Fibre is not just a 'filler' but an essential part of the ration – too little forage can result in colic, diarrhoea, laminitis, wood-chewing, tail-chewing and dung-eating.

GRASS

Horses have evolved to eat grass and good pasture contains all of the nutrients required by the horse, including carbohydrates (starch and sugars), protein, minerals and vitamins. The nutrient value of grass changes over the growing season; spring grass is very nutritious but as the season progresses, the grass matures and contains more fibre and less nutrients. Different species of grass also provide varying levels of nutrients to horses.

HAY

Hay is dried grass. Meadow hay is made from permanent, established pasture which usually contains many species of grasses and often some herbs and other wild plants. Meadow hay tends to be softer and have lower protein levels than seed hay, which is made from ryegrass-based leys grown specifically for hay. Seed hay is generally coarser than meadow hay and often contains higher levels of protein. Legume hays include clover and sainfoin and more commonly alfalfa (lucerne).

The nutrient value of hay will depend on:
• the nutrient value of the grass when the hay was cut
• how efficiently the grass was dried, turned and baled.

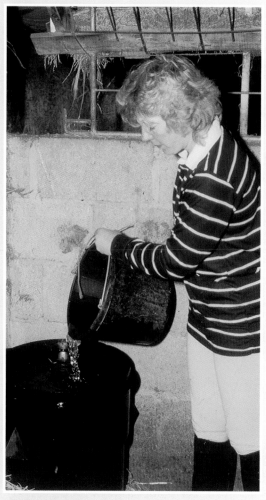

Whatever the management regime, constant access to fresh water is essential.

- A constant supply of fresh, clean water should always be available.
- If this is not possible, water the horse at least three times a day in winter and six times a day in summer. In this situation always water before feeding.
- Water a hot or tired horse with water that has had the chill taken off.
- If a bucket of water is left constantly with the horse, change it and swill out the bucket at least twice a day, and top it up as necessary throughout the day. Standing water becomes unpalatable.
- Horses that have been deprived of water should be given small quantities frequently until their thirst is quenched. They must not be allowed to gorge themselves on water.
- During endurance work water the horse as often as possible, at least every two hours. Hunters should be allowed to drink on the way home.
- If horses have a constant supply of fresh, clean water there should be no need to deprive the horse of water before racing or fast work. However, the horse's water can be removed from the stable two hours before the race, if thought necessary.
- A hot or tired horse should not be allowed to take a long drink. Allow only a few small sips until he has cooled off and his respiratory rate has lowered.
- Horses may dehydrate, losing large amounts of body salts and water, after heavy sweating or during long journeys on hot days. These salts can be replaced by adding electrolytes to the water or feed.

Properties of good quality hay:
- clean, fresh and sweet-smelling
- green
- free from dust and mould
- a ryegrass hay is potentially of a higher feed value than meadow hay
- if you can identify seed heads then the grass was cut late and the hay will be of lower feed value.

The most important factor is that hay is free from dust, mould and fungal spores; mouldy hay can cause irreparable damage to the horse's lungs. As long as hay is clean, any nutrient deficiency can be made up by feeding concentrates or supplements. Horses which suffer from respiratory problems may be fed hay which has been thoroughly soaked prior to being fed to the horse.

HAY ALTERNATIVES
The horse is designed to live on a high-fibre diet, so any shortfall of hay must be compensated for by adding another high-fibre feed, for example:

- haylage
- straw
- chaff
- sugar beet pulp
- high-fibre cubes.

Most of the hay alternatives mentioned have a better nutrient value than the hay they are replacing or supplementing and should be fed carefully; it may be necessary to reduce or change the concentrate ration.

HAYLAGE
Haylage lies between silage and hay in its feeding

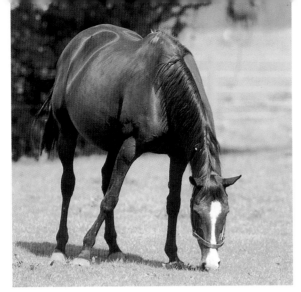

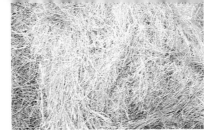
Meadow hay

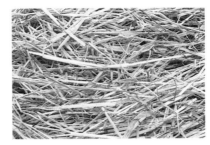
Seed hay

Grass – a horse's natural food.

value and digestibility. It is highly palatable and horses can take in large amounts of energy quite rapidly, so care should be taken not to overfeed. Haylage should be substituted for hay on a weight-for-weight basis; it contains a lot of water and is consequently heavy, so the horse will be receiving equivalent amounts of energy and protein from a smaller volume ration. The downside of this is that the horse will be receiving less fibre and the haylage will be eaten more quickly than the equivalent hay ration. Special closely-woven hay nets can be used to feed haylage in order to slow down the horse's rate of eating.

Before buying haylage find out how it was made and have it analysed to assess the quality. Correct fermentation is vital to preserve the haylage and also affects its suitability for feeding to horses. The following guidelines should be used:

- the dry matter should be between 45 and 65%, preferably 55-65%;
- the pH (acidity) should lie between 4.5 and

5.8 – above a pH of 6, the haylage will not be acidic enough to prevent the potentially lethal micro-organisms developing.

Some haylage is produced specifically for horses. Grass is cut and allowed to wilt until the moisture content is down to about 45% and then baled in the same way as hay. The bales are then compressed to about half their size and sealed in tough, plastic bags. Fermentation takes place which preserves the grass. Different types of bagged haylage are produced, for example alfalfa and high-fibre types are available.

STRAW
Good-quality oat straw in small quantities can act as a useful source of fibre for horses with sound teeth, but it is deficient in most nutrients. It is a good filler for fat ponies that do too well on hay. Hungry horses brought in on to straw beds may eat too much straw, which can lead to impactive colic.

COMPOSITION OF HAY AND OTHER HIGH-FIBRE FEEDS

FEED	CRUDE PROTEIN (%)	CRUDE FIBRE (%)	DIGESTIBLE ENERGY (MJ DE/KG)	DRY MATTER (%)
Hay	4.5-10	30-40	7-10	80
Haylage	8-14	30-38	9-11.5	55-65
Straw	3	40	6	88
Sugar beet pulp	7	34	10.5	Fed soaked
Alfalfa chaff	15-16	32	9-10	80
Alfalfa/straw chaff	10.5	38	7	80
High fibre cubes	9	20	8.5	85
Grassmeal	16	36	9-10	85

CHAFFS

Most straw-based, molassed chaffs are designed to bulk out the hard feed and to slow down the horse's rate of eating. Hay and alfalfa or straw chaffs have been designed as partial or complete hay replacers, to be fed pound-for-pound for good-quality hay. Alfalfa chaff is too 'high-powered' to be fed to most horses as a hay replacer, but is a useful 'top-up', especially for horses in hard work, being high in energy, protein, minerals and vitamins. This is the most common usage in North America, where chaff is better known as either A&M (alfalfa and molasses) or O&M (oat, straw and molasses).

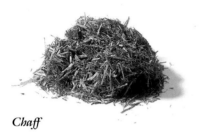

Chaff

SUGAR BEET PULP

Sugar beet pulp falls between a forage and a concentrate. Sugar beet is a root vegetable used as a source of sugar for human consumption. Once the sugar is removed, all that is left is fibre and pulp. Molasses is then added before it is dried and shredded or pelleted. Sugar beet is similar in energy value to oats but the energy comes from digestible fibre and not from starch, so making it less 'heating'.

Sugar beet shreds should be just covered in water and soaked for up to 12 hours. Cubes or pellets should be covered in 2-3 times as much water and soaked for up to 24 hours. Sugar beet should be

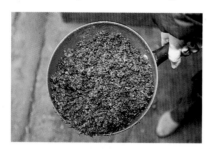

Soaked sugar beet

freshly made up every day as it can ferment, especially in warm weather. Horses can be fed up to 1.8kg (4 lb) dry weight of beet pulp per day; this amounts to about four scoops of wet sugar beet pulp. Unmolassed sugar beet pulp is now available, reducing the soluble carbohydrate level of the diet.

CONCENTRATES

Concentrate feedstuffs tend to be split into two groups:

- Straights or cereal grains
- Compound feeds.

STRAIGHTS

Straights refers to cereal grains such as oats, barley and maize. These are all carbohydrate sources containing high levels of starch. However, their mineral balance is poor, as they contain low levels of calcium and high levels of phosphorus, which is the reverse of the horse's requirements. The protein level may appear to be good, but the quality of the protein is poor, being low in lysine, an essential amino acid. Feed manufacturers use straights when manufacturing horse feed, but balance the deficiencies by adding vitamin and mineral pre-mixes and high-quality protein sources.

The horse is not designed to eat cereal grains, and so great care should be taken when feeding them. No more than 2.5kg (5.5lb) of grain should be fed at one feed, due to the horse's small stomach.

Straights may undergo various processes, before they are sold:

- extrusion – cooking at great pressure which breaks up the starch molecules and makes the feed more digestible.
- micronisation – flaking and toasting which again makes the starch more digestible.
- rolling – crushing the grain; once open to the air, the grain will start to lose its feed value and should be used within two weeks.
- steam cooking – passing the grain through heated rollers which cook and split it. Again the starch is made more available, increasing the digestibility.

	FEED	DESCRIPTION	NUTRITIONAL VALUE	FEEDING HINTS
Oats	Oats	Plump, shiny, clean, dust-free. Can be fed whole or crimped.	8-13% crude protein 11-14 MJ DE/kg 10-12% fibre 4.5% oil Low in calcium, B-complex vitamins, vitamin A and lysine.	Palatable, easily digested, 'safer' to feed that other cereals, high in fibre, low in energy, weigh light. Can make up all the concentrate ration. Avoid 'new' oats (less than 3 months old).
	Naked oats	Oats without the husk.	13% crude protein 16 MJ DE/kg 3% fibre 9% oil.	Energy-dense. Good for performance horses with poor appetites.
Barley	Barley	Plump, dust-free, rounder than oats. Fed rolled, steam-flaked, micronised or boiled. Cooked barley is more digestible and less likely to lead to starch overload.	8-10% crude protein 12-13 MJ DE/kg 5% fibre 2% oil Low in calcium, B-complex vitamins, vitamin A and lysine.	Provides more energy and lower fibre than oats and weighs more. Some horses are allergic to it; cooking may solve this problem. Can make up all the concentrate ration.
Maize	Maize	Can be fed whole, but usually steam-flaked and rolled.	8% crude protein 14-15 MJ DE/kg 3% fibre 4% oil.	The most energy-dense grain, palatable and digestible. Useful for poor-doers or horses with very high energy requirements. Not usually more than 25% of the concentrate ration.
Bran	Bran	By-product of flour production. Should be free-flowing with little dust. May be fed as mash; mild laxative.	15% crude protein 10 MJ DE/kg 11% fibre 3% oil Not very high in fibre. Low in calcium.	Palatable, weighs very light. Expensive, largely replaced by chaffs. No more than 10% of the concentrate ration. Should be supplemented with limestone flour.

FEED	DESCRIPTION	NUTRITIONAL VALUE	FEEDING HINTS
Oil	Sunflower, corn and soya oils are preferred.	0% crude protein 35 MJ DE/kg 0% fibre Very good energy source. Cod-liver oil provides vitamins A, D and E and essential fatty acids.	Increases vitamin E requirement. 300ml (0.5 pt) replaces 900 g (2 lb) oats.

APPEARANCE, NUTRITIONAL VALUE AND FEEDING HINTS FOR SOME PROTEIN SOURCES

FEED	DESCRIPTION	NUTRITIONAL VALUE	FEEDING HINTS
Linseed	Small, shiny, brown seeds.	22% crude protein 18 MJ DE/kg 7% fibre 31% oil Low-quality protein. Expensive. Largely replaced by soya bean meal.	Palatable, good coat conditioner. Must be boiled to destroy poisons. During boiling absorbs a lot of water and becomes a jelly. Mild laxative properties.
Soya bean	Raw beans contain toxin and must be heat treated. Can be either fat-extracted (protein source) or full fat (energy and protein).	44% crude protein 13 MJ DE/kg 6% fibre 1% oil Full-fat soya up to 20% fat.	Very high-quality protein for horses. Oil helps coat condition. Can be added to traditional hay and oat rations as sole protein source.
Peas and beans	Peas are now more common than beans. Fed micronised or steam-flaked. May be sold as mixed flakes with maize and barley.	24% crude protein 13 MJ DE/kg 6% fibre 5% oil Good source of lysine.	Palatable, often included in coarse mixes. Traditionally added to winter diet of horses.
Milk powder		34% crude protein 15MJ DE/kg 0% fibre 0.6% oil High in lysine.	Palatable. Energy not available to weaned animals. Expensive.

COMPOUND FEEDS

Compound feeds can be divided into three groups:
• High-fibre cubes
• Concentrate cubes or coarse mixes
• Balancers – cubes or coarse mixes, or protein concentrates.

High-fibre cubes are designed to replace all or part of the hay and concentrates in the ration and tend to be used for overweight ponies, when hay is scarce, or to supplement poor-quality grazing. They are also useful to maintain the condition of resting horses and ponies, when they can replace the concentrate ration. Such cubes should be fed with a good-quality chaff.

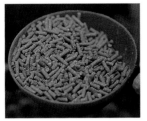
Cubes

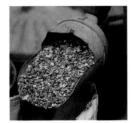
Coarse mix

Concentrate cubes or coarse mixes provide a balanced diet for all types of horses and are designed to be fed with forage and water. Different formulations are made for horses with different needs: high-protein feeds for growing stock, high-energy feeds for working horses and low-energy feeds for resting or those in light work.

Balancer cubes or mixes are higher in protein and designed to balance a straight such as oats. One of the most common is the 50:50 oats to oat-balancer mix. Half the concentrate ration is oats and the other half oat-balancer. The oat-balancer corrects the deficiencies in the oats and the combination results in a balanced ration when fed with forage.

All compound feeds must, by law, declare certain ingredients. The following information must be given:
• % by weight of crude oil
• % by weight crude protein
• % by weight crude fibre
• % by weight of total ash
• amounts of added vitamins A, D and E (shown as international units IU per kg)
• total selenium content if synthetic Se has been added (mg/kg)
• if an antioxidant has been added.
Some manufacturers now include digestible energy and digestible crude protein figures also, but this is not compulsory. Sell-by dates are also on the label, allowing the freshness of the feed to be assessed before purchase.

The advantages of feeding compound feeds include:

• the feeds contain everything the horse needs and do not require supplementation
• there are feeds for every type of horse
• the feeds are of consistent quality and are produced under conditions of strict quality control
• most products have a good shelf-life and an expiry date so that you can ensure the food is fresh

• they are virtually dust-free, making them suitable for feeding to horses with a dust allergy
• they are highly palatable – coarse mixes are specially designed to tempt fussy feeders and care must be taken not to overfeed them.

STORING CONCENTRATE FEEDS
All concentrate feeds should be stored in a feed room that is horse-proof and secure. The feed room must be dry, well-ventilated, cool and kept clean and hygienic. Any sacks of feed should be stacked on pallets and kept out of direct sunlight and heat. Open bags must be stored in vermin-proof containers. Use up all the old feed and clean out the bin before any new feed is poured in.

SUPPLEMENTS
Supplements are substances added to the horse's diet in order to balance it or correct a deficiency. Common supplements include:
• vitamins, e.g. biotin
• minerals, e.g. limestone flour
• broad-spectrum vitamin and mineral supplements, containing a range of micronutrients
• body salts (electrolytes).
A stabled horse is likely to require supplementation of vitamins A, D, and E, plus folic acid. A selection of B vitamins may be necessary for performance horses receiving a high level of concentrates and with limited access to grass. Of all the trace elements, inadequate intakes of copper, selenium, manganese, iodine and zinc are most frequently detected and should be included in a supplement.

When feeding supplements remember to:
• read the manufacturer's instruction beforehand
• use the measure provided and replace the lid tightly after use
• store in a cool, dry place and avoid exposure to strong sunlight
• buy an appropriate amount so that it can be used before its sell-by date
• remember compound feeds are already supplemented; if the horse is receiving the amount of cubes recommended by the manufacturers, it should not need another supplement
• few horses are receiving the maximum amount recommended by the feed manufacturer and may need a supplement to make up the balance
• introduce supplements gradually, taking about a week to build up to the full dose.

EXAMPLES OF COMPOUND FEEDS AVAILABLE

FEEDS FOR VARIOUS WORKLOADS	PROTEIN (%)	OIL (%)	FIBRE (%)	DIGESTIBLE ENERGY (MJ DE/KG)
Rest or light work				
Mix	8.5	2.2	15	9
Cubes	9	2	18	8.5
Light or medium work				
Mix	10	3.25	11	10
Cubes	10	3.25	15	9.5
Medium to hard work				
Mix	12	3.25	8	12
Cubes	11.5	3.25	12	11
Hard, fast work				
Mix	14	5	6	14
Cubes	14	4	9.5	13
Old age	11	4.5	11	11
Showing condition	12	4.25	9	12

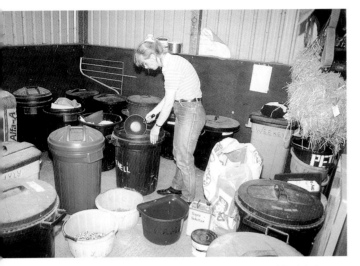

Organise the feed room so that each type of food is kept in a clearly- marked, damp-proof and vermin-proof container.

Remember, unless the horse has a specific problem, a supplement is only necessary if:

- the horse is being fed poor-quality feedstuffs
- high performance is required
- the horse is under stress, such as old age, illness or growth
- salt will need to be added to the diet if the horse does not have access to a salt lick
- body salts (electrolytes) are essential for performance horses and should be given whenever the horse has been sweating after work
- cereal-based rations must have limestone or dicalcium phosphate added to them.

ADDITIVES

An additive is a substance which is added to an already-balanced ration. Common additives include:

- enzymes – biological catalysts aimed to improve digestion by various means
- herbs – a natural alternative to supplements
- probiotics – 'live' bacteria to help re-colonise the gut after stress or antibiotics
- yeasts – improve the number of fibre-digesting bacteria in the hind gut.

RATIONING

Feeding horses is generally accepted as a combination of experience, knowledge and 'feel'. The quantity of feed a horse needs depends on many factors, including:

- condition
- age
- size
- health
- type
- breed
- work done
- reproductive status
- temperament
- environment.

WORKING OUT A RATION

The ration for a particular horse can be worked out by following four easy steps:

- estimate the horse's bodyweight and condition score
- decide on the horse's appetite
- decide on the ratio of roughage to concentrates
- calculate the ration.

A simple method of estimating the horse's weight is to place a weigh-tape around the girth and use the table below to give an approximate guide to the relationship between height, girth and bodyweight.

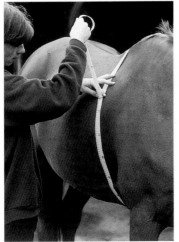

HEIGHT		GIRTH		BODYWEIGHT	
(hh)	(cm)	(cm)	(in)	(kg)	(lb)
11	111	135-145	53-57	200-260	440-572
12	122	140-150	55-59	230-290	506-638
13	132	150-160	59-63	290-350	638-770
14	142	160-170	63-67	350-420	770-924
15	152	170-185	67-73	420-520	924-1144
16	162	185-195	73-77	500-600	1100-1320
17	172	195-210	77-83	600-725	1320-1595

How much the horse weighs will also be affected by how much condition it is carrying. This will also affect how much you feed a horse – a thin horse will need more to eat than a fat horse.

CONDITION SCORING

'Condition scoring' is an objective way to assess a horse's condition. To condition-score a horse, stand directly behind it and note the amount of flesh covering the pelvis and top of the quarters. Compare your findings with the comments in the table below. Remember that hard-working horses such as endurance horses and eventers are usually kept in lower body condition than dressage and show horses.

CONDITION SCORE	QUARTERS	BACK AND RIBS	NECK AND SHOULDERS
0: Extremely emaciated	Deep cavity under tail and either side of croup. Pelvis angular. No detectable fatty tissue between skin and bone.	Processes of vertebrae sharp to touch. Skin drawn tightly over ribs.	'Ewe-neck' (neck shaped like a sheep's neck); very narrow; individual bone structure visible. Bone structure of shoulder visible. No fatty tissue.
1: Thin	Pelvis and croup well defined, no fatty tissue, but skin supple. Poverty lines (deep lines running down hindquarters either side of tail) visible and deep depression under tail.	Ribs and backbone clearly defined, but skin slack over bones.	'Ewe-neck'; narrow, flat muscle covering. Shoulder accentuated, some fat.
2: Moderately thin	Croup well-defined, but some fatty tissue under skin. Pelvis easily felt, slight depression under tail. Not obviously thin.	Backbone just covered by fatty tissue, individual processes not visible, but easily felt on pressure. Ribs just visible.	Narrow but firm. Shoulder not obviously thin.
3: Moderately fleshy	Whole pelvic region rounded, not angular and no 'gutter' (depression) along croup. Skin smooth and supple, pelvis easily felt.	Backbone and ribs well covered, but easily felt on pressure.	Neck blends smoothly into body. No crest except for stallions. Layer of fat over shoulder.
4: Fat	Pelvis buried in fatty tissue and only felt on firm pressure. 'Gutter' over croup.	Backbone and ribs well covered and only felt on firm pressure. 'Gutter' along backbone.	Wide and firm with folds of fatty tissue, slight crest, even in mares. Fat build-up behind shoulder.
5: Obese	Pelvis buried in firm, fatty tissue and cannot be felt. Clear, deep 'gutter' over croup to base of dock. Skin stretched.	Back looks flat with deep 'gutter' along backbone. Ribs buried and cannot be felt.	Very wide and firm, marked crest, even in mares. Shoulder bulging fat.

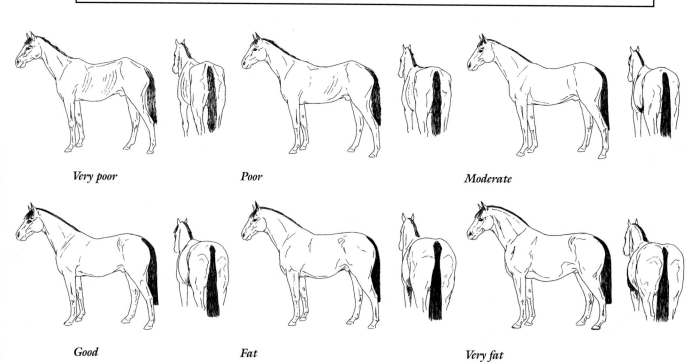

Very poor

Poor

Moderate

Good

Fat

Very fat

APPETITE

Appetite refers to the amount of food required per day. Most horses have an appetite of 2.5 per cent of their body weight. The table below shows the amounts of dry food a horse needs to eat every day in order to maintain condition and body weight and the amount of work it is doing.

Bodyweight	200 kg 440 lb	400 kg 900 lb	450 kg 1000 lb	500 kg 1100 lb	550 kg 1200 lb	600 kg 1320 lb
Moderate work level: appetite = 2.5% of bodyweight	5 kg 11 lb	10 kg 22 lb	11.5 kg 25 lb	12.5 kg 27.5 lb	13.5 kg 30 lb	14.5 kg 32 lb

RATIO OF ROUGHAGE TO CONCENTRATES

The horse in light work will need more hay and less energy feed, while the horse in hard work will need less hay and a greater proportion of high-energy hard feed.

A guide to the ratio of roughage to concentrates

Work level	Roughage %	Concentrate %
Resting	90-100	0-10
Light	75-80	20-25
Moderate	65-70	30-35
Hard	55-65	35-45
Intense	40-50	50-60

It is recommended that roughage should make up at least 50 per cent of the ration; however, the greater the physical activity, the less bulk the horse is likely to consume.

THE RATION

For our example ration, let us take a 16hh (162 cm) horse in moderate work:

- The horse weighs 500 kg (1100 lb)
- It will have an appetite of 12.5 kg (27.5 lb)
- It will be fed 30% concentrates and 70% roughage.

This results in a ration of 3.75 kg (8 lb) concentrates and 8.75 kg (19.5 lb) roughage.

Rations for a 16hh, 500kg horse at varying work levels

Work level	Hay	Concentrate	Comment
Resting	10-12 kg 22-26.5 lb	1-2 kg 2-4 lb	Amount depends on weather, amount of grass, etc.
Light	9-10 kg 20-22 lb	2.5-3 kg 5.5-6.5 lb	Low-energy cubes
Moderate	8-9 kg 17-20 lb	4-4.5 kg 9-10 lb	Medium-energy cubes
Hard	6.5-8 kg 14-17 lb	4.5-5.5 kg 10-12 lb	High-energy feed
Intense	5-6 kg 11-13 lb	6-7.5 kg 13-16.5 lb	Racehorse mix or cubes/naked oats

The next step is to decide what concentrates to feed depending on the horse's individual requirements and your personal preference. Once a ration has been made up for a horse and written on the feed board, it is vital to monitor the horse's reaction to the new ration:

- Does the horse eat up? If the horse is leaving food, it may be that you have over-estimated its appetite, the food is not palatable or the horse is feeling off-colour.
- Are the horse's temperament and performance affected?
- Is the horse gaining, losing or maintaining condition?

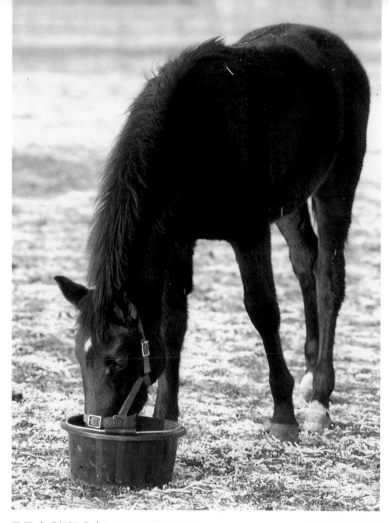

Concentrates may need to be fed in addition to hay to horses wintering out at grass.

PRACTICAL FEEDING

FEEDING BEHAVIOUR OF HORSES

Like all animals, horses can become protective at feeding time. This is particularly true in the field where the horse may feel that it is competing with others and may lash out or bite in an attempt to guard its feed. This means that the carer must be very aware and safety-conscious when feeding horses in the field and in the stable.

All horses are individuals and will have different feeding habits; some are always greedy, knocking over feed buckets in their enthusiasm, while others are more cautious, eating only when the yard is quiet. It is important that the horse owner is aware of these habits so that any change from normal behaviour can be noted and acted upon immediately. A change in the horse's eating and drinking habits is often an early sign of illness. Once a horse has settled into a feeding routine it is unwise to change the type, time and method of feeding suddenly.

FEEDING HORSES AT GRASS

Some horses at grass will need supplementary feeding with hay and concentrates, depending on weather conditions, type, size, age of horse and whether or not it is in work.

FEEDING, WATERING AND WORK

The amount of food a horse should have before exercise depends on the amount of physical exertion he is expected to make.

A racehorse will not be given any food for several hours before a race. A novice event horse may be allowed a feed and a small hay net on the morning of the competition, but no bulk food until after the cross-country phase.

At least four hours' digestion time should be allowed between a concentrate feed and hard physical exertion.

If a horse is normally allowed free access to water, there is no need to remove his water buckets before work.

Fluid and electrolyte balance is important and the horse must be watched for dehydration, which can seriously affect performance. Ensure the horse drinks, and provide electrolytes in the food or water. After performance, offer water to a horse in small quantities at regular intervals.

Tired horses are often over-faced by a large feed but this can be overcome by dividing the normal feed into two and feeding it at intervals. The horse's appetite will indicate how tired he is, and until he is eating normally his condition should be carefully monitored.

PRACTICAL FEEDING: HAY

A common-sense approach to the practicalities of feeding will avoid accidents and wastage.

Ideally, hay should be provided in the field in a large rack or feeder, which should be of a safe design and moved regularly. Racks should be placed in a well-drained spot away from the fence, with good clearance all round.

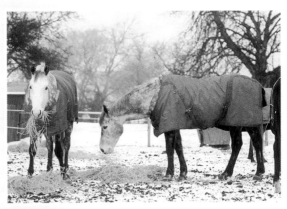

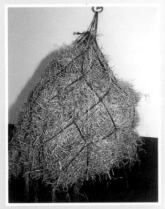

◀ *Tie a haynet securely, high enough that when empty, it does not trail where a foot can get caught in the net.*

Alternatives include haynets, which can be tied securely to a solid fence post or tree so they will hang just over the top of the horse's leg when empty. Or piles can be placed directly on the ground – wasteful but safe. With either method, provide at least one more 'feeding station' than there are occupants in the field, to avoid aggression and bullying. Place in a sheltered, well-drained position a minimum of 12 ft (4m) distance apart.

PRACTICAL FEEDING: CONCENTRATES

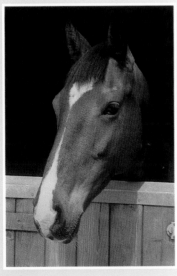

◀ *Avoid creating stress by, as far as possible, feeding all horses at the same set times each day. If one horse has to be fed at a different time, take it out of sight of the others for feeding.*

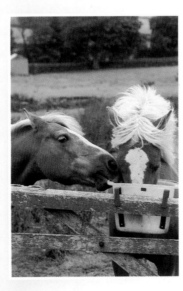

◀ *Some horses at grass will need additional concentrates depending on weather conditions, type, age, size and work done. Where horses are being fed outside an enclosed stable, allow plenty of space between them. Concentrate feeding should always be supervised, or dangerous arguments can ensue (see left).*

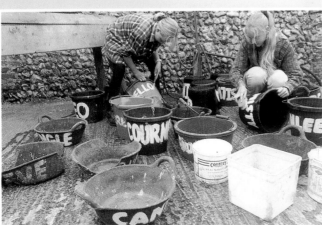

◀ *Clean buckets regularly to prevent a sticky residue building up that will contaminate fresh feed.*

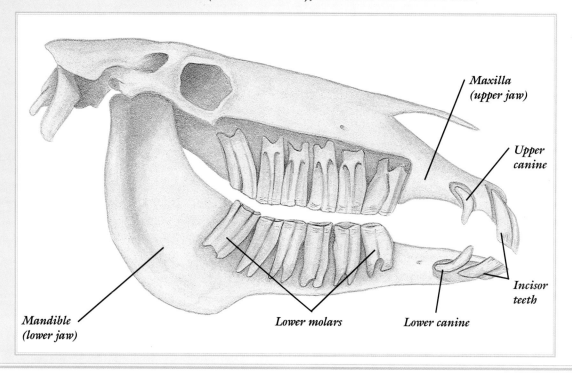

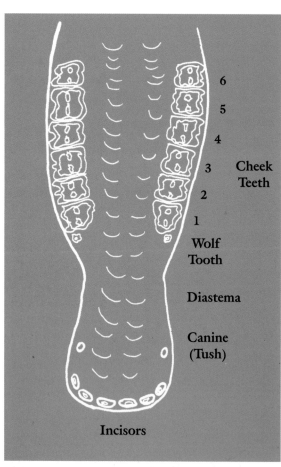

The upper jaw of the horse as viewed from inside the mouth, showing the molars (cheek teeth), wolf teeth, canines and incisors.

COMMON PROBLEMS OF THE DIGESTIVE SYSTEM

MOUTH AND TEETH PROBLEMS

Adult horses all have six incisor teeth at the front and six cheek teeth to each side of both the upper and lower jaws. The space between the incisors and the cheek teeth is called the diastema. In addition to incisors and cheek teeth there may be wolf teeth, situated just in front of the cheek teeth in the upper and lower jaws, and canines (tushes), which are situated in the middle of the diastema. Canine teeth are common in males and uncommon in females.

Equine teeth differ from human teeth in that, in the horse, the adult teeth grow throughout life. As the teeth are continually worn away by grinding on very fibrous food, continuous growth prevents them from rapidly being worn down. The characteristics (shape, angle and markings) of the teeth alter as horses grow older, and this is used in an attempt to 'age' horses. However, above six years old, ageing by teeth is very inaccurate, and the age given may be incorrect by several years (see Age Assessment by Dentition, Chapter Twelve) The upper jaw being slightly wider than the lower one, the upper cheek teeth are set slightly wider apart than the lower cheek teeth. As a result, the outer edges of the upper, and inner edges of the lower cheek teeth may not be worn down as quickly as the rest of the tooth, leading to sharp outer edges that need regular attention (see Teeth Care, Chapter Two).

LAMPAS

Cause: Inflammation of the hard palate in the upper jaw that occurs in young horses as the incisors of the upper jaw erupt.

Signs: Swelling and protrusion of the hard palate.

Treatment: None is necessary. This is a completely natural occurrence and will subside once the teeth have fully erupted. It is not due to a vitamin or mineral deficiency, as commonly believed.

PARROT MOUTH

Parrot mouth is the term given to the protrusion of the incisors of the upper jaw beyond those of the lower jaw.

Cause: This is a congenital defect, the cause of which is unknown, but it can be hereditary.

Signs: Protrusion of the upper incisors, visible when the lips are parted .

Treatment: In most cases the problem is merely cosmetic, and no treatment is required. In severe cases when the upper and lower incisors do not meet at all, surgery can be performed on foals.

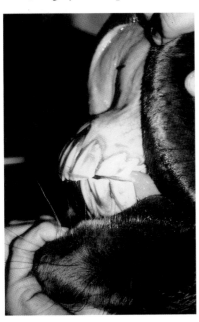

◀ *Parrot mouth*

QUIDDING

Quidding is the expression used when horses drop half-chewed hay or other fibrous material from their mouths. It is generally rolled up and coated in saliva, and appears the shape of a small cigar.

Cause: Any problem which causes pain and difficulty when chewing will cause a horse to quid. Commonest are sharp edges on the outside of the upper and inside of the lower cheek teeth that

develop because these areas are not worn down as quickly as the rest of the teeth. Tooth fractures, abscesses, wave mouth, shear mouth and step mouth (see later) can also cause quidding.

Signs: Dropping feed from the mouth, weight loss, possibly bad breath (halitosis).

Treatment: Sharp points may be removed by rasping by a veterinary surgeon. Regular rasping and checks on the teeth and mouth may also prevent other problems from developing.

WOLF TEETH

Wolf teeth do not erupt through the gum surface in all horses, and even when they do, they remain much smaller than the other teeth with much shorter roots. Despite causing few problems as a general rule, wolf teeth are sometimes blamed for bitting or head carriage problems.

Cause: Any difficulties are generally caused by the teeth, which are very small and sharp, pinching against the gums and causing pain.

Signs: May cause bitting problems or head-shaking.

Treatment: May be removed under standing sedation in a relatively simple procedure.

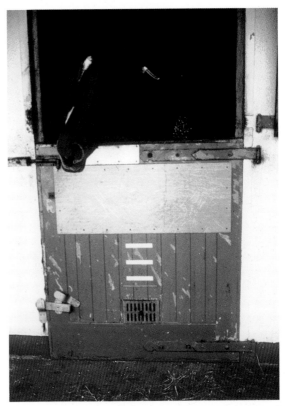

Partially-chewed hay dropped outside the stable door of a horse that quids.

INFECTED TEETH

Infection involving the teeth can occur in all ages of horses. In some animals there is little evidence of pain, but others may be very dull and uncomfortable.

Cause: Dental infections may occur due to fracture of teeth, defects in the development of the teeth, gum disease or tooth root infection.

Signs: Signs vary according to the tooth involved and the cause of the infection. Some horses may develop a high temperature and go off their food. Most horses will quid, and they often have bad breath and pocketing of food around the infected tooth. Some animals will have a one-sided nasal discharge, whereas others will have externally obvious facial swelling, sometimes with a tract discharging pus.

Treatment: Most infected teeth require removal, a procedure that needs specialist equipment and knowledge due to the long root of the horse's tooth. Removal may be performed with the animal standing under heavy sedation and analgesia. It often takes over an hour, and some cases will require a general anaesthetic. Repeated operations may be

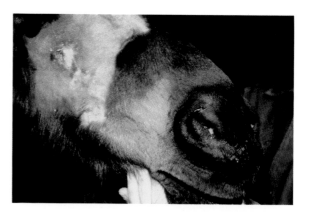

Pus drains from the nostril and facial swelling of a horse with an infection of the right-side third upper cheek tooth.

necessary. If the sinuses are also infected, insertion of flushing systems via holes in the horse's face and flushing for several weeks are sometimes required.

STEP MOUTH

In this condition there is a definite 'step' in the grinding surface of the cheek teeth, when viewed from the side.

Cause: Step mouth occurs when a cheek tooth is lost. With no opposite number to grind against, the tooth in the opposite jaw is not worn down and so becomes much longer than all the other teeth, creating a 'step' configuration.

Signs: No signs may be seen in mild cases, but in severe cases the horse's ability to chew is limited, and quidding and weight loss may be seen. If the step mouth is not treated, the continuing uneven wear of adjacent teeth will lead to the development of 'wave' mouth, as a result of the long tooth jamming in the gap left by the lost tooth.

Treatment: Prevention is better than cure. All horses which have lost adult teeth should be rasped regularly to prevent a 'step' from developing.

WAVE MOUTH

A more serious development from the step mouth condition. Here the cheek teeth do not form a continuous, flat, grinding surface when viewed from the side. Instead, they have a wave configuration, because of different amounts of wear on individual teeth.

Cause: Abnormal eruption of teeth, enamel hooks, shear mouth or any other condition causing uneven wear of teeth.

Signs: No signs may be seen in mild cases, but in severe cases the horse's ability to chew is limited,

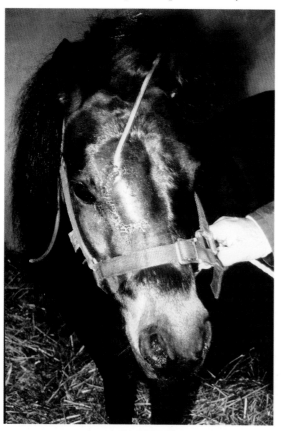

After surgery to remove an infected cheek tooth, a flushing system has been inserted.

and quidding and weight loss may be seen.
Treatment: Routine rasping will prevent wave mouth. If it does develop, rasping may correct it but full correction may not be possible in advanced cases.

SHEAR MOUTH

This is a condition where the grinding surfaces of the teeth develop an abnormally steep slope (greater than 15 degrees) when viewed from the front.
Cause: Shear mouth develops as a result of other, long-standing dental problems (such as enamel hooks, see below), which interfere with the horse's ability to chew normally. Thus an abnormal slope develops on the grinding surface as the teeth are worn away unevenly.
Signs: Sharp enamel points develop on the edges of the teeth, causing pain during chewing. This causes quidding and weight loss.
Treatment: Routine rasping will prevent shear mouth, and if it develops, rasping may correct it. However in advanced cases it may never be possible to correct fully.

ENAMEL HOOKS

Hook-like formations commonly occur on the front of the upper cheek teeth and back of the lower cheek teeth .
Cause: Hooks develop when the upper and lower cheek teeth do not overlap completely, but the upper teeth protrude in front and lower teeth behind. Without regular, correct rasping, these hooks may develop. Often the hook at the front is noticed and removed by rasping, but the one at the back is missed and may grow very long.
Signs: Hooks interfere with the horse's ability to grind its food properly, so causing quidding. If they are present for a long time they may cause abnormal wear of other areas, resulting in wave or shear mouth.
Treatment: Regular rasping will remove hooks before they form properly. Large hooks can be removed using specialist dental shears, but this procedure does carry a risk of the affected tooth fracturing.

ERUPTION CYSTS

Cysts are sometimes seen in young horses as the cheek teeth erupt.
Cause: Cysts develop around the apex (root) of the teeth as they erupt into the mouth. The most common site is around the apex of the second or third cheek teeth, especially in the lower jaw.
Signs: Large, bilateral, firm, painless swellings on the bottom of the lower jaw or occasionally the upper jaw, overlying the cheek teeth.
Treatment: These are a normal feature of tooth eruption in the horse and treatment is neither necessary, nor in fact possible. Cysts do not cause discomfort and will reduce in size as the animal ages.

Normal

Tooth Loss and 'Stepmouth'

Hooks on the First Upper and Last Lower Cheek Tooth

'Wavemouth'

Normal (Aproximately 10-15° angle)   'Shearmouth' (Greater than 15° angle)

Cheek   Tongue   Cheek   Tongue

Normal configuration of the molar (cheek) teeth of the horse, and some common abnormalities of wear.

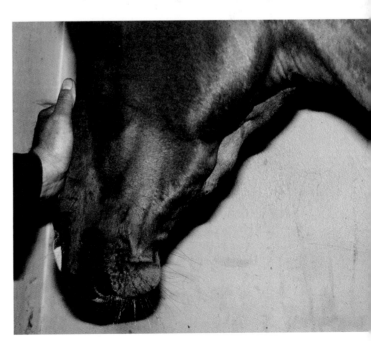

Eruption cysts on the lower jaw of a young horse.

DIGESTIVE DISORDERS

DEHYDRATION

Dehydration occurs when loss of fluid from the body, via faeces, urine, sweat and water vapour in exhaled air, exceeds fluid intake from food and water. As dehydration occurs, fluid is lost from the blood, which becomes more concentrated. When the fluid lost from the blood is not replaced, the volume of blood in the body decreases. Blood carries oxygen and nutrients to the body, and removes waste products. If there is less blood, it is unable to circulate to all of the tissues as frequently as normal. Consequently, the heart beats faster in an attempt to circulate the blood around the body more quickly, attempting to compensate for the decreased blood volume. The animal is described as being in 'shock'. Eventually, if this situation cannot be reversed, the horse will die.

Causes: Dehydration may occur as a consequence of colic, diarrhoea, choke, excessive sweating, poor appetite or blood loss. The commonest causes of dehydration in the horse are colic and diarrhoea.

An average adult horse (15.2 hh) produces approximately 125 litres of saliva and digestive juices each day. These usually pass through the small intestine as it digests food, and are then reabsorbed in the large intestine. In surgical colic cases where the intestines are blocked, fluid is continually produced in saliva and digestive juices but is prevented from reaching the large intestine by the blockage and so cannot be re-absorbed. Instead it sits in the small intestine causing dehydration and pain as it stretches the intestinal wall. In cases of diarrhoea, inflammation of the large intestine reduces its ability to re-absorb fluid, and so the horse passes out very loose, watery faeces (diarrhoea).

Prolonged exercise, such as in endurance rides, may cause excessive amounts of fluid to be lost in sweat, particularly if the weather is very hot. This will cause dehydration, if not replaced. In addition, whenever large amounts of blood are lost, the amount of fluid in the body is markedly depleted and dehydration and shock follow.

Lack of appetite will cause dehydration through the failure to take in fluid. This also occurs in choke, where fluid is also lost in saliva, which cannot be swallowed.

Signs: As dehydration develops, affected animals will become progressively duller and more shocked. The amount of urine produced will decrease as the body tries to conserve fluid, and urine will also become

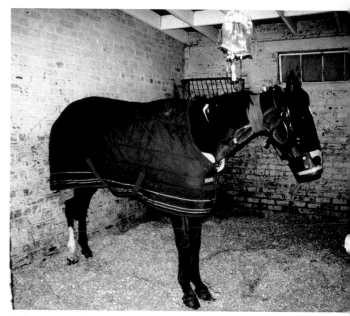

Serious cases of dehydration require fluids to be given intravenously via a drip.

more concentrated. Animals will have a tacky or dry mouth, and their lower limbs and ears will become cold.

Treatment: Treatment involves replacing the fluid which is lost. The fluid contains water and electrolytes, and it is important that both are replaced, using specially formulated solutions. In mildly affected animals where there is no evidence of choke or intestinal blockage, it may be possible to replace fluids by inserting them directly into the stomach via a stomach tube. All other conditions require sterile fluids to be administered directly into the bloodstream via a drip. Volumes involved may be huge, and in horses with severe diarrhoea 100-200 litres of fluid may need to be given via a drip each day!

CHOKE

Choke occurs when solid material becomes blocked in the oesophagus (food pipe), preventing food and saliva from passing into the stomach and intestines.

Cause: A horse may choke on any substance, but the most common cause is feeding sugar beet which has not been adequately soaked. As the sugar beet is mixed with saliva and swallowed, it swells and blocks the oesophagus. Choke may also occur if apples, carrots or parts of other root vegetables are swallowed whole, or if an animal swallows something unusual such as a stick or plastic bag. Most animals recover from choke completely, but if

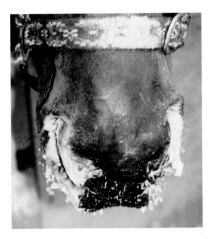

The frothy nasal discharge of a horse with choke contains saliva.

the oesophagus is badly damaged it may develop scar tissue which narrows it, predisposing the animal to choking on normal feed such as hay.

Signs: Signs develop rapidly. Affected animals are dull, with coughing, retching and spasm in the musculature of the neck as the horse tries to clear the blockage. Saliva and food pass back out of the mouth and down both nostrils. As time progresses a large amount of saliva is produced and the breath will smell sour.

It may be possible to feel thickening in the neck at the site of the blockage in the oesophagus. There is a risk that food and saliva is inhaled into the lungs if the choke persists, causing pneumonia to develop leading to further coughing, dullness, increased respiratory rate and raised temperature. If choke persists, the horse will become dehydrated.

Treatment: Fortunately, most horses manage to clear the oesophageal obstruction within 10-15 minutes without suffering any ill effects. However, if the choke persists beyond this time, a vet should be called. Treatment with a sedative to calm the animal down, muscle relaxants to relieve the oesophageal spasm, and antibiotics to protect against pneumonia will cure most cases. Occasional animals require the insertion of a tube into the oesophagus to the level of the obstruction and gentle flushing to clear it. This may be done in the standing animal under heavy sedation but often requires a general anaesthetic.

If the animal is dehydrated, fluid therapy via a drip (or stomach tube after the obstruction has cleared) is necessary. Animals which develop severe scarring may be vulnerable to repeated episodes of choke and need a refined (pureed) diet to prevent this. If scarring is suspected it can be checked by passing a small camera called an endoscope into the oesophagus.

COLIC

Colic is a general term used to describe abdominal pain in the horse. The abdominal cavity contains the gastro-intestinal tract (GIT) from stomach to rectum; the liver; the urinary tract containing kidneys, ureters, bladder and urethra; and the reproductive organs in the mare. It is lined by a thin membrane called peritoneum. Although 'true colic' refers to pain relating to the GIT or peritoneum, pain in the liver, urinary tract and reproductive organs may appear similar. Some diseases unrelated to the abdominal cavity, such as laminitis and azoturia, may also be mistaken for colic.

The severity of signs shown by horses with colic is highly variable. Whereas some animals may behave very violently, rolling, kicking and getting cast, others may simply appear dull and off their food. Most cases of colic do resolve with appropriate medical therapy, although some animals require surgery. The sooner surgery is performed, the better the prognosis for survival. Thus all animals with colic should be examined by a veterinary surgeon as soon as possible.

INITIAL EXAMINATION

Presented with a horse with suspected colic, your vet will first conduct a basic clinical examination. Most horses with colic may be in pain but, are generally speaking, relatively healthy. Those requiring surgery, however, are at risk of developing shock, and much of the examination will be directed toward detecting the early signs of this.

In most cases of colic the horse's temperature remains normal (38.0C, 100.5F). Horses with advanced shock will have a decreased temperature and their lower limbs and ears will feel cold, but a high temperature is uncommon. Both pain and shock will cause the heart and respiratory rates to rise. If the heart rate is elevated from its normal range (36-44 beats per minute) due to pain, it seldom rises above 60 beats per minute. In advanced shock, however, it may reach as high as 150 beats per minute. In contrast the respiratory rate, which in a normal horse may be between 6-16 breaths per minute, can be markedly elevated due to pain alone, as high as 60 breaths per minute, and may even be higher than the heart rate.

Your vet will spend some time listening to the horse's gut sounds using a stethoscope. The intestines make noise as the muscle in their wall contracts and moves food along. Horses normally have quite loud gut sounds. In colic these may be markedly increased and it may be possible to hear them from the far side of the stable. This is generally a good sign – if gut sounds are decreased this may mean that the gut has twisted and thus stopped working and making any noise. Or it may simply mean that your horse is constipated!

RECTAL EXAMINATION

Before conducting a rectal examination the horse should be properly restrained, to prevent it from injuring itself, the handler or the vet (see Chapter Two, Methods of Restraint).

When performing a rectal examination only the intestines at the back of the abdominal cavity (approximately 40 per cent of the total) can be felt, in addition to the spleen, left kidney and bladder and the uterus and ovaries in a mare. A normal small intestine cannot be felt, but the large colon can often be identified. During rectal examination your vet is trying to identify whether the guts have twisted or displaced. If this has happened they may inflate with both gas and fluid, rather like a balloon. In severe cases this may even be visible as external swelling of the abdomen.

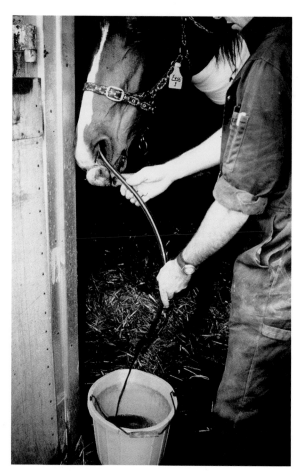

Draining fluid from the stomach, using a stomach tube.

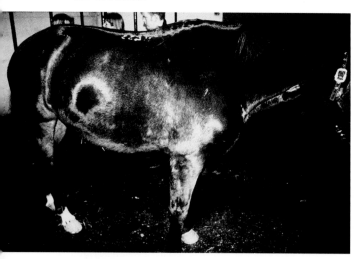

If the gut has become twisted or displaced, gas build-up in the intestines can cause marked distension of the abdomen.

STOMACH TUBING

Horses are unable to vomit and if fluid accumulates within the stomach, it may become so full that it bursts, spilling food into the abdominal cavity. Should this occur, it is impossible to save the horse. Vets will therefore pass a long tube up the nose, down the foodpipe (oesophagus) and into the

stomach when examining a horse with colic and attempt to siphon off any fluid or gas which has accumulated to prevent stomach rupture. This test would yield very little (less than two litres) or no fluid in a normally healthy horse.

If a horse is constipated, liquid paraffin and Epsom salts may be given via the tube directly into the stomach in an attempt to clear the obstruction.

PERITONEAL TAP

The peritoneum is a thin, invisible membrane lining the abdominal cavity and covering the intestines. It produces a small volume of clear yellow fluid which looks rather like human urine, that lubricates the abdominal cavity and prevents the abdominal organs from sticking to each other. If the gut twists and dies off, blood, bacteria and gut contents may leak into the abdominal cavity, causing the peritoneal fluid to appear cloudy, pussy or bloody. Your vet may take a sample of the peritoneal fluid ('tap' the peritoneal fluid) from your horse's abdomen, by placing a

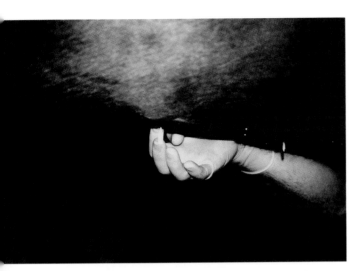

By placing a needle through the abdominal wall, a sample of peritoneal fluid can be taken.

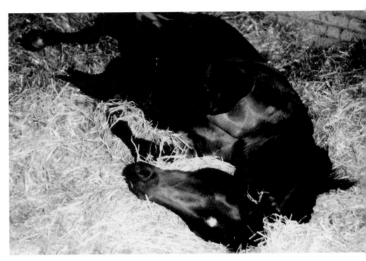

A horse with colic is usually in severe pain and may thrash around in the stable, kick at its abdomen and attempt to roll.

needle into the bottom of the abdomen and collecting the fluid as it drips out. In some fat ponies this may be difficult and a very long needle (10cm/4 ins) may be necessary to get through the fat and into the abdominal cavity.

BLOOD SAMPLES

Blood samples may be examined for signs of shock in horses with colic, but extensive tests are not generally necessary. When infection or liver disease are suspected, or the cause is unknown, further examination of blood samples may be useful.

IMMEDIATE CARE

Despite detailed examination it is often impossible to establish the exact cause of the colic. The horse should be treated with analgesics and regularly re-evaluated to monitor recovery and avoid any recurrence. Withdrawing all food from horses with colic is advisable, until after the problem has resolved. Horses at grass or on a straw bed may be moved to shavings or paper bedding, or muzzled to prevent them from eating grass or bedding. Fortunately most cases do resolve with medical treatment, even if the exact cause has not been diagnosed.

TYPES OF COLIC

SPASMODIC COLIC

As the name suggests, the intestines of horses with spasmodic colic develop muscular spasms or 'cramps', causing pain. This is one of the commonest types of colic in horses.

Cause: The cause of spasmodic colic is unclear. In many animals it seems to develop for no apparent reason, although as some excitable animals may develop spasmodic colic with the slightest of changes in their daily routine, it could be regarded as a symptom of increased stress levels. It has been suggested that some cases may be due to the migration of worms through the intestinal wall, causing 'hyper-excitability' of that portion of intestine and 'cramps'. A single worm may be all that is required to trigger such spasms, which therefore may occur in horses which are receiving regular and appropriate worming treatment.

Signs: Some horses with spasmodic colic may show very severe pain and thrash around the box. It is often possible to hear rumbling gut noises from quite a distance and animals may produce several piles of faeces in quick succession following the onset of colic. The respiratory rate may be markedly elevated, but heart rate is not usually very high. Rectal examination, stomach tubing and peritoneal tap will all yield normal results.

Treatment: Injection of a 'spasmolytic' drug to relax the intestines will eliminate signs of pain within 10-15 minutes, usually faster.

PELVIC FLEXURE IMPACTIONS

The pelvic flexure is the narrowest part of the large colon. It is the place where the large colon doubles back on itself, producing a similar shape to a toilet

U tube. Not surprisingly, this is the site where food accumulates if a horse becomes constipated. Pelvic flexure impactions and spasmodic colic are extremely common causes of colic in the horse.

Cause: Pelvic flexure impaction is essentially constipation, and is most common in horses which eat their straw bedding. It often occurs in autumn and winter as horses are brought in off grass to stables but is also fairly common in animals which are quite fit and in a lot of work but which then receive an injury requiring them to be completely box rested.

Signs: Some horses show only mild pain, but go off their food, whereas others are violently colicky. Pain is often intermittent. Faecal output will be markedly reduced, and faeces are drier than normal. Heart and respiratory rates may be elevated, consistent with pain, but will return to normal during pain-free periods. Gut sounds vary from normal to reduced. A large pelvic flexure filled with stodgy faeces will be felt on rectal examination, but peritoneal fluid will be normal and little or no fluid will be obtained from the stomach when the stomach tube is passed.

Treatment: Liquid paraffin and/or Epsom salts (usually mineral oil in North America), with added water, are given via stomach tube in an attempt to lubricate the faeces and draw water into them. Severe impactions, which may have developed over several days, could require the administration of fluids via a drip into the vein in order to rehydrate the animal. Pain relief may be provided by the use of bute (phenylbutazone) or a similar drug.

TYMPANIC COLIC

Similar to human indigestion, tympanic colic occurs when the intestines become distended with gas.

Causes: The over-production of gas within the intestines, commonly the result of gorging on new grass in the spring. If a horse is turned out onto grass for long periods after being stabled over winter, it may not be able to digest this quantity of grass and may produce excessive quantities of gas. Likewise, any sudden feed change may induce tympanic colic. Mistakenly providing mouldy or spoilt feeds is another common cause.

Signs: Gas within the intestines causes stretching of the bowel wall. This is very painful and thus animals often colic violently. Heart and respiratory rates may be as high as 60-70 beats or breaths per minute and gut sounds are often absent since the muscle in the stretched intestinal wall is unable to contract. On rectal examination, balloon-like distension of the intestines may be felt and large amounts of gas may be freed when a tube is passed into the stomach.

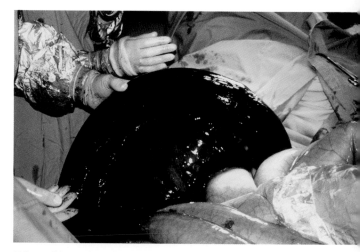

Diseased intestines during surgery. The loop of dark red/purple small intestine at the top of the picture is dead and must be removed. The four loops below are very distended by gas and fluid.

Peritoneal tap is normal and faecal production is variable, although large amounts of wind may be passed!

Treatment: Liberation of gas from the stomach following 'tubing' may cause all pain to subside. Some light exercise such as walking out in hand or lungeing for 10 minutes at the trot may help the animal to 'pass wind' and the colic to resolve. However painkillers (analgesics) and intestinal relaxants may be necessary.

There are many other causes of colic, and as already described, many cases go undiagnosed, but the pain abates and the horse gets better. Among these are worms, enteritis (both may also cause diarrhoea) liver disease, bladder stones, kidney disease, poisoning, stomach ulcers, over-eating, and other unknown causes.

SURGICAL COLIC

Those cases of colic requiring surgery may have a huge range of causes and often it is not possible to fully diagnose the cause before the examination of the horse's intestines at surgery. The sooner the need for surgery is diagnosed, the better the chances of success. If in doubt, it is better to transport the horse to a hospital for continual monitoring. Then, if surgery is necessary, it can be performed immediately, so avoiding the delay involved in transport. The greater the delay, the poorer the prognosis.

Causes: The intestines of the horse are very poorly designed and have an amazing ability to twist around themselves, telescope upon themselves and develop blood clots which cut off blood supply. Poor worm control and irregular feeding may predispose to colic, but often no trigger factor can be found.

Signs: Usually horses with a surgical lesion will show obvious signs of colic, with pawing, rolling and kicking at the abdomen. However, as the affected gut dies off, so do the nerve fibres which transmit the sensation of pain, and so the animal's pain may actually decrease. As this occurs, shock and dehydration begin to set in and the horse will become very dull. The heart and respiratory rates will continue to rise and may become very fast, and gut sounds will usually disappear. Although the horse may pass faeces in the first few hours, it generally stops after this.

Remember that if a horse is found with colic first thing in the morning, it may have started the night before. As it only takes 4-8 hours in some cases for the gut to die off and rupture, all signs of pain may have passed when the colic is discovered (although there is usually evidence of disturbed bedding) and the horse will be dull. If the gut ruptures, the horse cannot be saved. When rupture occurs, the horse will usually be extremely dull, sweat excessively ('dripping in sweat'), feel very cold and be very reluctant to move at all.

In many cases of surgical colic, abnormalities can be felt on rectal examination. However, it does take time for gas and fluid to build up within the intestines after a twist has occurred, and so abnormalities may only become apparent after several examinations. Some animals with a surgical problem will produce large volumes of fluid and gas when a tube is passed into the stomach, but this is not always the case. Peritoneal fluid may change colour, but this can take several hours, and if one piece of gut has telescoped into another, the fluid leaking from it may not pass into the abdominal cavity, and so peritoneal fluid may remain normal.

Treatment: Obviously surgery is necessary. This may involve simply flipping a piece of intestine back into the correct position; or it may require large amounts of bowel to be cut out, with drainage of fluid and gas which has accumulated from the pieces which remain. Thus colic surgery may take several hours. Once it is completed, the horse is not 'out of the woods', and may require over a week of intensive care. During this time there are many potentially life-threatening complications. The muscle in the wall of remaining intestine, which was stretched by the accumulation of fluid and gas, may stop working and contracting after surgery. This is called 'ileus' and is a very serious complication which may cause the horse to deteriorate to a worse state than before surgery. Infection may also occur. Horses will not be able to

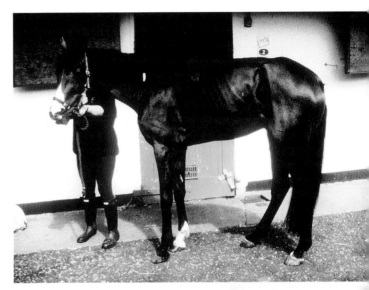

Even with intensive care, many cases of chronic grass sickness do not survive.

eat for several days and may be very dehydrated, especially if ileus occurs. Such cases may require large volumes of fluids to be administered via a drip (see Dehydration).

If a horse pulls through the first few weeks, at least two months' box rest, followed by at least two months in a paddock, are usually necessary before they can be ridden again. Should infection develop at the surgical site, the abdominal wound may partially break down forming a pouch containing intestines, which can be palpated under the skin. This is called an incisional hernia.

GRASS SICKNESS (EQUINE DYSAUTONOMIA)

Grass sickness is a disease which causes damage to the part of the nervous system which controls involuntary functions. Damage occurs throughout the nervous system, but some of the most obvious signs are due to dysfunction of the GIT. To the author's knowledge, no cases have been seen in Ireland or North America.

The condition can be seen in any age of horse, but is most common in two to seven-year-olds. The peak incidence of the disease is between April to July, and as the name suggests, it occurs in horses which have access to pasture. Most affected horses are at grass full-time or during the day, but it is occasionally seen in horses which only graze for a few minutes each day. Animals which have recently (within the past two months) moved on to a field are at higher risk of developing grass sickness, as well as animals which have been stressed (recently purchased, mixed with

strange horses, travelled long distance, etc.). Fatter animals are at higher risk for developing the disease.
Causes: The cause of grass sickness is unknown. The disease is not contagious, however, and it is thought that a toxin (possibly produced by a fungus) may be responsible for the signs seen.
Signs: There are three forms of grass sickness: acute, sub-acute and chronic.

In **acute** grass sickness, horses show violent colic. The heart rate may be very high, and the abdomen obviously distended. Stomach tubing may yield large volumes of foul-smelling green fluid, and intestinal distension may be felt on rectal examination. Some horses will show patchy sweating and fine muscle tremors. The horse will have difficulty swallowing (dysphagia) or choke as attempts are made to eat. The results of a peritoneal tap will be normal, unless the gut has ruptured, in which case gut contents will be obtained. The horse will be constipated and may only survive for one or two days.

The symptoms of **sub-acute** grass sickness are similar to acute, but less intense with a slower onset and longer duration of illness. Only small amounts of dung will be passed, often coated in a white membrane which looks like a cobweb. Horses will rapidly lose weight, their appetite will be reduced, and when they do attempt to eat they may have difficulty swallowing. Few survive longer than one week.

In **chronic** grass sickness, violent colic is not seen. Signs tend to develop slowly, sometimes over several weeks. Few changes will be felt on rectal examination and stomach tubing will yield no, or very little, fluid. The heart rate is usually elevated to about 60 beats per minute and gut sounds are very much reduced. The appetite will be very poor, and patchy sweating and muscle tremors are obvious. Horses often appear very sleepy, with droopy eyelids. They may stand with all four legs together like an elephant on a tub, and have very snuffly breath sounds due to a 'snotty nose'.
Treatment: Horses with acute grass sickness will not survive and should be euthanased on humane grounds as soon as the diagnosis is made. Most cases of sub-acute grass sickness will also deteriorate rapidly and require euthanasia.

Some horses with chronic grass sickness may survive if they receive intensive nursing care, although weight loss will be severe. Treatment should only be attempted if the horse is able to swallow and prepared to eat, is able to pass faeces and does not have too severe abdominal pain. It involves laborious and time-consuming support by frequently offering small quantities of palatable, easily-digestible food and trying to tempt the appetite. Plenty of attention and

'TLC' is the mainstay of support as medical treatment is limited. This regime needs to be maintained for many weeks and it is often over a year before a return to work can be considered. Even with the best of care many horses with the chronic form of the disease will not survive.

PERITONITIS

Inflammation or infection of the peritoneum, the thin membrane which covers the intestines and abdominal cavity.
Causes: Peritonitis usually occurs secondary to the leakage of bacteria into the abdominal cavity. This may occur in surgical colics where gut dies off and becomes 'leaky'; following worm damage to intestines; or in mares, if the uterus (womb) is torn during foaling. Very rarely, injuries to the abdominal wall will penetrate all layers and introduce infection.
Signs: Peritonitis is a very painful condition. In contrast to most cases of colic, movement itself causes pain, so most horses with peritonitis are reluctant to move, and if they do so, will have a very stiff, stilted, gait. The presence of infection will cause temperature, heart rates and respiratory rates to rise, and gut sounds will often be reduced. Roughening of the surface of the intestines may be felt on rectal examination, but often no abnormalities will be found. Passage of a stomach tube will not usually yield fluid, although the fluid obtained after peritoneal tap will often be bloody and pussy.

As the disease progresses, the animal will be dull, be reluctant to eat, and will often lose weight dramatically.
Treatment: Surgery may be necessary to remove dead bowel or close tears, e.g. in the uterus. Prolonged courses of antibiotics, anti-inflammatory drugs and wormers may be necessary, and dehydrated cases may require fluid therapy (see Dehydration, above). Some cases of peritonitis may not survive, and treatment is often prolonged and expensive.

DIARRHOEA

Diarrhoea is uncommon but potentially life-threatening in horses.
Cause: There are many causes of diarrhoea, but the most common is damage to the intestines from cyathostomes (small redworms). The disease may be referred to as 'cyathostomiasis'. Bacterial infections causing diarrhoea are less frequently seen but may be highly contagious. Foals develop diarrhoea as they begin to eat solid food. This usually (but not always) coincides with the mare's first season after foaling ('foal heat') and thus is called 'foal heat diarrhoea'. A

contagious viral diarrhoea is also seen in foals. Occasionally, tumours and inflammatory bowel disease may also lead to diarrhoea.

Whatever the cause, all cases involve inflammation of the large intestine, reducing its ability to absorb fluid from the gut contents. As excessive amounts of fluid faeces are produced, dehydration develops unless the horse compensates by drinking more water.

Signs: In mild cases of diarrhoea there will be increased amounts of loose faeces, but the horse will remain bright with a good appetite. However, severe cases will be extremely dull and produce excessive amounts of faeces with the consistency of water ('hose-pipe diarrhoea'). These animals will rapidly develop shock, with high pulse and respiratory rates, cool lower limbs and ears, and may die within hours of the onset of the disease. Fortunately such cases are rare.

'Foal heat diarrhoea' is an entirely natural phenomenon. The foal will remain healthy and alert, the diarrhoea will resolve within a few days and no treatment is necessary. In contrast, viral and bacterial diarrhoea may produce severe signs, as in adults, and require intensive treatment.

Treatment: Fluid therapy is an important part of treatment of diarrhoea and severe cases may require huge volumes to be administered via a drip (see Dehydration). In addition anti-inflammatory drugs may be used to reduce the inflammation in the intestines. In cases of 'cyathostomiasis' wormers may be administered. Antibiotics are not used in many cases of bacterial diarrhoea since they may kill off the 'good' bacteria in the gut, allowing over-growth of the 'bad' bacteria and causing diarrhoea to worsen. Instead, probiotics may be given. These are drugs containing 'good' bacteria to try to re-populate the gut and eliminate the 'bad' bacteria. Natural yoghurt has a similar effect.

POISONING

RAGWORT

Ragwort is one of the most common sources of poisoning to horses. It is a bright yellow weed, seen very commonly in pastures and on road-side verges.

Cause: Ragwort causes liver disease. The fresh plant is unpalatable to horses and will rarely be eaten, but if it is present in a dried form in hay, it cannot be detected and will be readily taken in. Ingestion of a large amount over several months is necessary before signs of poisoning become apparent, but this can easily occur if the plant goes undetected.

Signs: Dullness, depression and lack of appetite, with weight loss are the most common signs. Other signs of liver disease may also be seen (see below).

Treatment: The damage to the liver is irreversible, so treatment is aimed at modifying the diet to reduce the work of the liver.

ACORN

Acorns and oak leaves are unpalatable to horses, and will only be eaten if there is no other feed or grazing available, so fortunately poisoning is rare. Nevertheless it is advisable to fence off access to oak trees growing on pasture land.

Cause: Acorns are poisonous when digested. Their main effects are on the GIT, kidneys and blood.

Signs: Severe colic and bloody diarrhoea are the commonest signs. In some cases animals may be found dead.

Treatment: There is no antidote available for the poison in acorns. Treatment is aimed at purging the gut contents (using liquid paraffin administered via a stomach tube) to prevent further absorption of the poison. Fluids are given via a drip.

LEAD

Lead poisoning is also uncommon in horses.

Cause: Animals rarely have access to lead, but poisoning may be seen in horses which lick lead-based paints or batteries. Paddocks should always be cleared of any rubbish that could be a source of lead.

Signs: Lead attacks the nervous system, causing weakness, incoordination, inappetance and weight loss. Horses may be unable to swallow or neigh and may tremble. In severe cases fits may be seen.

Treatment: This is aimed at removing lead which has accumulated in the body. Drugs known as 'chelating agents' will remove lead from body stores, allowing it to be excreted in the urine. In mild cases this will allow recovery, but in advanced cases the nerve damage may be too severe.

LIVER DISEASE

The liver is a very important organ, responsible for the processing of proteins, fats, carbohydrates, vitamins and red blood cells. It plays an essential role in detoxifying drugs and products of the body's metabolism and in making factors involved in blood clotting. The liver has a large 'functional reserve'. This means that 70-80 per cent of the organ can stop working before signs of liver disease are seen, resulting in many cases of liver damage going undetected. When liver damage is recognised, a large amount of the liver is affected and this damage may have been going on undetected for months or years.

POISONOUS PLANTS

Horses on good-quality pasture rarely eat harmful plants, but fields and hedgerows should still be checked regularly. Depending on the location and species, such plants should either be securely fenced off, or pulled up by the roots and burned. Take care using herbicide spray and be sure to inspect hay, as many plants are more palatable, yet more poisonous, when dry.

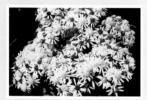

Ragwort

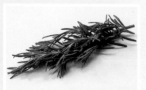

Yew

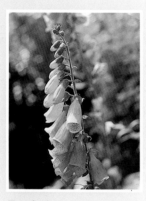

Foxglove

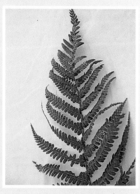

Bracken

Plants that are poisonous to horses include:

ragwort
oak (including acorns)
yew
wild clematis (Old Man's Beard)
ground ivy
columbine
hemlock
henbane
cowbane
hellebore
bracken
woody/black/deadly nightshade
lesser/greater celandine
St John's wort
soapwort
sandwort
water dropwort
pimpernel
flax
purple milk vetch
kidney vetch
lesser periwinkle
laburnum
horsetails
conifers
rhododendron
privet
laurel
larkspur
monkshood
potato (when green,
including leaves & stems)
poppy
lupin
iris
buttercup
chickweed
buckthorn

broom
hemp
white/black bryony
thornapple
meadow saffron
darnel
bulbs of daffodil/hyacinth/
snowdrops/bluebell
magnolia

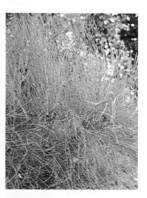

Broom

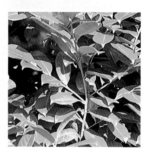

Laurel

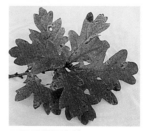

Oak

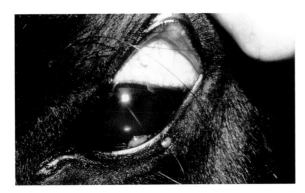

▲ *The area above the eye, the sclera, is normally white. Here, liver disease has led to jaundice, tingeing the sclera yellow.*

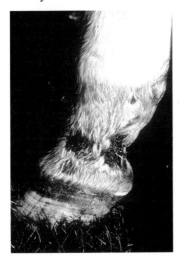

◄ *Abnormal skin lesions are a common symptom of liver disease.*

Thus many cases of liver disease are irreversible once recognised.

Cause: The commonest cause of liver disease in the British Isles is ragwort poisoning (see above). Blockage of the bile ducts by stones may cause disease, but is very rare. Bacterial infection of the liver also occurs rarely. Parasites may migrate through the liver, usually causing mild disease. In some cases the cause of liver disease is unclear.

Signs: Signs of liver disease are varied due to the wide variety of functions of the organ. Dullness, depression, poor appetite and weight loss are the most common symptoms. Colic and diarrhoea may also be seen.

Some horses may develop jaundice (yellowing of the skin) but because of the hair of the coat this can be difficult to see. Others may bleed excessively from small cuts or gums, because blood-clotting proteins are not being produced. Some animals develop 'sunburn', even when the sun is not very intense, and

others behave abnormally, pressing their heads against wall, 'star gazing', circling constantly or falling over. Occasionally affected horses will fit.

Treatment: Usually the liver damage is irreversible and treatment is aimed at reducing the amount of work that the liver has to do. This is achieved by feeding a highly-digestible diet, supplementing vitamins, protecting from excessive sunlight and resting the animal. If parasites or bacteria are the cause, wormers or antibiotics may be given. Some animals may stabilise and improve with this treatment but others continue to deteriorate and require euthanasia.

URINARY DISORDERS

The urinary system comprises two kidneys, connected via two urethers to the bladder, which drains via the urethra. With the exception of CO_2 removed by the lungs, it is responsible for the extraction and removal of all waste products from the body and is closely involved with the body's complex balancing of water, acids and salts.

Disorders of the urinary system are rare in horses, though are more common in mares than in males. When they do occur, however, they can be serious. The adult horse will normally urinate between 2-10 litres per day.

Owners should be aware of the signs of potential problems:
• signs of pain on urination: excessive grunting/ straining, restlessness
• abnormal frequency of urination, quantity, or thirst
• abnormal urine colour (normal is pale yellow/amber, with no darkness or blood-staining).

RENAL FAILURE
The kidneys filter blood and form urine, which contains nitrogenous waste, acids and water. They play a vital role in controlling body water levels, altering the amount excreted according to the horse's water intake. The organ continues to function even when 70 per cent is damaged.

Causes: Failure can be caused by a drop in blood pressure (e.g. from dehydration, haemorrhage, shock, heart disease), blockage of the urine flow at the urethra or bladder(e.g. from stones), or toxins (from plants, metals, drugs or following azoturia).

Signs: Urine initially becomes highly concentrated, though may then become very dilute following initial acute phase. Tenderness felt by vet on rectal palpation.

Treatment: Depends on cause and severity.

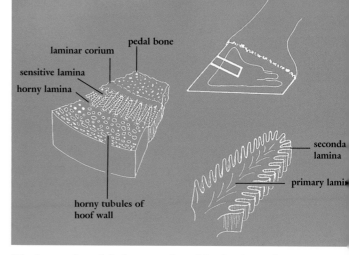

The interaction of the horny and sensitive laminae of the foot.

BLADDER/KIDNEY STONES (CALCULI)

Calcium carbonate 'stones', formed from mineral substances from the urine, can develop anywhere in the urinary system, but are commonly found in the bladder or kidneys.

Cause: Imbalance in pH levels of urine. (Most common in areas with high mineral-content in water).

Signs: Straining to urinate. Urine dribbling, possibly 'scalding' vulva and legs of mares. Slight colic symptoms.

Treatment: Surgical removal of stone. Management should be re-assessed to prevent recurrence. Carefully wash and dry scalded areas of skin and apply medicated cream.

CYSTITIS

Inflammation of the bladder – relatively rare in equines.

Causes: Bacterial infection. Secondary complication of conditions (e.g. bladder stones or paraylsis) where bladder function is impaired.

Signs: Horse strains to urinate frequently but with little success. May be dribbling and scalding of skin around vulva/inner legs. Urine may be blood-stained.

Treatment: Dependent upon identifying cause. Antibiotics may be required. Clean, dry and apply medicated cream to affected skin.

POLYNEPHRITIS

Causes: Inflammation and degeneration of the kidney, commonly found in mares following foaling where bacteria have passed up the urethra. Infection can come from the bloodstream (e.g. in foals where umbilicus becomes infected).

Signs: Weight loss, lethargy, weakness, swelling of abdomen and legs, halitosis (bad breath). Excessive thirst. Blood analysis shows anaemia, electrolyte imbalance and increased urea levels.

Treatment: In early stages, condition may respond to antibiotics and correction of body salt imbalances.

POLYNEURITIS EQUI

Paralysis of the bladder (see Chapter Six).

LAMINITIS

Laminitis is among the most common causes of equine lameness. Most cases are entirely due to mismanagement and are thus avoidable. As the condition is extremely painful, laminitis is a major welfare issue. Although there are gaps in our understanding of the disease, we do now know enough to prevent 80 per cent of cases happening in the first place and to achieve successful treatment of 80 per cent of those which do occur.

In the normal foot, the horse is suspended by two sets of interlocking laminae, the dermal or 'sensitive' laminae attached to the outer surface of the pedal bone, and the epidermal or 'insensitive' laminae which line the inside of the hoof capsule. So the horse is quite literally 'hung' within his hooves – he does not stand in them as we do in our boots (see Chapte Four).

It is important to be able to differentiate between four conditions, all of which have previously been lumped together under the term 'laminitis':

- laminitis
- acute founder
- sinkers
- chronic founder.

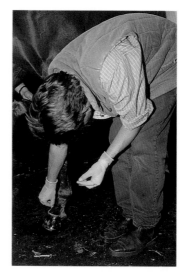

A careful examination of the lower leg, coronary band and foot helps identify the type of laminitis involved. Accurate diagnosis is essential.

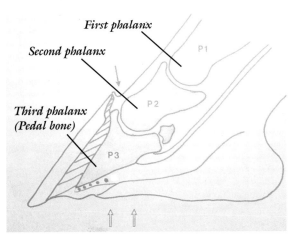

Cross-section of a foundered foot showing sinking of pedal bone.

First phalanx

Second phalanx

Third phalanx
(Pedal bone)

P1

P2

P3

Research has shown that being able to tell these four conditions apart is the most useful skill when it comes to applying the correct treatments at the right time and in being able to predict whether the animal will recover. No special techniques such as X-rays or blood samples are needed to differentiate between these four conditions – just the ability to feel with your fingers and use your eyes.

Laminitis can cover the full range of severity from an animal which simply shows a mild lameness at trot, to one which is lying down groaning and sweating. It is common for the condition to be misdiagnosed and confused with anything from sore shins, arthritis, navicular disease, tetanus, colic, azoturia or injuries to the back or hind legs.

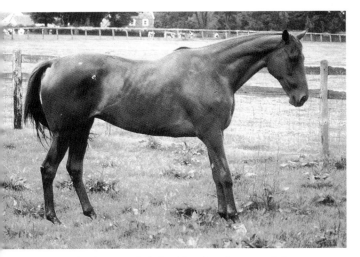

The characteristic 'rocking horse' stance of the laminitic, desperate to relieve the weight from its toes.

RECOGNISING THE SIGNS

LAMINITIS

All laminitis cases have abnormally strong pulsation in the arteries which supply the feet. The feet may be hot, cold or a normal temperature, so feeling for heat in the feet is a waste of time. These cases have the characteristic stance with the animal taking its weight on its heels and relieving its toes. Remember that although the front feet are the most commonly affected, any number or combination of feet can be affected. For example, if both hind feet are affected the horse will stand with the hind feet forwards under the belly and the front feet pulled backwards.

Laminitis cases have sore feet, so will tend to shift their weight from one to another continually. Nevertheless, the feet will look normal – no long toes nor high heels, nor growth rings on the hoof wall which are wider at the heels than around the toes.

ACUTE FOUNDER

These have all the symptoms of laminitis cases but also have depressions just above the coronary bands on the affected feet. The depressions can be felt with your fingers: they start in the central part of the coronary band above the toes and, as the condition worsens, they extend backwards towards the heels. The deeper the depressions and the further they extend sideways, the worse the founder. This occurs because in founder cases the bond between the interlocking laminae in the front part of the foot has started to fail and the pedal bone is beginning to move down within the hoof capsule. The weight of the horse is overcoming the cohesion between the two sets of laminae. As it moves down, it pulls the overlying skin with it, which is what causes the coronary band depression that you can feel.

SINKERS

These horses are the most severely affected. Cases do not always show the typical heel-loading stance, but rather stand flat-footed and are very reluctant to move at all. If they are forced to move, depending on the severity, they will walk slapping their feet down or may rush forward dangerously and run into anything in their path. They have strong digital pulses and may have stone-cold feet. All sinkers have depressions which extend all the way round the coronary band, right back to the bulbs of heels.

Sinker cases have lost all connection between the laminae all the way around the foot, so these poor animals are indeed standing in their hooves as we stand in our boots.

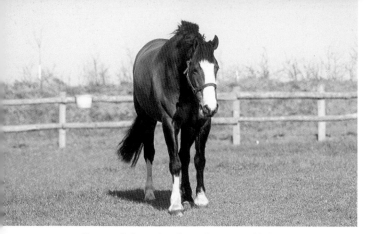

Over-weight animals or those on a high sugar or starch diet are at greatest risk from laminitis. Medium-quality pasture is more than sufficient for equines.

CHRONIC FOUNDER

These cases are characterised by having distorted feet as a result of having suffered acute founder in the past. They have growth rings which are wider at the heels than around the toes, on the walls of the affected feet. The toes tend to become overgrown so that the front walls of the feet appear concave when viewed from the sides. The heels grow more quickly than the toes and the soles of the feet appear flat or, in severe cases, convex. The white lines around the toes are wider than normal and susceptible to infections. Some chronic founder cases remain lame all the time, with recurrent attacks of acute lameness. When their feet are X-rayed they have severe changes both in the lining of the hoof walls, and part of the pedal bones will have dissolved away. Other chronic founder cases, which were less severely affected during the acute founder stage, can live a pain-free life and perform quite satisfactorily as general riding animals given regular and correct foot dressing and shoeing.

Remember that chronic founder cases can also have concurrent laminitis, acute founder or rarely, sinking.

CAUSES OF LAMINITIS

We know that there are particular sets of circumstances which commonly precede the onset of laminitis.

OBESITY/OVER-EATING

It is a fact that fat animals are at higher risk than thin ones. So keeping your horse in a lean, fit condition and preventing him from becoming obese will go a long way to preventing the disease. It is the sugar and starch part of the diet which causes laminitis, not, as was once thought, protein.

When a horse over-eats on a sugary feed, be it fresh grass, cereals, coarse mixes or nuts, not all the carbohydrate can be digested in the small intestine. Part of the meal overflows in the caecum and colon where it induces a change in the population of microbes which normally live there. The sugary fluid encourages the growth of microbes which do not normally live in the large colon and as these increase in number, they produce acid which kills off the normal microbes. As these die, toxins are released into the gut from the bodies of the bacteria. The normal bacteria are there to complete fibre digestion for the horse and produce a variety of essential micro-nutrients, so their loss is serious. The increased acidity in the large bowel is thought to damage the mucosal lining which allows the uptake of toxins and acid into the blood stream.

This is where the understanding of the mechanism of dietary laminitis becomes a bit thin. As yet, we do not know how such damage to the gut and the changes within the bowel cause the changes we see in the horse's feet. What we do know is that the normal blood flow within the foot is disrupted: there is a great increase in the total flow to the foot, but reduced perfusion of the laminar tissues. Whatever the precise mechanism, we know that there is damage to the two interlocking sets of laminae which normally hold the horse suspended within his feet. We know that the damage to the laminae begins up to 40 hours before the horse shows any lameness.

TOXAEMIA

Any form of toxaemia can lead to laminitis. Many illnesses – pneumonia, pleurisy, diarrhoea, infection of the uterus and retention of foetal membranes after foaling, can all result in the production of bacterial toxins which enter the horse's blood circulation. Similarly the ingestion of plant toxins, fungal or chemical toxins can predispose to laminitis.

SIDE-EFFECTS OF CERTAIN DRUGS

Some drugs, including wormers such as pyrantel, or corticosteroid drugs, have the potential to cause laminitis as a serious side-effect. In the UK, corticosteroid drugs, often used to reduce fluid accumulations or to treat sweet itch or chest complaints, all carry a warning that they can induce laminitis. In the author's view, these drugs should only be used as a last resort and, if they are used, the owners should be made fully aware that in some cases, the laminitis which follows can be so severe that the horse has to be euthanased.

TRAUMATIC LAMINITIS

This follows fast work on hard surfaces. Another form occurs in horses which show lameness after nailed-on shoeing. These animals have poor horn quality which cannot cushion the sensitive tissues from the concussion of hammering on the shoes. The lameness may persist for up to two weeks. This problem can be

treated successfully by adding the supplement
Farrier's Formula to the diet.

WEIGHT-BEARING LAMINITIS
If an animal becomes severely lame on one leg due,
for instance, to a fracture or infection, it takes all its
weight on the other leg. When this continues for
more than 24 hours, the weight-bearing foot can
develop laminitis. This occurs commonly in hind legs.
Often all the attention is given to the 'bad' leg and the
damage to the opposite foot is overlooked until it is
too late to treat successfully.

HORMONAL CAUSES
The common hormonal causes of laminitis are
thyroid insufficiency, Cushing's Disease and oestrus-
dependent laminitis. The first two can be diagnosed
by blood testing and treated successfully by
medication. Some mares show laminitis when they
are in season and these cases can be a problem to treat
in the long-term. There are drug therapies which
suppress oestrus or, as a last resort, the mare could be
spayed.

COLD WEATHER LAMINITIS
Very occasionally, horses will show laminitis when
they are left out in cold weather. This is thought to be
due to a reduction in blood flow to the feet. Fitting
insulating leg wraps can prevent this condition, which
should be differentiated from bruising to the soles
when the horse's feet become balled-up with snow.

STRESS LAMINITIS
This occurs rarely – there are usually other reasons
why the horse has developed laminitis. However, the
stress of travelling, particularly in hot or cold
conditions, and the stress of working or vaccination
can induce laminitis.

POOR SHOEING
Fitting shoes which press on the sole can cause
laminitis. Additionally, neglecting the feet of chronic
founder cases by allowing the toes to grow too long
and the heels too high, can cause recurrent attacks of
lameness.

TREATMENT
Always call the vet if any form of laminitis is
suspected, as he is the only one able to help you
diagnose and manage your horse with the use of
specific drugs. Treat laminitis with just as much
urgency as colic. Do not rely on advice from
unqualified people nor buy potions over the counter

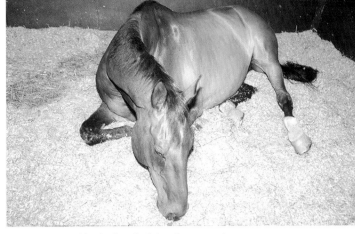

Shavings provide the best bed for the recovering laminitic.

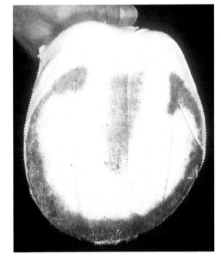

Frog supports help take the strain off the laminae. A roll of bandage has been laid along the frog and taped in place to act as an arch support for the foot. The frog support must not be too thick, or the horse will be more lame. This horse has been walked along a black mat to show the areas of weight-bearing.

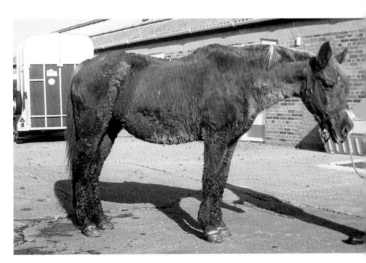

A tumour of the pituitary gland, frequently the cause of laminitis in a horse or pony with Cushing's Disease. Note the abnormally long, thick coat. These cases fail to shed their coats in spring. Other symptoms include diabetes, weight-loss despite an increased appetite, swelling above the eyes, a tendency to sweat excessively, and a pendulous abdomen.

from tack shops and feed stores – none are of any use. To prevent your horse from becoming a cripple you need professional help.

- Firstly diagnose whether your horse is a case of laminitis, acute founder, sinking or chronic founder, using the criteria above.
- Discover what caused the laminitis. If you do not know this, you have no hope of treating or removing the cause.
- Move the horse to a stable with a deep bed of clean, dry whitewood shavings covering the entire floor area to a depth of 18ins (45cm). If the horse is a long way from the stable, transfer it by trailer or box rather than walk it.
- Your vet will want to fit frog supports to the feet. Correctly fitted frog supports make 90 per cent of the laminitis and acute founder cases much more comfortable immediately. Supports help take the strain off the laminae and reduce the risk of the horse foundering. Whether you remove the shoes or not depends on the shape of the soles. If the soles are concave, the shoes may be removed, if flat or convex they are best left on. If the horse is severely lame, do not fight with it to remove shoes, just fit thicker frog supports.
- The vet will want to prescribe a drug called acepromazine which will help to normalise the blood flow to the feet and reduce the animal's anxiety. Also a limited dose of bute (phenylbutazone) as a painkiller. If you call the vet quickly, he will be able to use another drug called heparin to help prevent blood clotting in the small blood vessels in the laminae. He may wish to take blood and urine samples from the horse to help him decide what caused the laminitis and whether the horse needs any specific treatments.

Under no circumstances should the horse be force-walked. On the contrary, he should be encouraged to lie down in a comfortable bed. Shavings are the bedding of choice as the horse will not eat them and they are nicely cushioning to the feet. If the horse is down for some days, shavings are less abrasive to the skin than sand.

I recommend that even laminitis cases be stabled for one month following the return of soundness without painkillers. This gives the feet time to heal and gives you time to gradually diet the horse. Remember you should never starve horses – with or without laminitis. The recommended treatments for acute founder, sinking and chronic founder are outside the scope of this chapter but can be discussed with your veterinarian.

FEEDING THE LAMINITIC

Assuming that the animal is fat and is suffering a dietary-induced laminitis, then you should only feed him forage. This means hay, cut grass (not lawn mowings), alfalfa, clean straw or any combination of the four. There are good proprietary feeds available such as a Fibre Blend, Hi Fi Lite and Alfa A, any of which will satisfy the dietary requirements of laminitis cases when fed in combination with Farrier's Formula supplement, and yet achieve a gradual weight loss.

Feeding any form of cereals will only exacerbate the imbalance in the hind-gut bacteria and provide too many calories. All horses are individuals when it comes to feeding; the same diet will put weight on some animals, keep others at maintenance and cause others to lose weight. As a rough guide, you may feed the following to achieve a gradual weight loss in stabled or yarded horses and ponies. You will never diet horses if they are at grass, unless you fit them with a grazing muzzle.

SAMPLE DIETS

A fat Shetland pony fed twice a day, each feed to consist of:

$1/2$ lb Hi Fi or Fibre Blend
1 pint soaked sugar beet shreds
1 measure Farrier's Formula
with $1^1/2$ lbs good-quality hay three times daily.

A fat 14 hh pony fed twice a day, each feed to consist of:

1 lb Hi Fi or Fibre Blend
2 pints soaked sugar beet shreds
2 measures Farrier's Formula
with $2^1/2$ to 3 lbs good-quality hay three times daily.

A fat 16 hh horse fed twice a day, each feed to consist of:

$2-2^1/2$ lbs Hi Fi or Fibre Blend
3 pints soaked sugar beet shreds
$2^1/2$ measures Farrier's Formula
with 3-4 lbs good-quality hay three times daily.

If your horse is not fat and has laminitis, then ask your vet to check him out for parasitism, liver or kidney disease and, most importantly, Cushing's Disease. All too often a horse is dieted in an effort to avoid laminitis, but still gets the condition. In fact,

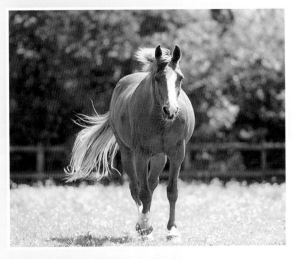

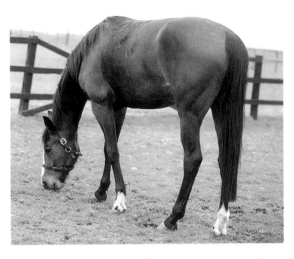

▲ *Fat animals are at a much higher risk of contracting laminitis than lean ones. Do not allow your horse or pony to get over-weight or obese. Avoid sugar- and starch-rich feed, whether fresh grass, cereals, coarse mix or nuts.*

▲ *Avoid turning out onto lush grazing, for example cattle pasture or fields which have been fertilised. Laminitis is best controlled by using dieting paddocks where the amount of grass consumed can be restricted. Alternatively fit a grazing muzzle as a preventative measure.*

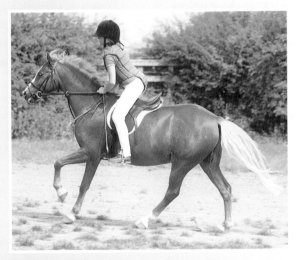

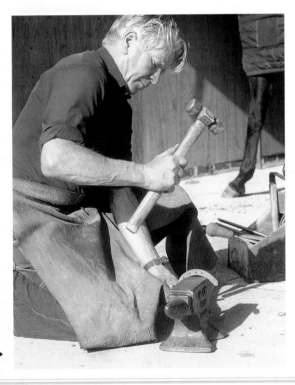

▲ *Give regular, steady exercise to keep the horse or pony in lean, fit condition and promote healthy circulation. Avoid working on hard ground.*

Have the feet regularly attended to by a good farrier. ▶

the horse has Cushing's Disease. The laminitis in these cases is due to a pituitary gland tumour and has nothing to do with their diet.

SHOEING THE LAMINITIC
Shoeing for the laminitic depends on the precise diagnosis. The treatment plan will vary, from correct foot trimming to re-establish the hoof capsule in line with the pedal bone, to the fitting of specialist

shoes(such as the heart bar). It is crucial that the farrier works only in conjunction with a competent veterinary surgeon. Having initially taken the appropriate X-rays, a treatment is selected appropriate to the particular type of laminitis involved and its cause. A further period of settlement will undoubtedly take place and regular re-assessment is required that should involve both farrier and vet.

4 THE HORSE IN MOTION

There are some truly wonderful sights in this world and to a horseman or horsewoman, one of these is the horse in motion. To watch the natural collection and extension of a horse trotting in a field, or that feeling of the horse underneath fall into frame while riding, is indescribable. It is part of, or possibly the heart of, the allure of all equestrian pursuits.

There will always be an unknown factor, element or 'mystique' about the motion of the horses. What makes an Olympic champion, dressage horse, cutting, or reining horse, jumper, gaiter or the powerful draft animal, goes far beyond the mechanics of bone and muscles. Possibly this 'unknown' can be attributed to the spirit of the horse. The rest – the legs, the bones, the muscles, and their co-ordination – is what is known and is what we will talk about in this chapter.

BONE

The bones of the body are composed of very hard, densely compacted bone, called cortical bone, and softer, less dense bone, called spongy bone. Cortical bone adds strength and rigidity, while spongy bone adds compression and elasticity. The amount of each compared to the other varies from bone to bone and is dependent on the function of that particular bone. This is most evident when comparing the differences between the long bones of the leg, which are long, hollow and have very thick cortical bone, to the bones of the head and chest which are flat, short, and have a thin cortical layer with a thick spongy centre. The long bones of the leg bear the majority of weight and are essential for motion; therefore they are thicker and harder in order to carry the load. The flat bones are more responsible for blood production and are part of the framework that gives the body shape. For this reason they have less cortical bone and greater spongy bone. All bones have a thin outer layer called the periosteum that supplies the bone with blood, nerves and is the initial site of healing and remodelling.

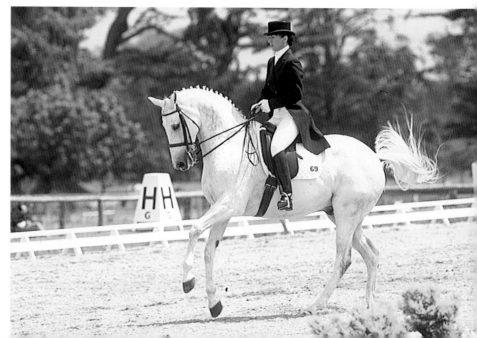

Poetry in motion. The mechanics of muscle and bone are only part of the inspirational sight of a horse in perfect control of his body and movement, whether in the field or the arena.

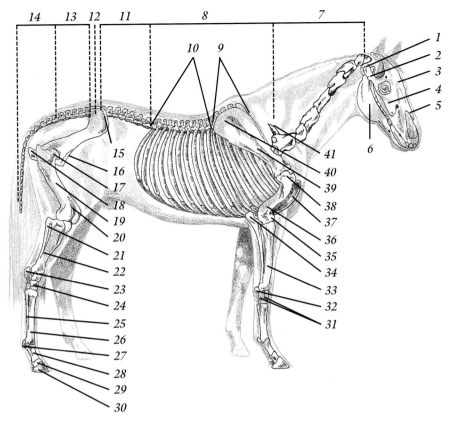

THE SKELETON OF THE HORSE

1. Occipital bone
2. Zygomatic arch
3. Frontal bone
4. Maxilla (upper jaw)
5. Nasal bone
6. Mandible (lower jaw)
7. Cervical (neck) vertebrae
8. Thoracic vertebrae
9. The 8 'true' ribs attaching to sternum
10. The 10 'false' ribs joined to one another by cartilage
11. Lumbar vertebrae
12. Tuber sacrale (point of croup)
13. Sacrum, usually 5 vertebrae fused together
14. Caudal (tail) vertebrae
15. Tuber coxae (point of hip)
16. Pelvis
17. Hip joint
18. Tuber ischii (point of buttock)
19. Femur (thigh bone)
20. Patella (knee cap) and stifle joint
21. Fibula
22. Tibia
23. Calcaneus, forming point of hock
24. Hock joint
25. Small metacarpals (fore-limb), small metatarsals (hind-limb), (splint bones)
26. Large metacarpal (fore-limb) large metatarsal (hind-limb)
27. Sesamoids at fetlock joint
28. Proximal phalanx (long pastern, os suffraginis)
29. Middle phalanx (short pastern, os coronae)
30. Distal phalanx (coffin bone, pedal bone, os pedis)
31. Carpal joint (carpus, knee)
32. Accessory carpal bone (pisiform)
33. Radius
34. Olecranon (point of elbow)
35. Elbow joint
36. Humerus (upper arm)
37. Sternum (breast bone)
38. Shoulder joint
39. Scapula (shoulder blade)
40. Scapula cartilage (cartilage of prolongation)
41. First thoracic vertebra with its strong spinous process

Put all the bones together and they form the frame of the body known as the skeleton.

The equine skeleton is divided into two separate parts:
• the axial skeleton (the skull, spine, ribs and sternum)
• the appendicular skeleton (the limbs).

THE AXIAL SKELETON
The spine is designed to support the considerable weight of the abdomen, and is relatively rigid compared to that of other athletic animals. It is made up of individual bones called vertebrae, that fit together to form a chain that surrounds and protects the spinal cord.

The spine is made up of five sections. There are seven vertebrae in the neck (cervical), 18 or 19 in the upper back (thoracic) and six in the loins (lumbar). The last lumbar vertebra articulates with the five fused sacral vertebrae that join to form a single bone at the top of the pelvis. Between 15 and 20 vertebrae (caudal or coccygeal) form the tail.

Vertebrae vary in detail according to their

position, but have a basic shape that consists of a body and arch, a pair of transverse processes at the side, and two pairs of surfaces where the bone articulates with its neighbours. When lined up, the shape creates a channel to house the spinal cord, with a gap at each junction between vertebrae allowing nerves and blood vessels to pass through.

Muscles and ligaments attach to the vertebral processes, and each vertebra is joined to its neighbours at its articular facets, where a cartilage disc allows for slight, but very limited, compression and flexibility. The spinous processes stick up like a shark's fin from each vertebra in a line and can be felt beneath the skin. The tranverse processes, however, are surrounded by muscle and can only be felt in a severly emaciated horse.

The spine is designed in a series of curves which, in the way of a suspension bridge, gives it enormous strength to carry the weight that hangs beneath it. What it is not designed for is to support weight on top, as it is expected to do when carrying a rider. Although there is a degree of lateral and vertical flexibility, enabling the horse to bend around circles and round over a jump, both the shape and articulation of the vertebrae and the way the surrounding muscles work, do restrict flexibility of the spine and make it vulnerable to damage when subjected to unnatural stress or trauma. (See Chapter Nine for problems involving the back.)

THE APPENDICULAR SKELETON
The appendicular limbs attach to the axial skeleton at two points – the shoulders (the pectoral girdle) and the pelvis (pelvic girdle). The fore-limb is connected to the body by a series of muscles and ligaments along the thorax, to the scapula. There is no real bony joint between the shoulder joint and the vertebral column. This allows for large flexibility of the shoulder, and reciprocal movement between the lower limb and the shoulder. This makes up for the lack of flexibility in the spine. The muscles of the shoulder move the shoulder forwards as the lower leg moves back. Since the body is connected to the shoulder, this action creates forward movement. In contrast, the hind-limbs are attached by bone at the pelvis.

The horse's front leg from the knee down has all the same bones and ligaments as the human hand. The horse has evolved in such a way that it now walks on the tip of the third finger. This tip gradually became dominant and the two fingers on either side became smaller and smaller and closer

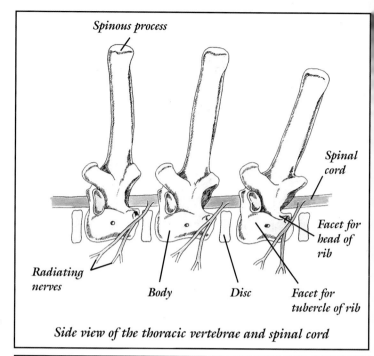

Side view of the thoracic vertebrae and spinal cord

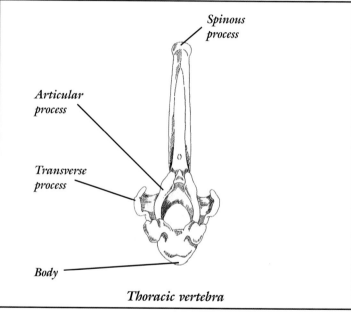

Thoracic vertebra

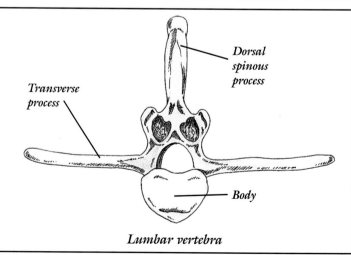

Lumbar vertebra

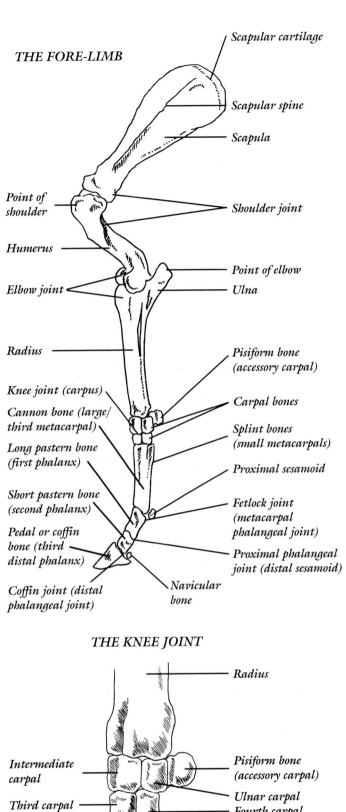

THE FORE-LIMB

to the centre finger, until all that was left was the metacarpal bones that now form the horse's splint bones. The outer two fingers, compared with the human thumb and little finger, vanished completely. The horse's carpus (knee) is the human wrist, the cannon bone is the third metacarpal bone, the fetlock the first knuckle, the long pastern the first phalanx, the pastern joint our second knuckle, the short pastern bone the second phalanx, the coffin joint the last joint of the finger and the coffin bone the third phalanx. The hoof is really a modified finger nail.

The hind-leg developed in a similar fashion and from the hock down can be compared to a human foot. This evolved from the centre toe, with the hoof being a modified finger nail, the pedal or coffin bone the third phalanx, the short pastern bone the second phalanx, the long pastern bone the third phalanx, the cannon bone the middle or third metatarsal bone, the splints the remnants of the second and fourth fingers (the second and fourth metatarsal bones), and the hock a modified ankle called the tarsus. The stifle is the same joint as the knee in humans.

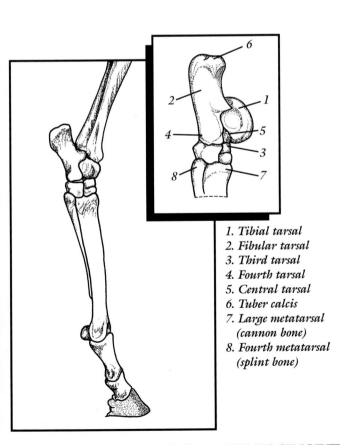

1. Tibial tarsal
2. Fibular tarsal
3. Third tarsal
4. Fourth tarsal
5. Central tarsal
6. Tuber calcis
7. Large metatarsal (cannon bone)
8. Fourth metatarsal (splint bone)

THE HIND LIMB (inset) THE HOCK JOINT.

THE KNEE JOINT

THE FUNCTION OF BONE

Bones have three main functions: they create the framework for the body, produce blood cells and produce motion. Bone also stores magnesium, calcium and phosphorous ready to be used during pregnancy or lactation.

The leg bones of the horse are engineered for efficient, fast movement, capable of bearing the forces of the leg hitting the ground, carrying the weight of the horse and acting as levers against which the muscles work. The long bones of the leg are hollow, making the bone light, yet have a very thick, strong cortex, enabling them to withstand heavy concussion.

JOINTS

A joint is the site where two bones meet. The amount of movement and structure vary depending on the site and bones involved. The joints created by the ribs meeting the spinal canal, for example, or the joints created by the bones of the head, have minimal or no movement and little structure, while other joints, such as those in the leg, have a wide range of movement and a very intricate structure.

These joints all have the same basic components. The joint capsule is a strong, fibrous outer covering, lined inside by the synovial membrane. The synovial membrane is composed of cells called synovytes that produce synovial fluid, a thick viscous liquid composed mainly of hyaluronic acid, that fills and lubricates the joint. At the junction of the joint capsule and the bones is a rich supply of blood vessels that provide the joint with its circulation. The ends of the bones that the joint forms around have a thick layer of cartilage and cartilage-producing cells called chondrocytes.

THE MAJOR JOINTS OF MOTION

Carpus   Referred to commonly as the 'knee', this joint is actually the equivalent of the human wrist. It is composed of three small joints, the top one of which is completely isolated from the lower two, which do communicate with each other.

Stifle   Equivalent to the human knee, this joint is made up of two joints, one created by the femur and patella and the other by the femur and the tibia.

Hock   Named the 'tarsus' by anatomists. Equivalent to the human ankle, this joint is composed of four smaller joints.

Fetlock   Equivalent to the human first knuckle. Commonly referred to as the 'ankle'.

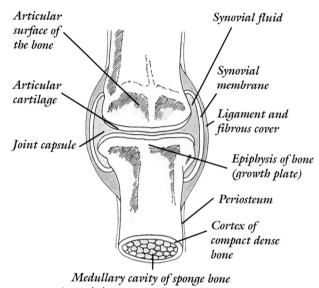

The structure of a joint, showing a section through a long bone

THE FUNCTION OF JOINTS

The joints create the junction between two bones. In the leg their main function is intricately involved in the motion of the horse. In general, joints of the leg flex or extend. Flexion occurs when the angle of the joint decreases or closes. Extension of the joint occurs when the angle of the joint increases or opens. Some joints, such as the fetlock, are structured so that they can flex in two directions. The forward flexion of the fetlock functions to add elasticity to the leg whilst bearing weight.

MUSCLE

There are two types of muscle in the body – smooth and striated. Smooth muscle is composed of spindle-shaped cells, interlaced together, that contract in a wave or circular fashion. It is mainly present in blood vessels and the intestines. Striated muscle is composed of straight, rectangular-shaped cells aligned in long fibres, which cause the shortening of the muscle when contracted. This is the type of muscle cells that make up all the skeletal muscles of the body.

THE FUNCTION OF MUSCLE

Throughout the body, the major muscle groups work in pairs or groups to create forward and backward movement, stabilise joints and dampen motion to create smooth movement of the body. Forward and backward motion, or opposite motion of the leg, is accomplished by reciprocal muscle action. Here, muscles are paired on either side of the bone and as one muscle flexes the other relaxes to allow movement.

Extensor muscles cause the extension of a joint, while flexor muscles cause the flexion of a joint. Overall, muscles on the front of the leg tend to pull the leg forward and the muscles at the back of the leg pull the leg back, pushing the body forward and creating forward propulsion. The front limbs create lift and forward movement of the body, while the main function of the hind limbs is propulsion of the body forward.

TENDONS AND LIGAMENTS

Tendons and ligaments are composed of long strands of collagen fibres aligned parallel to each other. A good comparison would be baler twine that is not twisted. The twine itself is composed of several smaller, parallel strands of twine. The strength of the tissue (tendon and ligament) comes from this collective alignment of parallel fibres.

There is very little blood supply to tendons or ligaments. These tissues get their nutrition by diffusion, which means that nutrients must travel from the outside of the tissue to the inside by moving around the cells. Many tendons and ligaments are surrounded by a fibrous covering or 'sheath' that protects and provides blood supply and lubrication.

Tendons connect muscle to bone. Ligaments connect bone to bone or bone to tendon. In general, tendons cause movement of a joint, whilst ligaments add strength and support to a joint or structure. The major tendons of the legs are the deep digital flexor tendons, superficial flexor tendons, the suspensory ligament and check ligaments.

THE FUNCTION OF TENDONS AND LIGAMENTS

The main function of a tendon is to create the movement of a joint and to support the structures it is connected to. One end of the tendon is connected strategically to a joint while the other end is

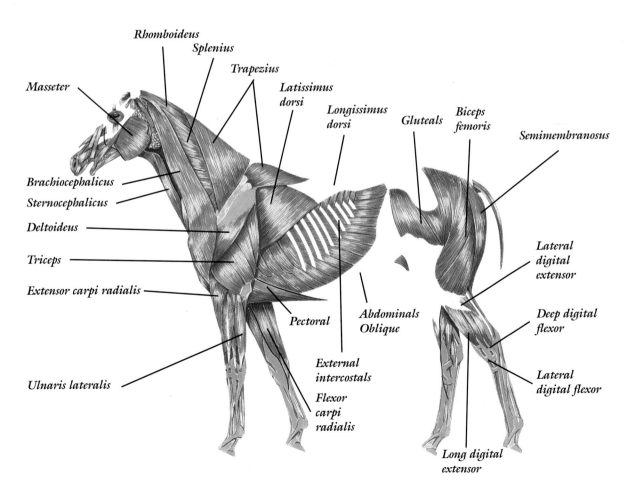

THE MAJOR SUPERFICIAL MUSCLES OF THE HORSE

THE MAJOR MUSCLE GROUPS
THE FORE-LIMB

MUSCLE	ORIGIN/INSERT	NATURE	FUNCTION
Brachiocephalicus muscle	*origin* – front of humerus, *insert* – head of the horse	extends the shoulder joint	pulls leg forward, paired with the latissimus dorsi muscle
Latissimus dorsi muscle	*origin* – back of humerus, *insert* – the back along the area of the withers	flexes the shoulder joint	pulls the leg back, pushes body forward, paired with brachiocephalicus muscle
Serratus thoracis	*origin* – back of shoulder, *insert* – onto the neck	flexes the shoulder joint	moves shoulder-blade down and back, helps push leg forward, paired with serratus cervicis
Serratus cervicis	*origin* – front of shoulder, *insert* – onto the neck	extends the shoulder joint	moves shoulder-blade up and forward, helps push leg back and body forward, paired with S.thoracis
Pectoral muscle	*origin* – centre of the humerus, *insert* – sternum	keeps leg close to body	makes the humerus centre of rotation of the fore-leg
Extensor carpi radialis muscle	*origin* – bottom of the humerus, converts into extensor carpi radialis tendon, *insert* – front of third metacarpal (cannon) bone	extends carpal joint	straightens leg, bringing foot forward preparing foot to land at end of flight phase
Biceps brachii	*origin* – front of the shoulder blade, *insert* – humerus	stops shoulder joint flexion	contracts during weight-bearing phase to keep leg extended and moving forward
Triceps muscle	*origin* – point of elbow, *insert* – top of humerus and shoulder blade	keeps elbow joint extended	contracts during weight-bearing phase, keeps leg extended and aids serratus cervicis to move leg back, body forward
Deep digital flexor muscle	*origin* – point of elbow converts to deep digital flexor tendon, *insert* – back of coffin bone	helps keep leg straight during weight-bearing phase, works with check ligament	contracts at end of weight-bearing phase to help move leg back, body forward and lift hoof off ground, shortens leg

THE HIND-LIMB

MUSCLE	ORIGIN/INSERT	NATURE	FUNCTION
Iliopsoas muscle	*origin* – femur, *insert* – pelvis	flexes hip joint	pulls leg forward
Biceps femoris	*origin* – back of pelvis, *insert* – top back of femur	directly flexes stifle joint, through reciprocal apparatus flexes hock and fetlock	shortens leg during flight phase to increase efficiency of motion
Gluteus medius	*origin* – pelvis, *insert* – top back of femur	extends hip joint	main muscle responsible for moving back, body forward
Hamstrings (tendinosis muscles)	several muscles *origin* – top of pelvis, *insert* – front side of stifle joint	no real flexion of extension of joints	main function is to pull leg back, push body forward
Quadriceps femoris	*origin* – front half of pelvis and top of femur, *insert* – front of stifle joint	extends stifle joint	causes upward movement of patella aiding in locking the stifle, part of the stay apparatus of hind limb
Tensor fasciae latae muscle	*origin* – front of pelvis, *insert* – quadriceps femoris muscle	extends stifle joint	works with Q.femoris muscle to lock stifle, the stay apparatus of hind limb
Peroneus tertius muscle	*origin* – front bottom of femur, *insert* – hock joint	connects stifle and hock joints	creates one half of reciprocal apparatus, if one joint flexes the other must flex
Superficial digital flexor muscle	*origin* – bottom back of femur converts into superficial digital flexor tendon, attaches to point of hock, runs down back of cannon bone, *insert* – pastern	mostly tendon	other half of reciprocal apparatus, pulls taut when stifle flexes, helps flex hock, flexes fetlock, shortens leg

THE TENDONS AND LIGAMENTS OF THE LOWER LEG

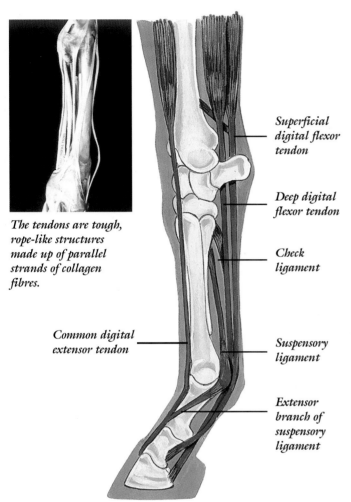

The tendons are tough, rope-like structures made up of parallel strands of collagen fibres.

Common digital extensor tendon

Superficial digital flexor tendon

Deep digital flexor tendon

Check ligament

Suspensory ligament

Extensor branch of suspensory ligament

THE HORSE'S FOOT

The horse's foot is a highly-specialised, wear-resistant structure that is designed to support the bodyweight and absorb concussion. It is made up of two distinct parts:
• insensitive structures (external)
• sensitive structures (internal).

INSENSITIVE STRUCTURES
The equine equivalent to a human fingernail, the foot is the extension of the superficial layer of skin, or epidermis. The hoof capsule itself derives from the **coronary corium**, which is situated immediately beneath the coronary band. There the highly vascular corium has a membrane covering, of which little teat-like projections called papillae are responsible for the development of the horny hoof capsule.

The hoof capsule consists of tubular horn created from hair follicles called horn tubules. Thousands of individual horn tubules are bonded together with a substance known as inter-tubular horn. The tubular horn becomes flattened and overlapped to add strength. It is noticeably thickest at the toe for extra protection, and gradually thins towards the heel to allow for dynamic flexibility. A hardening process called keratinisation then takes place, enabling the outer hoof capsule to become the hard structure, or **wall,** with which we are all familiar.

At the heel, the hoof wall becomes inverted to form the **bars** of the foot. This adds strength to the hoof and increases the bearing surface of the horny wall.

connected to muscle. When the muscle contracts it causes movement of the joint. Extensor tendons cause extension of a joint and flexor tendons cause flexion.

Ligaments function mainly to add strength and stability to a joint, bone or tendon or to resist the movement of these structures. This resistance of movement that both tendons and ligaments create is most important during the stance phase of motion, when the forces on the leg are the greatest and tend to cause over-flexion.

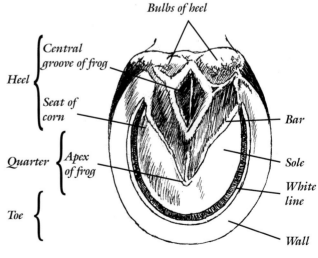

Bulbs of heel

Central groove of frog

Heel

Seat of corn

Quarter

Apex of frog

Toe

Bar

Sole

White line

Wall

UNDER-SIDE OF THE FOOT

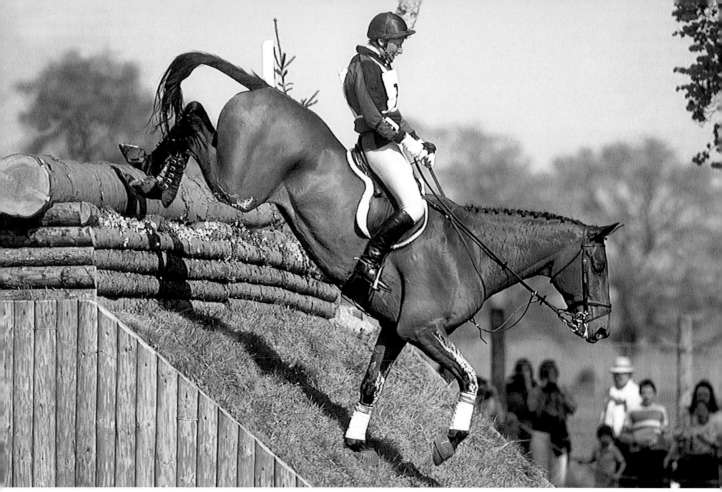

Athletic activity puts tremendous strain on the structures of the lower leg, in particular the tendons, which enable extension and flexion of the joints, and the ligaments, which add strength and stability and restrict over-flexion.

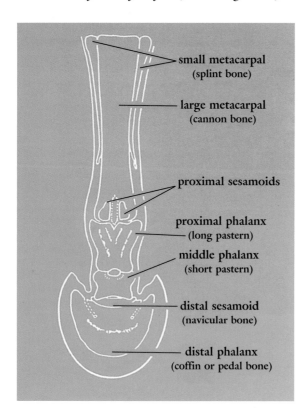

small metacarpal
(splint bone)

large metacarpal
(cannon bone)

proximal sesamoids

proximal phalanx
(long pastern)

middle phalanx
(short pastern)

distal sesamoid
(navicular bone)

distal phalanx
(coffin or pedal bone)

The bones of the foot

By virtue of its shape and position, the **frog** plays an important role in the integrity, shape and dynamic function of the foot. Its rubbery texture and shape assists in dissipating dynamic energy during weight-bearing.

The **horny sole**, like that of the horny wall, is derived in the same way from the tubular horn, except that here the horn tubules are more widely spread, allowing for more inter-tubular horn to be developed. It is this primary difference in development that allows the sole to exfoliate, so constantly reproducing and redeveloping. Vaulted in shape, not unlike the bridge of the human foot, the sole gives extra strength and support to the limb.

The **horny laminae**, which encompass the internal aspect of the hoof wall, are vertical, leaf-like projections, which descend from the coronary groove to the ground surface. These non-sensitive laminae inter-digitate with the sensitive laminae of the distal (third) phalanx, or pedal (coffin) bone.

SENSITIVE STRUCTURES
Each horny structure has its corresponding sensitive structure. All of these are highly vascular and possess their own nerve supply.

The **sensitive sole** (corium of the sole) is situated

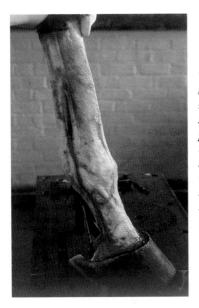

The hoof is a continuation of modified skin that surrounds and protects the pedal bone (third, or distal phalanx), navicular bone and part of the short pastern bone (second phalanx).

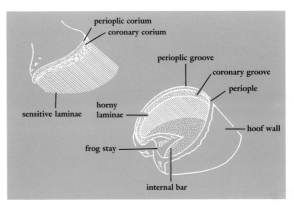

▲ *The structure of the hoof capsule.*

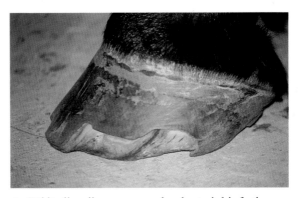

▲ *White line disease occurs when bacterial infection becomes established in the soft horn at the junction between the insensitive and sensitive laminae.*

on the solar aspect of the distal phalanx (pedal bone). As with the coronary corium, it has a velvet-like appearance and also contains the papillae which develop the tubular horn of the sole.

The **sensitive laminae** (laminal corium) are vertical, fleshy protrusions that cover the anterior surface of the distal phalanx. Each primary sensitive laminae has secondary leaves, which inter-leaf with their horny counterpart, thus encapsulating the distal phalanx.

The **sensitive frog** forms a proportion of the digital cushion within the posterior aspect of the foot and it is covered with a corium which produces the horny frog. Thicker than that of the sole, this corium is a mirror-image of the horny frog.

Situated above the coronary band, the **perioplic corium** produces the periople, which in turn produces a layer of horn that protects the coronary band. It extends around the band, but thickens considerably towards the heels and where it extends to protect the bulbs of the heel.

The **digital cushion** is a large fibro-fatty mass which, through its position, actually forms the bulbs of the heels that are clearly visible at the very back of the foot. It is a major absorber of concussion within the foot. The fibro-fatty composition of the digital cushion renders it virtually insensitive, enabling it to absorb dynamic energy by being deformed and compressed during weight-bearing.

Two vertical wing-like plates of fibro-cartilage called **lateral cartilage,** situated either side of the foot, assist in the dissipation of dynamic energy. Attached to the lower wing of the pedal bone and

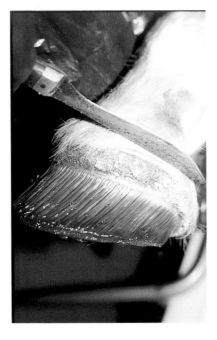

◀ *The sensitive laminae are vertical, fleshy protrusions that encapsulate the pedal bone. The coronary corium can be seen above the laminae.*

extending to above the coronary band, these lateral cartilages can sometimes ossify (turn to bone), producing a common condition is known as sidebone (see page 116). This can affect one lateral cartilage (known as unilateral sidebone), or both, when it is known as bilateral sidebone. Normal cartilage can be felt in the standing horse and should yield to thumb pressure. Once sidebone is advanced, the elasticity of the cartilage is lost, and it can clearly be felt as a hard prominence above the coronary band.

The **white line** is a soft horn which acts as a junction between the horny wall and horny sole. It forms a useful indicator of the thickness of the individual's horny wall. Being soft, it has the ability to expand, and so assists as an expansion joint between the wall and the sole. Bacteria can become established within the white line, however, leading to the development of the condition known as 'white line disease'.

LIMB & HOOF CAPSULE ASSESSMENT

The influence of the general conformation and quality, regular after-care by a competent farrier results in a normal, functional hoof. As is the case of conformation in general, certain specific criteria can be used to determine whether a foot is correctly 'balanced'.

WEIGHT DISTRIBUTION
An understanding of the mechanical influence of weight distribution in the horse is essential when considering the specific conformation of an individual's limb and hoof.

The weight distribution of the horse is divided up proportionally. With the head and neck placed forward of the centre of gravity, 60 per cent of the total bodyweight is transferred through the fore-limbs. Upright columns have therefore developed in the fore-limb to support this extra weight. To assist weight distribution, round fore-feet give the front feet a larger bearing surface.

The weight of the remaining 40 per cent of body mass is distributed through the hind-limbs. As propulsion is confined to the hindquarters, the hind-limb has developed to act as a lever, with a large muscle mass at the top. The more oval-shaped hind feet reduce the likelihood of interference during movement.

RELATIONSHIP BETWEEN LIMB AND HOOF
When looking at hoof conformation and balance, it is important to draw a relationship between hoof capsule and limb. Ideal limb conformation is when, viewed from the front, a vertical line will bisect the limb centrally from the knee to the ground surface. The outline of the limb and hoof capsule should be symmetrical and no deviation should occur at the fetlock or pastern joint. Medial-lateral balance of the hoof should be clearly visible.

HOOF-PASTERN AXIS
The hoof-pastern axis is assessed by viewing the limb and hoof from the side. A vertical line from the point of the shoulder should bisect the knee and fetlock centrally. A second line is then drawn to bisect centrally from the centre of the fetlock through the pastern and hoof capsule. This is known as anterior-posterior balance.

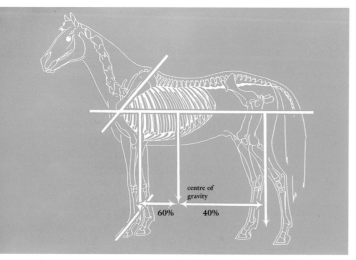

centre of gravity

60%   40%

▲ *The distribution of weight through the skeleton.*

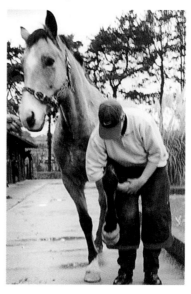

The farrier must make a careful assessment of the alignment of each limb and hoof.

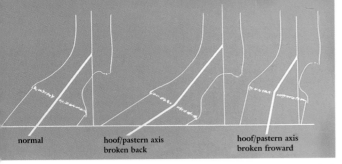

normal   hoof/pastern axis broken back   hoof/pastern axis broken froward

▲ *The effect of variations in the hoof-pastern axis. Ideal conformation depends on the individual horse and limb.*

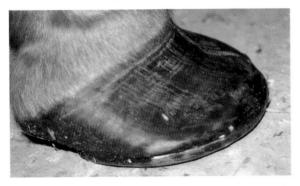

▲ *The long, sloping foot of the 'broken' hoof-pastern axis shows how the hoof capsule becomes distorted and weakened and the bodyweight is transferred backwards on to the heels, creating tension on the tendons and ligaments.*

With the influence of the Thoroughbred extending into both general and specific breed requirements, there has been a tendency to breed horses with a slightly longer, more sloping pastern. The ideal pastern angle in the fore-limb, of 50 to 55 degrees, can in some instances be increased to such an extent that the angle becomes 'broken-back'. As a result, a long, sloping foot is allowed to develop naturally. Bodyweight is subsequently transferred backwards, to dissipate within the posterior third of the foot. Natural pressure, continually displaced behind the centre of gravity, results in distortion of the hoof capsule, with a long toe and low, weak heel. The horse then walks on the heel, breaking down the horny structures.

Where the hoof-pastern axis is severely broken-back, tension is created on both the tendons and the ligaments. Tension on the digital flexor tendon over a long period of time can develop into pathological changes such as navicular disease, due to the increased pressure on both the navicular bursa and bone.

With the horn tubules subjected to increased pressure within the heel area, the circulatory system can also be affected. The horn begins to break down, and eventually little or no horn is produced at the heels. Lack of pressure at the front of the foot allows the toe to extend forwards. In extreme cases, a resistance here can be clearly seen on the dorsal wall at approximately half the distance between the coronary band and the ground surface. Horn tubes being stretched at the toe then begin to bend and fracture, causing visible cracks within the hoof wall.

The white line is also affected, being stretched and extended at the toe. Weakened and torn, it can then be easily penetrated by bacteria, causing such conditions as seedy toe and white line disease.

WEATHER CONDITIONS

Climatic changes can affect horses' feet. Excess moisture during long wet spells can cause the feet to become saturated and, under pressure, the horn will re-modify its shape. Alternatively, long dry spells can cause the foot to dry out and crack. In extreme cases it will shrink, causing superficial cracks within the wall. These can cause a problem when shoeing as the foot can be rendered smaller and periods between shoeing shortened.

DIET

There are many products available relating to foot care, but no substitute for a healthy, balanced diet. If deficiencies are present, dietary supplements are available containing biotin methionine, copper and zinc, which have been scientifically proven to assist in horn production.

When considering using oil or grease in an attempt to advance better horn quality, it should be noted that in prolonged dry weather, as mentioned above, the horn requires moisture. Daily use of an oil-based product would prevent any moisture from being absorbed through the horn. A non-oil-based moisturising solution would be more effective under these conditions.

KEEPING FEET HEALTHY

Being a living structure, the hoof requires regular attention to maintain strong, healthy horn. The connective horn tissue can separate and begin to break down if proper care is not kept up. Under-foot conditions also affect the frog in a number of different ways.

An increasing number of horses are now kept in stabled situations and as a result are more likely to suffer with foot problems, mostly associated with bacteria or fungal spores. Bedding must always be kept dry, as bacteria or fungal spores from wet or dirty bedding will soon invade the horn structure, creating an infection. The fungus, an anaerobe, thrives in a warm, moist environment and so any infection of this type will very quickly lead to more acute conditions.

Infection can be prevented by regularly cleaning out the feet.

THE 'HOT' SHOEING PROCESS

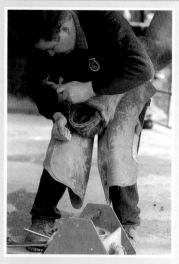

◀ *The buffer and driving hammer are used to cut the clenches of the old shoe, which is then levered off with pincers. Cleanly-cut clenches should mean no hoof wall is torn as the shoe is removed.*

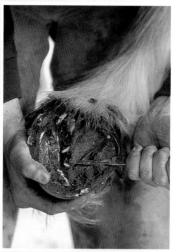

◀ *The foot is prepared for the new shoe by cleaning out the sole and frog, and assessing their condition and the shape and balance of the foot. Wall over-growth is removed using the drawing or toeing knife or hoof cutters. If necessary, rough sections of the frog or sole are trimmed. The rasp is used to create a level bearing surface.*

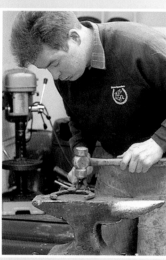

▲ *The farrier chooses a shoe of the correct size, weight and type for the individual horse and the work it does. Manufactured shoes with ready-made nail holes and 'fullering' (the groove that minimises weight and adds grip) are now most commonly used. After heating in the forge, adjustments can be made to the shape of the shoe on the anvil to give a good fit. If only slightly worn, old shoes are sometimes replaced after the horn is trimmed and the foot prepared (known as 'removes' or 're-fits'). Whilst still hot, the shoe is taken to the foot on the pritchel and fitted. The light searing of the horn indicates the extent to which the foot and shoe are in contact. Any alterations necessary to the shape or heel length of the shoe can then be made.*

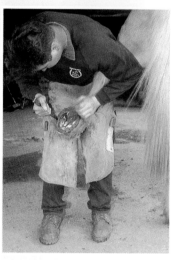

▲ *After cooling in water, the shoe is nailed on using nails designed to continue to fill their hole throughout wear. Correct choice of size is important to avoid early loosening of the shoe. The toe nail is generally driven in first. Three nails are generally used on the inside and four on the outside. The shoe is secured by the turning over and twisting off of the clenches – the ends of the nail which protrude from the hoof wall – and its toe clips (fore-shoes) and quarter clips (hind-shoes).*

The foot is finished by using the driving hammer to ▶ embed the clenches into a small indentation created in the hoof wall. The clips are tapped back to lie flush with the wall. Finally the rasp is run around the lower edge of the wall where it meets the shoe, to reduce the risk of cracking.

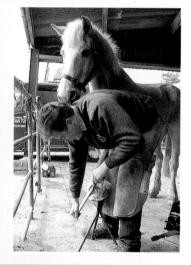

ROUTINE CARE: THE UNSHOD FOOT

- The feet should be cleaned out daily to remove dirt and debris from the sole and lateral and central clefts. Use this opportunity to assess the condition of the feet, paying particular attention to the frog and heel areas. This will prevent bacteria from infecting the horn over long periods of time.

- Wash mud and stable dirt off the sole and hoof wall regularly, as these prevent the horn from 'breathing'. Hoof oil or other non-medical preparations should not be over-used. Oil-based products effectively create a barrier between the hoof wall and the environment, preventing the absorption or evaporation of moisture.

- Check that the white line has not been penetrated by foreign bodies such as stones or gravel. If it has, pick this out carefully and wash the foot out with clean water. Check the sole for penetrations. Flat-soled horses, and those kept on stony pastures, are particularly vulnerable to puncture wounds.

- Watch for any cuts or abrasions to the coronary band. If over-looked, these can lead to more acute problems at a later stage.

- Have excess horn trimmed on a regular basis, as wear rarely matches growth rate.

ROUTINE CARE: THE SHOD FOOT

Unlike the unshod foot, the shod foot requires more care than simply attention to maintain healthy horn. Penetration of the wall during nailing allows the horn to divide and, in more serious cases, to split. Bacteria can enter the wall via the old nail holes and be over-looked, leading to serious conditions such as white line disease and other abnormalities.

- Maintain a regular shoeing regime that suits each horse's individual requirements. Normally this would involve attention every 4 to 6 weeks.
- Pick out feet on a daily basis, paying particular attention to the sole, frog and heel areas. Check there are no foreign bodies present, or debris lodged under the shoe, especially between the frog and the heels of the shoe.
- Check the coronary band for abrasions or cuts, and the bulbs of the heels for any bruising or cuts due to over-reaching or treads.
- Look for any cracks or splits in the hoof wall.
- Check the nails are tight and the clenches are still embedded into the hoof wall. Loose shoes can contribute to corns and are at risk of coming off (being 'cast').
- Note any uneven wear of the shoes and report any concerns to the farrier at the next shoeing appointment.

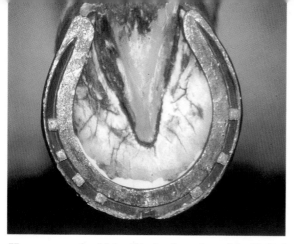 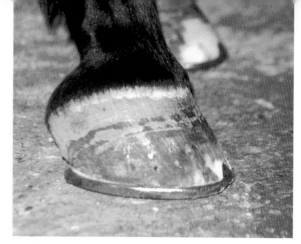

Horse owners should familiarise themselves with all the features of good farriery.

THE WELL-SHOD FOOT

The advance of equestrian sport, and upturn in owner-rider education, has meant that the judgement that a foot has been 'well-shod' purely by the fact that the shoe has stayed on for six weeks has long since gone. Owners and riders are now aware that each case should be taken on its merits, depending on a number of issues, and that styles of shoeing vary depending on individual requirements. Certain basic principles of farriery must be adhered to, however.

- Initial assessment of the foot before shoeing should consider firstly conformation (both of a general nature and individual foot conformation).
- Correct trimming of the foot before applying the shoe is of paramount importance and its effect on the soundness of the horse should never be under-estimated. The initial assessment should also take into account the individual's work requirements. Two identical horses with varying job descriptions may require different styles of shoeing. For example, a dressage horse expected to work for long hours on an artificial surface will have different requirements to a stable-mate who hunts twice a week. As the dressage horse's exercise takes place almost entirely under strictly controlled circumstances, shoeing can be tailored to assist with whatever the owner requires. In contrast, the hunter is likely to encounter less than ideal conditions that vary from week to week. The main shoeing criteria here is one of safety, assisting in the prevention of injury through interference and finally, to ensure that the shoes remain on.
- A shoe should be selected that is appropriate in type and weight for the size of the horse and nature of the work it is expected to do.
- The fitting and shape of the shoe should have taken into account any conformational errors of the foot. It is possible to enhance the shape of the hoof capsule through the way the shoe is fitted.
- The shoe must be adjusted to fit the foot rather than the foot to the shoe. There should be no excessive rasping of the foot at the toe, (known as 'dumping') or over-trimming of the frog and sole. The frog should make contact with the ground surface.
- A level bearing surface must be created. There should be no daylight between the foot and the shoe, particularly at the heels.
- The foot should be reduced in length at both toe and heel and, as required, on both sides. The heels of the shoe should not be too long nor too short, although length here can vary due to individual conformation of the feet.
- The correct number and size of nails used is important. The number will vary depending on the size of the foot. Traditionally seven were used – four on the outside and three on the inside – but this has only confused the situation. By and large, most farriers will use six nails on a normal foot – three on each side. This can increase to eight in large horses, and decrease to as little as four in miniature animals. The ideal is to use the smallest amount of nails possible whilst still ensuring the shoe is well secured. As horn separates when penetrated by a nail, nail size is therefore important relative to the size of the foot. Nails should sit neatly into, and fill, the nail holes, and be driven well home.
- Nails should exit the hoof wall, as far as possible in line and at approximately a third to half the distance between the coronary band and the ground surface. Clenches should be slightly longer than their width and be well 'seated' so that they remain strong. If clips are fitted these should also be let into the hoof wall at the same angle and be flush when finished. It is common practice to fit shoes with two clips at the toe quarters of the hind feet. This enables the shoe to be fitted just under the toe, helping to prevent injury.

Good farriery can only be achieved taking into account all of the above, although individual requirements may give reason for the farrier to modify some of these points. The horse owner can assist the farrier by giving any relavent information

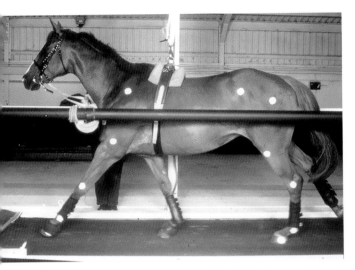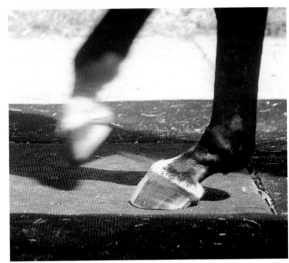

The advance of technology has allowed far deeper understanding of equine biomechanics, through the use of force-plate analysis (right) and video cinematography of horses working on treadmills.

and should be encouraged to take an interest in the daily management of the feet and arranging shoeing on a regular basis.

FUTURE TRENDS

Whilst the basic criteria for shoeing the horse remain unaltered, there are occasions when attention to detail is required when shoeing for specific purposes.

There are two quite separate and distinct aspects to remedial shoeing of any kind.

Firstly, it must be borne in mind that *corrective* shoeing can only be achieved if the skeletal structure has not reached maturity. The nature of the deformity will dictate how effectively it can be treated.

Where *remedial* work is appropriate, the advancement of modern technology has led to the widespread use of other materials as an alternative to the traditional metal shoe. Plastic and rubber compounds have been successfully employed over the years to assist in the treatment of certain conditions. This has led to a large range of glue-on products, mainly associated with the treatment of developmental conditions in young horses. Careful preparation and application can help in the re-alignment of deformed limbs. Other advances in products that assist in the protection of the sole have meant that we now have many styles and varying consistencies of sole pads – a far cry from the leather pad once invariably used to protect the foot from injury!

The advance of foot-related products and their use in farriery has arisen directly to meet the demands of both horse and rider. One of the areas of equine research that has developed in leaps and bounds within recent years, is that of biomechanics. Research programmes at several leading universities are contributing to a much greater understanding of equine biomechanics. Horses can be worked on a treadmill with video cinematography linked to computer software which can calculate the length of stride and measure angles of articulation, comparing each limb with its opposite number. Force-plate analysis allows the horse to be trotted in-hand whilst accurate measurements are made of the point at which the foot engages the ground surface, the amount of vertical loading through the limb, and the point at which the horse's foot leaves the ground.

Such detailed analysis will undoubtedly assist our understanding of conformation and how horses should be shod to assist with certain limb deformities. It also gives us an opportunity to experiment with other styles of shoeing, such as the rolled toe, long heels, short heels, wedged heels, bar shoes and four-point shoeing etc., by allowing us to see the effects of these techniques demonstrated through scientific data rather than simply personal interpretation. This data can then be used educationally, to promote good foot care and aid the correct development of foot care and farriery products.

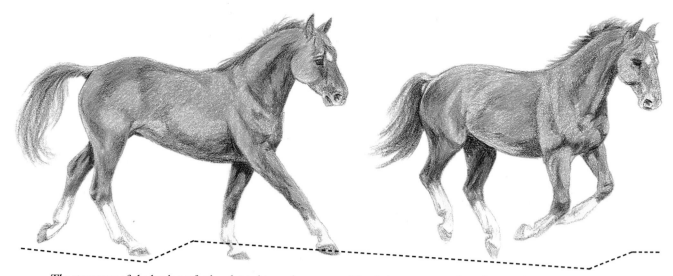

The structure of the leg is perfectly adapted to saving energy. Muscle is concentrated at the top of the leg, leaving the lower leg light in weight. Flexion of the fetlock and knee joints help to minimise the up-down movement required with each stride. The flattened trajectory this creates is even and effortless in comparison to speedier animals, such as the cheetah, who flex their backs to create huge bounding strides, but are rapidly exhausted.

MOTION

DESCRIPTION OF MOVEMENT

TRACKING
This term describes the proximity of the landing site of the hind-limb in relation to that where the fore-limb had just been. Since the hind-limb is mainly responsible for the propulsion of the horse, it is desirable for the hind-limbs to 'track up'. Positive advancement occurs when the hind-leg tracks past the point where the fore-limb has been. Negative advancement occurs when the hind-limb falls short of where the fore-limb has been.

FOOT FLIGHT
This describes the direction and pattern of the foot as it moves through the air. The leg is designed to flex while moving through the air in order to decrease the energy needed to move it forward. The energy needed to move the leg is related to the length of the leg. During flight the leg is bent, the leg length thereby shortened and the energy required decreased. The result is an arc-shaped flight pattern.

STANCE PHASE
The time that the leg is on the ground.

FLIGHT PHASE
The time that the leg is in the air.

BREAK-OVER
The end of the stance phase and the point of last contact of the hoof with the ground as it is being lifted into the flight phase. The break-over point is composed of the ground and the toe of the hoof.

CENTRE OF GRAVITY
The point of the horse where, if the body was suspended from rope, the front and back halves would balance. Located just behind the withers, it is the point of the concentrated weight of the horse. Since the centre of gravity is closer to the fore-limbs, more weight is carried by the 'forehand' of the horse (see page 98).

STAY APPARATUS
The co-ordination of tendons, muscles and ligaments that develops to stabilise the leg and allow the horse to sleep standing up.

The front stay apparatus is composed of many of the tendons and ligaments of the fore-limb. Stabilisation of the fetlock is created by the flexor tendons, the sesamoidean ligaments and the suspensory ligament.

Extra strength is added to the deep digital tendon by the carpal check ligament. The flexor tendons support the fetlock from the back, and the suspensory ligament, front extensor tendons and the sesamoidean ligaments support the joint from the front, preventing flexion of the joint.

The carpus is stabilised by the radial check ligament and the configuration of the bones of the carpus.

The hind stay apparatus is also composed of many tendons, ligaments and muscles, but the main component is the ability of two muscles, the *quadriceps femoris* and the *tensor fasciae latae*, to pull the patella (knee cap) over the medial trochlear ridge (inside ridge) of the femur.

This 'locks' the stifle, and through the reciprocal apparatus of the hind leg, also 'locks' the hock and fetlock joints.

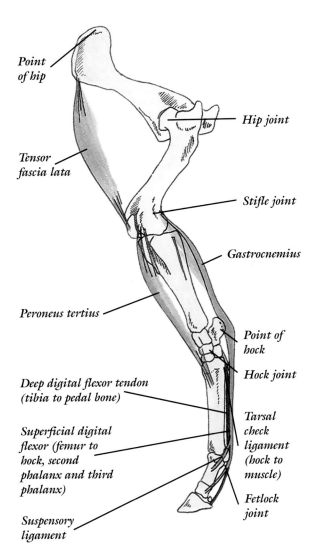

Point of hip

Hip joint

Tensor fascia lata

Stifle joint

Gastrocnemius

Peroneus tertius

Point of hock

Hock joint

Deep digital flexor tendon (tibia to pedal bone)

Tarsal check ligament (hock to muscle)

Superficial digital flexor (femur to hock, second phalanx and third phalanx)

Fetlock joint

Suspensory ligament

The stay apparatus of the hind leg

RECIPROCAL APPARATUS OF THE HIND LIMB

Joins the stifle and hock and fetlock joints, such that if one is flexed the other is also flexed. The apparatus is composed of the *peroneus tertius,* running down the front of the leg connecting the front of the stifle joint to the front of the hock joint, and the *superficial deep flexor muscle* and tendon, running down the back of the leg connecting stifle joint to hock and fetlock.

THE DYNAMICS OF MOVEMENT

In its simplest form, the body is moved by forward advancement of a limb – as the limb is pulled back,

the body is pushed forward. The hind-limbs supply the propulsion or forward movement of the horse. The fore-limbs aid in forward movement and add upward lift to the body. This is required to increase distance travelled by adding a second force – an upward force – to the movement, creating projectile motion.

Consider throwing a ball straight forward from you and compare the distance travelled by that ball to one thrown into the air. The ball thrown into the air will travel farther because another force, the force of upward movement, has been added to the forward movement of the ball, increasing the overall energy and so the distance travelled. In physics this is known as 'vector dynamics'. This upward lift by the front limbs is very important in the performance of the horse, especially in sports such as dressage, eventing and jumping.

FORE-LIMB MOVEMENT

Forward movement of the leg begins with contraction of the *brachiocephalicus* muscle and relaxing of its paired muscle, the *latissimus dorsi,* causing the humerus to be pulled forward. At the same time, the *serratus thoracis* contracts and moves the shoulder back.

As the leg moves forward, the elbow and knee flex, shortening the leg and creating the foot flight. As the leg nears the end of the flight phase, the *extensor carpi radialis* contracts, straightening the leg in preparation for landing. As the leg starts to come down, the *serratus cervicis* contracts and its paired muscle, the *serratus thoracis,* relaxes, moving the shoulder forward and swinging the leg back. Also at this time the *brachiocephalicus* relaxes and the *latissimus dorsi* contracts, pulling the leg back.

When the hoof is fully on the ground (stance phase) the carpus is straight, the fetlock is dorsi-flexed and the shoulder is still moving forward. At this time the force of gravity from the centre of gravity is acting on the joints to try to flex them. The *biceps brachii* muscle stops the shoulder joint from flexing, the *triceps* muscle keeps the elbow joint from flexing and the flexor tendons and the suspensory ligament support the fetlock from over-flexion and stop the pastern and coffin joints from flexing.

Forward movement of the shoulder continues to push the leg back to the point of break-over, where the deep flexor muscle contracts and lifts the leg up. Speed is determined by the speed of the leg swing back.

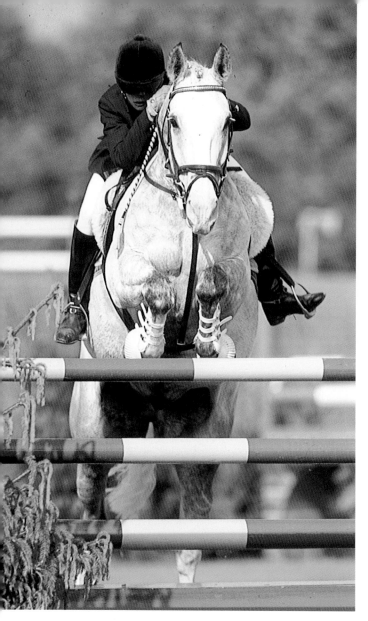

The upward lift of the front limbs is crucial to performance in dressage, eventing and jumping horses.

HIND-LIMB MOVEMENT

The hind-limb has the same bases of motion as the fore-limb. The limb swings forward and as it is pulled back, the body is pushed forward. The limb is pulled forward by contraction of the *iliopsoas* muscle. This also causes flexion of the stifle joint and of the hock and fetlock, through the reciprocal apparatus. The leg is pulled back by the *gluteus medius* and is aided by the hamstrings and other smaller muscles. Also at this time the *quadriceps femoris* muscle contracts, extending the stifle. Through the reciprocal apparatus, this causes extension of the hock and relaxation of the superficial tendon, allowing the fetlock to dorsi-flex and the hoof to come forward, preparing it for impact on the ground. Once in the stance phase, the muscles continue to pull the leg back, causing the body to be pushed forward.

GAITS

The three most common gaits of the horse are the walk, trot and canter. Many breeds have a modified four-beat gait that may vary in speed and style. Some breeds of horse, most notably the Standardbred, also have a two-beat gait known as the 'pace'. (See panel opposite).

Gaits are described according to the speed, beat (sound made by the hooves as they land), order of the hooves as they land and length of stride. Fore and hind-limbs that are on the same side of the horse are termed 'paired' - for example, left front and left hind. Fore and hind-limbs that are opposite each other are termed 'diagonal' – for example, left front and right hind.

COMMON DISORDERS OF THE LOCOMOTIVE SYSTEM

TENDONITIS (BOWED TENDONS)

Causes: Tendons and ligaments are composed of long strands of collagen fibre aligned parallel to each other. The strength of the tissue (tendon or ligament) comes from this collective alignment. When a horse 'bows' a tendon or ligament, this fibre pattern is disrupted, either by over-stretching of the fibres (strain) or a full tearing of the fibres.

The most common sites of tendon injuries are the deep and superficial flexor tendons, the suspensory ligament, the distal check ligament and the annular ligament. All of these compose the support structure of the fetlock. Injury to them occurs from hyperextension (over-extension) of the fetlock joint and over-exertion of the tendon or ligament, causing tissue breakdown. Extension of the fetlock joint occurs as the leg hits the ground. The harder the leg hits the ground or the deeper the footing, the more the joint extends. With this in mind, it can be appreciated how the majority of these injuries occur in athletic horses especially those that race, jump, rein or cut.

Signs: The area becomes inflamed, appearing hot, painful and swollen. Often lameness, ranging from mild to severe, accompanies the injury.

Treatment: Traditionally, treatment of these injuries has been aimed at reducing inflammation in the early phases of the injury by cold therapy (hosing or icing the leg), poultices, anti-inflammatory drugs such as bute or banamine, and rest. Other therapies aimed at speeding up healing include surgeries such as tendon splitting, check ligament desmotomy (cutting the check ligament) and complementary

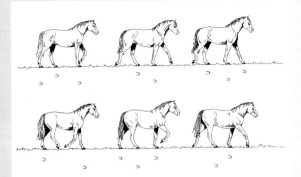

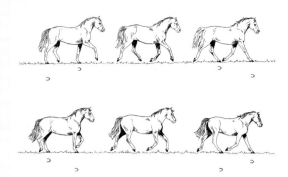

THE WALK

A walk is a regular four-beat gait. The movement is considered lateral, because one set of paired legs hit the ground first, followed by the opposite set of paired legs. For example: (1) left hind, (2) left front, (3) right hind, (4) right front.

THE TROT

A trot is a two-beat gait in which diagonal legs land on the ground at the same time: (1) left hind-right front (2) right hind-left front.

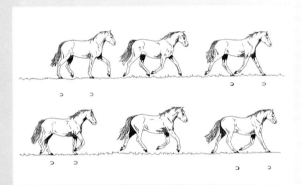

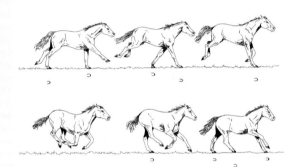

THE PACE

A pace is a two-beat gait where paired legs land on the ground at the same time: (1) left hind-left front (2) right hind-right front.

THE GALLOP

This is also a four-beat gait, each cycle of hoof-beats being separated by a suspension period: (1) left rear, (2) right rear, (3) left front, (4) right front, followed by a period of suspension in which all legs are off the ground. The hind leg that began the sequence is considered the leading hind leg, and its diagonal fore-limb is considered the leading fore-limb. The leading fore-limb describes the 'lead' of the horse. In the above example, therefore, the left hind and right fore-limbs are considered the leading limbs and the horse is described as being in the 'right lead'.

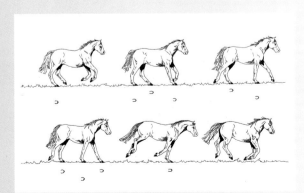

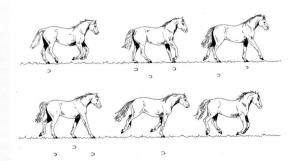

THE CANTER

This is a three-beat gait and is considered a collected form of the gallop. The leading legs land independently of each other and the opposite diagonal legs land on the ground at the same time. For right canter: (1) left hind, (2) right hind-left front, (3) right front. (see diagram on right). Left canter is shown in diagram on the left.

Self-inflicted injuries can occur by accident. Habitual injuries, however, are usually the result of poor conformation or action, immaturity, lack of balance or condition, or inappropriate shoeing that makes the horse knock himself when he moves and are known as 'interference'. (See Chapter Eight for *Leg protection*).

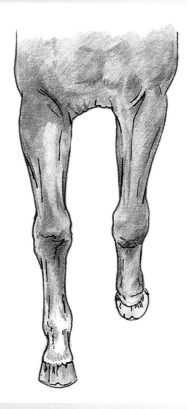

▲ *Correct, straight movement.*

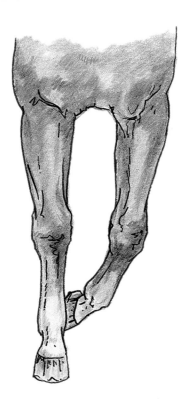

▲ **Brushing** *One fore-leg or hind-leg strikes the opposing fore-leg or hind-leg. An injury to the inside of the knee or hock caused by the inside toe of the opposite leg is known as a* **speedicut**. *This is rare, being most common in racehorses and polo ponies, but is serious as it often causes a fall.*

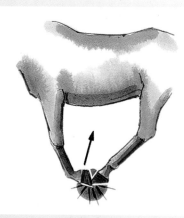

Forging *Common problem with young and unbalanced horses, or when the feet are allowed to become too long. As the front foot is picked up, the toe of the shoe is clipped by the toe of the hind shoe coming forwards. Some horses also have a tendency to over-step with the hind feet and tread on the heel of the front shoe, pulling it off and causing an abrupt halting of the stride.*

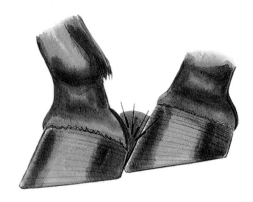

Over-reaching *A hind foot 'over-steps' and treads on to the heel of a front foot. A higher over-reach is termed a 'strike' and may sometimes cut into the tendon. A 'tread' is a wound on the coronet region caused by the horse stepping on himself or being trodden on, generally during travelling.*

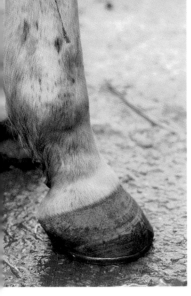

The characteristic swollen appearance of a 'bowed tendon'.

therapies such as magnetic, laser and ultrasound therapy. In all cases, time is still the number one treatment. Most tendon and ligament injuries take at least six months to heal, and some as long as a year or more.

There is very little blood supply to tendons or ligaments. These tissues get their nutrition by diffusion, which means that nutrients must travel from the outside of the tissue to the inside by moving around the cells. This is a very slow process and is one of the reasons why healing of these tissues is so slow. The amount of healing time required depends on the amount of fibre damage present. The best way to determine the extent of damage present is ultra-sonography of the affected tissue. Obviously the more damage present, the more healing time is required.

Whether the horse returns to full work or not depends on the strength of the affected tendon once healed. If fibres are strained but not torn, the parallel fibre pattern will not have been disrupted and once healed, the tendon or ligament still has the majority of its strength. If fibres have been torn, however, the fibre pattern will have been disturbed. The strength of the healed tissue depends on how closely the scar tissue aligns itself into parallel strands of fibre, rather than into a haphazard cross-linking formation. This scar tissue is what weakens the tendon or ligament and makes it more susceptible to re-injury.

Treatment is therefore also aimed at helping the forming scar tissue to align correctly. In the past this has been accomplished by controlled exercise and time. Mild to moderate use of the damaged healing tissue helps align the scar tissue and also decreases the formation of adhesion (scar tissue from the healing area to the surrounding tissue). The drug 'Bapten' or BAPN (beta amino-propionitrile fumatate) inhibits healing collagen fibres (scar tissue) from forming cross-links, which means the fibres heal in a parallel strands, making the healed tissue very strong. This drug has been

very successful with horses returning to full work and involves a series of injections into the newly-damaged area. It is not effective on old injuries that already have scar tissue present, or for strains, but it can be used for new tears in the tissue. This drug does not speed up healing and still requires strict veterinary supervision, controlled exercise, and time. However, it does allow a high quality of healing and also hope for horses whose careers might have been destroyed by these types of injuries. At present, this drug is not licensed for use in the UK, although it looks promising for the future. Currently, adequan (a polysulphated glycosaminoglycan) has been used with some success.

SWEENEY

Causes: Sweeney disease occurs when the suprascapular nerve is damaged, causing atrophy of the supraspinatus and infraspinatus muscles. In essence, the shoulder nerve is damaged and the shoulder muscle degenerates. Muscles need nerve stimulation, and if it is not present then the muscle degenerates to the point where it appears to have disappeared on the animal. It is thought that the nerve is damaged by direct trauma (a direct blow to the shoulder) or is pulled and strained by a backwards thrust of the leg (the leg slipping back). The nerve runs around the front of the shoulder bone, making it susceptible to this type of injury. This was once a very common problem in the large pulling horses that might slip on wet streets while pulling a load.

Signs: Initially, the horse may appear lame and, with time, the muscles of the shoulder deteriorate, leaving what appears to be the shoulder bone covered by skin.

Treatment: Little treatment is available for this problem. Stopping the damage of the nerve through anti-inflammatory drugs such as bute and banamine is the basic treatment. There is a possibility that the nerve can regenerate itself. This takes a long time however, possibly as much as 10-20 months. Signs of regeneration are return of muscle mass and more normal movement of the leg. Regeneration of the nerve is not common.

Some people believe that once the nerve has been damaged, the lack of muscle tone allows an outward pull of the shoulder and more strain on the nerve, causing still more damage to the nerve. A surgery has been developed to try and decrease this strain by removing the underlying bone and any surrounding scar tissue around the nerve.

In horses, the length of time in which muscle atrophy is reversible (i.e., the muscle's ability to regenerate if its nerve supply is re-established) has not yet been established. In humans this is about 20 months. This condition should therefore be monitored for at least six months to gauge what the outcome will be.

AZOTURIA (RHABOMYLASIS/SETFAST/ TYING UP) See Chapter Two and Chapter Nine.

RINGBONE
Causes: Ringbone, or phalangeal exostosis, is new bone development into the pastern joint (proximal interphalangeal joint or PIP joint) and the coffin joint (distal interphalangeal joint or DIP joint). This is caused by irritation, rupture or tearing of the lining of the bone (the periostium) where the joint capsule or tendons and ligaments attach. The body responds to this low-grade irritation by laying down bone, in an effort to stabilise the area. This is called periostitis and can happen for a variety of reasons, which include:

• chronic, long-term unbalanced shoeing
• poor conformation
• hard work, causing twisting and pulling of the joint and related structures
• trauma to the area.

Ringbone is described as 'high ringbone' when it involves the pastern joint, 'low ringbone' when it involves the coffin joint, 'articular ringbone' when the bone growth has moved into the joint, and 'peri-articular ringbone' when the bone growth is around the joint. The condition is additionally described as 'true' when new bone formation extends across the joint and restricts movement, and 'false' when only the shank of the bone is involved, so there is no restriction.
Signs: The result of this bone growth is almost always lameness, its severity depending on the amount and location of the bone growth. Ringbone is a progressive disease that can cause such severe lameness that euthanasia is chosen to relieve the horse from its suffering.

The most painful type is the articular ringbone, either high or low, because this affects the joint itself, creating an arthritic condition; this is the reason why many people also refer to this problem as arthritis. The bone growth can be mild, showing as a little bone spur on the X-rays, or very severe, causing the whole joint to fuse. The degree of lameness can also

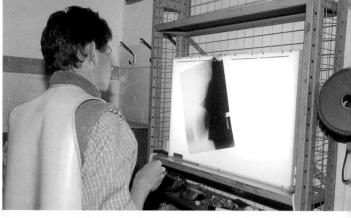

X-rays are a vital diagnostic tool for most skeletal and bone problems, including ringbone, navicular and arthritic conditions.

vary and does not always correspond with the severity of bone growth seen on the X-rays.
Treatment: There are several treatments, usually involving a combination of corrective shoeing, medical management, joint therapy, modified work and, in severe cases, surgery. The aim of treatment is pain relief, reduction of inflammation, decrease in the bony production or increase in bone production, causing fusion of the joint.

Initially, it is very important to analyse the horse's gait, conformation and shoeing to try and determine what might be causing the problem. Horses that land on their hooves abnormally (either on the outside of the hoof wall or inside of the hoof wall), have poor conformation (toed in, toed out, etc.), or are shod unbalanced, are more prone to developing ringbone.

The arsenal of treatments for this problem is vast and each case must be considered individually. Initially, pain relief and anti-inflammatory treatment is given by the use of non-steroidal anti-inflammatory drugs (NSAID), usually bute or banamine. Corrective shoeing is implemented and involves balancing the hooves, shortening and rolling the toes and fitting special pads to absorb shock. Some horses have responded very well to very thick cushy pads such as Poly Hoof or Honey-comb pads. These absorb the concussion at the pad and minimise the concussion for the horse, but are very difficult to keep on the hoof. Because the pads are so compressible, the nails tend to loosen up and the shoe falls off, or the hoof wall begins to crumble around the nail holes from the loosened nails. Horses using these pads must have a very strong, healthy hoof wall.

Selective use of softer shoe materials such as aluminium can assist. Ridden work should avoid hard surfaces, including roads.

The affected joint is often treated with anti-inflammatory drugs (steroids) and hyaluronate (synthetic joint fluid). This treatment is very effective in reducing the inflammation in the joint and replenishing the damaged joint fluid, making the joint more comfortable. Intravenous hyaluronate

(Legend) is also used for the same effects. Oral chondrotin sulphate/polyaminoglycan supplements have also been used. Although it is debatable whether these supplements in fact work or not, anecdotal reports indicate that they may help some horses. Exercise is recommended as much as possible, but work-load must be modified accordingly. Exercise can range from hand walk only, to walk/trot under saddle, to back to regular work, depending on the individual case.

In theory, once the joint has completely fused, the pain associated with the bone production resolves. Surgery, therefore, is aimed at fusing the joint and is accomplished by attaching plates to the joint or driving pins through the joint. However, surgery is not commonly used.

LOCKING PATELLA
Causes and signs: This condition is also termed 'upward fixation of the patella' or 'locking stifle'. Medically speaking, the patella becomes fixed on the medial trocheal groove, between the middle and medial patellar ligaments, causing the stifle and hock joints to become 'fixed' in extension. In plain terms, think of the stifle as the same as your knee. The knee cap or patella is held in place by three ligaments and some grooves in the long leg bone, the femur. When a horse 'locks' its stifle, the knee cap slips out of its normal location to the inside of the joint and is stuck between the inner two ligaments and the femur.

Locking the stifle is a normal procedure for the horse, used when sleeping standing up (the stay apparatus). It becomes abnormal when the horse is unable to shift the patella back into its normal location. There are a few reasons why this might occur. Some people believe there is a certain conformation (straight hind limb) that makes horses more prone. Another belief is that some type of traumatic incident (accident) causes the patella to lock. And finally, it is thought that the ligaments and muscles of the stifle may become weakened from the lack of use, allowing the patella to become locked and, because of their weakened state, the ligaments and muscles are unable to move the patella back into place.

If the patella locks frequently enough, the joint capsule and the surfaces of the patella or joint could become irritated or eroded causing lameness, so it is often necessary to correct this problem.
Treatment: When the stifle first becomes locked it can often be unlocked by backing up the horse. To prevent the stifle from locking, efforts must be

aimed at strengthening the muscles and ligaments of the stifle. This can be done by consistent exercise, particularly riding up and down hills. If this fails to work, some people believe that the area around the ligament should be injected with iodine (called internal blistering) which would cause an inflammatory reaction and scar tissue formation. This extra scar tissue formation is thought to add strength to the stifle and prevent the patella from becoming locked. Sometimes the locking becomes a significant enough problem that it becomes necessary to cut the medial patellar ligament.

FIBROTIC MYOPATHY
Causes: A fibrotic myopathy is an area of scar tissue that forms in one of the three muscles that form the back area of the haunches (rear upper portion of the hind leg). These muscles are called the *semitendinosus, semimembranosus* and *biceps femoris*. The scar tissue forms as a result of some type of trauma to these muscles, most commonly from sliding stops, catching a hind foot in a halter or intra-muscular injection. Sometimes this area can become calcified.
Signs: Since the muscle has changed from being very pliable to a tight band of scar tissue, the leg loses some of its range of motion, creating a characteristic 'goose-stepping' movement of the affected hind limb. As the leg moves forward and down, it stops just before it lands on the ground and is then slammed down or pulled back a little before hitting the ground. In essence, the leg cannot stretch forward enough and is pulled to the ground prematurely.
Treatment: Unfortunately, once scar tissue has formed it can be very difficult to remove. The treatment of choice for this problem is surgical

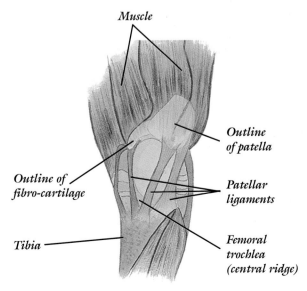

Muscle

Outline of patella

Outline of fibro-cartilage

Patellar ligaments

Tibia

Femoral trochlea (central ridge)

The patella and associated ligaments

correction by removing the scar tissue or cutting the tendon of the affected muscle. This releases the tension on the muscle belly, so the stretching is not so pronounced and the gait becomes more normal. Sometimes this surgery does not totally correct the problem, resulting in an improved but not completely normalised gait, and the horse's leg will never be able to fully stretch out again.

SPLINTS

Causes: The splint bones lie on either side of the cannon bone and are connected to the cannon bone by the interosseous ligament.

A 'splint' occurs in one of two ways:
• a sprain or tearing of the interosseous ligament
• trauma to the outside of the splint bone.

Interosseous ligament damage occurs most often from unbalanced pressures on the leg. This can easily occur as the horse is making sharp turns jumping, reining or cutting, or if the hoof is unbalanced. Trauma to the splint bone usually occurs from the horse hitting its leg or getting kicked.

Signs: Splints occur most frequently on the cannon bone just below the knee and appear as a hard or semi-hard lump. When they first happen they can be warm, swollen and painful to the touch. As they heal, they typically get smaller and harder but usually never go away completely. The horse is left with a permanent lump at the site.

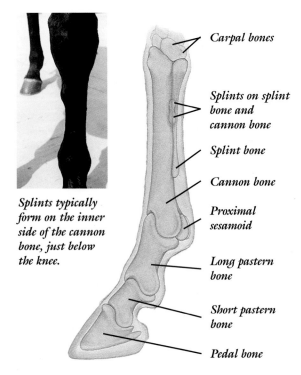

Splints typically form on the inner side of the cannon bone, just below the knee.

Carpal bones

Splints on splint bone and cannon bone

Splint bone

Cannon bone

Proximal sesamoid

Long pastern bone

Short pastern bone

Pedal bone

Area of splint formation. The splint affects both adjacent bones. It is an ossification (bony growth) that causes a callous, which fixes and reunites with the bone.

Treatment: A splint usually takes 6 to 12 weeks to heal, during which the horse's work must be restricted to the flat to minimise the stress on the leg. Most heal without a problem and any lameness subsides. Some do remain sensitive or become big enough to cause interference with the other structures of the leg (particularly the suspensory ligament), causing long-term problems.

ARTHRITIS

Causes and signs: Arthritis means 'inflammation of the joint'. The most common type of arthritis is what is collectively named 'degenerative joint disease' or DJD. This starts as an inflammation of the joint capsule and can progress into erosion of the cartilage and fusion of the joint. A cycle of inflammation develops. The inflammatory cells within the joint release destructive chemicals, causing deterioration of the normally thick joint fluid into thin fluid, irritation of the joint surface cartilage and irritation of the joint capsule. Once the fluid becomes thin, the joint surfaces are not as protected and they become irritated, causing yet more inflammation. The joint capsule reacts to this inflammation by developing synovitis, long finger-like villi on its surface that have a decreased ability to develop joint fluid.

This synovitis stops the joint capsule from replenishing its deteriorated joint fluid and adds to the inflammatory situation. Eventually the cartilage begins to erode. The body reacts by laying down more bone and the degeneration of the joint occurs.

Once the joint starts to develop bone, this type of arthritis is called 'osteo-arthritis' (from the Latin *osteo-* meaning 'bone' and *-itis* meaning 'inflammation'). This is a more serious type of arthritis that causes more severe lameness and requires more treatment. It can also end the career of some athletes. In the beginning the bone development is mild and appears as small spurs off the edges of the bones. As the disease progresses, the joint space begins to decrease and bone begins to fill in the joint until the whole joint fuses into one big wedge of bone. Once the joint fuses, the pain and lameness usually go away.

Young and old horses can be affected by arthritis and the causes vary. Initially, the inflammation of the joint is caused by some kind of trauma, either from a direct blow to the joint or from stress on the joint from work. Poor conformation, hard work, trauma and old age are some principal causes of arthritis. Racehorses tend to show more fore-limb arthritis, mainly in their carpi, and show horses to show more hock arthritis (spavin). Very young horses (even two to three years old) may have severe hock arthritis, either from being started at too young an age or being genetically prone to this problem.

Treatment: There are several treatments for arthritis and their use depends on the severity of the problem. All are aimed at stopping the cycle of inflammation and restoring the health of the joint fluid and joint-surface cartilage. Bute is given as an anti-inflammatory and pain-killer. Yucca, a herb, is a natural anti-inflammatory that is effective in mild forms of arthritis. Hyaluronic acid is the main component of joint fluid and is available in a synthetic form. It is often given intravenously for arthritis and is very effective as an anti-inflammatory, also helping to replenish the depleted joint fluid. It can also be injected directly into a joint.

Often, in more severe forms of arthritis, hyaluronic acid and anti-inflammatory steroids are injected into the joint. Adequan is a form of injectable polyaminoglycan, which is a major building block of cartilage that can be injected into the muscle. From there it is absorbed by the blood and taken to the joints where it helps the ailing cartilage. Adequan may also be injected into the joint with steroids. There are also feed supplements, chondrotin sulphates and glucosamine (also building blocks of cartilage), and while these are still not fully proven to be effective in the treatment of arthritis, many horses with mild forms appear to benefit from these supplements.

BONE SPAVIN

This is a form of osteo-arthritis of the hocks, where 'bone spurs' form on the edges of the bones making up the hock joint. Lameness often accompanies bone spavin. Treatment is as for arthritis – see page 112.

OSTEO-CHONDROSIS

Osteo-chondrosis (OCD) is a debilitating disease of the developing bone in youngsters. It is increasingly common, particularly amongst pure-bred horses bred for a specific purpose, e.g. Thoroughbreds, warm-bloods or heavy draft breeds.

OCD occurs when there is a defect in the conversion of cartilage to bone, a process that starts in the foetus and continues until maturity. Cartilage also covers bone in joints to allow ease of movement and OCD most commonly occurs in highly-mobile joints such as the shoulder, stifle, hock and fetlock. The affected cartilage separates from the bone, leaving it exposed. Movement causes fissures (tiny cracks) in both bone and cartilage and may lead to fragments breaking away. More joint fluid is produced, leading to swelling. Where defective cartilage collapses into the bone, cysts can occur in

weight-bearing areas. OCD in the growth plates of the long bones (e.g. cannon bones) is termed physitis.

Causes: Causes appear to include a genetic predisposition to the condition, nutritional imbalances (suggestions include excessive carbohydrates, calcium: phosphorus imbalance, insufficient copper, imbalance of trace elements or minerals). There is conflicting evidence as to whether an accelerated or interrupted growth rate is involved.

Signs: Although it appears during the first six months of life, signs may not show until later. The affected joint is usually swollen and the youngster is lame. The joint may be affected on one or both sides. Poor muscle development or odd-shaped hooves are secondary changes. X-rays will confirm diagnosis.

Treatment: In the early stages, correct nutrition and controlled exercise may manage the condition. Any detached fragments or flaps of bone can be removed by key-hole surgery. Most horses recover sufficiently to be worked, but prognosis depends on the seriousness and which joint is affected. Preventive measures include a considered choice of stallion, advice on a balanced diet for the pregnant mare and the foal (avoiding over-supplementation), plenty of natural exercise for mare and foal and careful observation of the foal to detect any signs at an early stage.

WINDGALLS AND BOG SPAVIN

Causes and signs: Trauma such as a fall, kick or severe concussion from heavy work can cause the joint to respond by producing more joint fluid and stretching the joint capsule, making the joint appear as if it has developed lumps around it. These are known as bog spavins in the hocks and as windgalls (or 'windpuffs') in the fetlock.

Treatment: Lameness rarely occurs, or if it does it is mild and is treated with rest and possibly anti-inflammatory drugs such as bute. Once the joint capsule is stretched it rarely shrinks back to its original shape. Therefore, even if the excess joint fluid is drained from the joint, the windgalls or bog spavins simply return once the joint capsule replenishes the joint fluid.

NAVICULAR DISEASE

Cause: Deterioration of the navicular bone from concussion and trauma. The navicular bone is located inside the hoof between the coffin joint and the deep flexor tendon. Its function is to keep a constant angle of attachment of the deep flexor tendon to the coffin bone, thus reducing the wear and tear on the flexor tendon. As a result of its location and function, the navicular bone is subject to tremendous forces from the flexor tendon and the bones of the coffin joint. As the horse bears weight on the leg, the deep flexor tendon is pulled taut, pushing up on the navicular bone which in turn is pressed up against the coffin bone and the short pastern bone, the bones that make up the coffin joint.

In the normal situation this is stressful on the navicular bone. Altered conditions of the hoof further increase the stresses on the navicular, causing deterioration of the surfaces and centre of the bone, inflammation of the navicular bursar, and adhesions between the navicular bone and the deep flexor tendon. Upright pastern conformation, small hooves compared to body size, broken-back pastern angles (see page 98), and concussion from jumping and sliding stops have been theorised to cause this disease. Some researchers believe that there may be an inherited component, either directly in the form of weak navicular bones or indirectly by poor conformation, creating the necessary predisposing factors. There has also been speculation on a lack of adequate blood supply to the bone itself creating deterioration from lack of oxygen (ischemic necrosis). Navicular disease is very prevalent in the American Quarter Horse but has also been seen in many other breeds.

Signs: The hallmark symptom of navicular disease is heel pain, located in the back third of the frog. All other symptoms revolve around this one singular constant. Initially, a horse may display intermittent front-limb lameness that resolves with rest but returns with exercise. Lameness is usually in both front limbs with one being more lame than the other, the lameness shifting back and forth between right and left legs or both legs being equally lame.

Horses with this problem typically have a stiff, short-strided, quick gait and land toe-first in an attempt to keep weight off the painful heel region. If both front legs are involved a true 'head bob' may not have been seen. Instead, these horses are uncomfortable to ride, feeling 'choppy', and often stumble.

The appearance of the hooves may be 'boxy', displaying contracted, high heels, and excessively worn-down toes. These horses are often positive to flexion tests (holding the coffin joint in flexion for one minute then jogging off, causing increased lameness if the area is painful).

Final diagnosis is usually determined by diagnostic

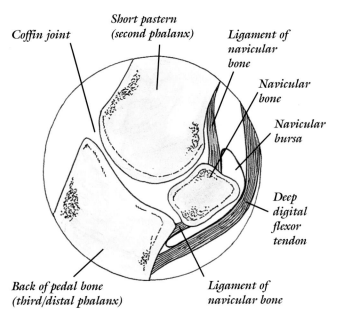

The important structures of the foot, showing in detail how closely they fit together at the rear of the foot. Poor lower limb and foot conformation, or bad shoeing, that results in over-long toes and collapsed heels, will increase pressure on the navicular bone, as the deep digital flexor tendon pushes the bone more tightly against the coffin joint.

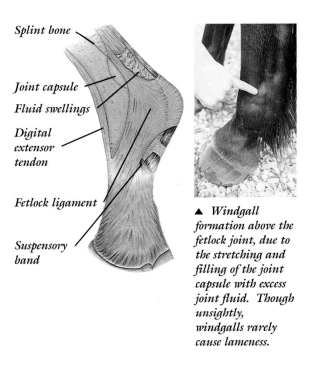

▲ *Windgall formation above the fetlock joint, due to the stretching and filling of the joint capsule with excess joint fluid. Though unsightly, windgalls rarely cause lameness.*

The formation of a tendinous windgall. A tendinous windgall is a distension of the flexor sheath surrounding the tendons as they run over the back of the fetlock. An articular windgall is a distension of the fetlock joint itself: the joint capsule fills with fluid, creating a swelling found between the cannon bone and suspensory ligament.

114

BONY AND SOFT TISSUE ENLARGEMENTS

Lumps, bumps or localised swellings on the legs are common, particularly in active horses. Some, though unsightly, do not cause lameness, although they may indicate past injury or disease or conformational weakness. Any new swelling should be investigated, particularly if there is heat and lameness present, as it may indicate injury or infection involving a joint, tendon or ligament.

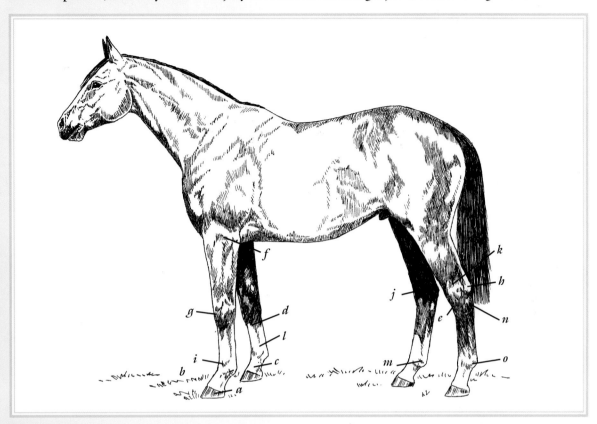

Bony enlargements can be caused by concussion or direct injury and are the result of ossification of cartilage or the production of excess bone in the trauma area.

a. sidebone
b. low ringbone
c. high ringbone
d. splint
e. bone spavin

Bursal enlargements are isolated, fluid-filled sacs that may occur naturally at potential pressure points, or as a result of enlargement of a tendon sheath by excess synovial fluid.

f. capped elbow
g. capped knee
h. capped hock
i. windgalls
j. bog spavin
k. thorough pin

Other swellings of soft tissue or joints could indicate a sprain, fracture, infection, arthritis or osteo-chondrosis and veterinary attention should be sought to investigate the cause. Damage to any of the tendons and ligaments of the lower leg will produce heat and swelling and should be regarded as serious.

l. sprained tendons
m. sprained suspensory ligament
n. curb
o. sesamoiditis

- **Curbs** are a sprain of the ligament running over the tendons at the back of the leg. They are almost always the result of faulty conformation.
- A **capped hock** is generally caused by management factors such as insufficient bedding. Although unsightly, this is not an unsoundness and does not affect performance.
- **Thoroughpins**, which are puffy areas through the hocks on the inside and outside, do not cause lameness but are considered blemishes.
- **Spavins**, on the inner, lower part of the hock, are an unsoundness. This may cause imperfect flexion of the hock, or make the animal drag its toe along the ground.

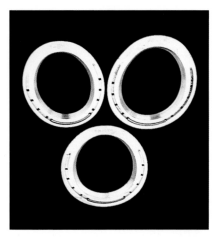

Aluminium egg-bar shoes: The egg-bar continues around the heels, giving added protection to the heel region, navicular bone and its associated structures.

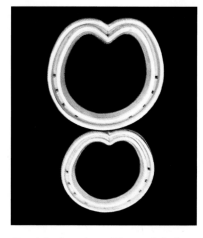

Straight-bar shoes: The straight-bar also enlarges the ground-bearing surface at the heels and enables the widest part of the frog to bear some weight. Protruding less far behind the foot than the egg-bar, it is less likely to be pulled off.

nerve blocks and radiographs (X-rays) of the navicular bone. Diagnostic nerve blocks of the heels (short-term local anaesthesia of the nerves that causes the area to become numb) resolves the lameness. Radiographs of the navicular bone reveal deterioration of the bone in the form of 'lollipop' lesions or increased vascular channels, decreased bone density, and holes in the centre of the bone.

Treatment: Once deterioration of the bone has occurred, there is no way to repair it. Instead all efforts are aimed at slowing down the process, reducing inflammation, increasing blood flow and relieving pain in the heel area. Initially this is achieved by therapeutic shoeing and medications. Shoeing traditionally consists of applying full bar or eggbar shoes, to give support to the heel area and improve distribution of the horse's weight. Also, used are pads to reduce concussion, dental impression in the caudal third of the frog to spread heels and increase circulation, occasionally wedge pads to elevate the heels and relieve stress on the deep flexor tendon, and finally shortening the toe to ease break-over.

Medications usually consists of phenylbutazone to relieve pain and decrease inflammation in the area. In more severe cases, the coffin joint may be treated with injections of cortical steroids and synthetic joint fluid (hyaluronic acid) to decrease inflammation and pain and replenish joint fluid damaged from inflammation. The navicular bursa (a fluid-filled sac between the navicular bone and the deep flexor tendon) can also be injected with coricosteroids in an attempt to halt destruction of the tissues. Oral medications such as isoxaprine and pentoxythiolline, thought to increase the blood-flow to the navicular area, have been used. Their efficacy is being questioned, but many swear by their use.

Management practices employed to help these horses have included turning them out on pasture, minimising indoor stabling, and altering their work-load, ideally by decreasing or stopping jumping work. Cutting the nerves to the heels has been a widely available and practised treatment, but many are now advising against this practice. Often the nerves grow back, and occasionally the lack of sensation of pain causes over-use of a damaged deep flexor tendon and navicular bone, resulting in a ruptured tendon or fractured navicular bone.

Overall treatment varies dramatically depending of the stage of the disease, geographical region, vet, farrier, and the horse itself. No one treatment seems to be the panacea, and every horse is different, calling for tailoring of the management and treatment accordingly.

SIDEBONE

Cause: Two lateral cartilages exist either side of the foot, encapsulated within the hoof. These are attached to the wings of the pedal bone and assist in the dissipation of energy created during weight-bearing. Certain types of conformation of the lower limb, such as a short, upright hoof-pastern axis, naturally create more concussion through the foot and limb. Over a period of time, this can cause the cartilage to ossify.

Signs: The natural elasticity of the cartilage is lost, compromising the internal structures of the foot during weight-bearing. The horse may not show lameness, however, or may have a short, pottery stride.

Treatment: Lameness can be treated with anti-inflammatories. Where a fragment of cartilage has broken off, this can be removed surgically.

PEDAL OSTITIS

Pedal ostitis describes inflammation of the periosteum covering the pedal bone. There continues to be debate within the veterinary profession as to whether this condition really does exist. What is in not in doubt is that the periosteal inflammation can be detected on an X-ray.

Causes: An increase in concussion over a long period of time.

Signs: Extreme cases will show acute lameness, generally in both front feet but sometimes in one foot only.

Treatment: Treatment is aimed at reducing concussion and attempting to make the foot more comfortable through the use of aluminium shoes. In severe cases aluminium eggbar shoes can be fitted.

CORONARY BAND INJURY

Injury to the coronary band should always be regarded as serious, as it can lead to complete separation of the horn tubules, eventually manifesting as a dorsal wall crack. Stabilisation at an early stage and fitting with an appropriate shoe will limit further damage.

CRACKS

The hoof capsule is subjected to enormous pressure during weight-bearing. If horn tubules are allowed to bend, superficial cracks (often termed 'sandcracks') will begin to appear in the dorsal wall of the hoof. If left untreated, these can culminate in a complete separation, leaving a deep crack that reaches down into the sensitive structures.

Causes: Poor foot conformation, leading to broken-back hoof-pastern axis (long toes and low, weak heels). Irregularly-shaped hooves or poorly-positioned limbs (e.g. toes in, or toes out) also predispose to cracking due to uneven weight distribution. Horn may also be weakened from lack of foot care, injury to the coronary band (see above) or excessive moisture loss.

Treatment: The cracks cannot be 'knit' together, but only healed in time by healthy horn growing down from the coronary band. Immobilisation of the crack is of paramount importance to prevent further damage. The foot can then be fitted with an appropriate shoe, such as a bar shoe, to improve weight-distribution. Regular washing with antibacterial solution is needed to ensure the crack does not become infected. Dietary supplements containing vitamin A, biotin and zinc will encourage strong new horn growth.

CORNS

Corns are bruised areas of the foot caused by the shoe putting pressure on the 'seat of corn' area, the angle where formed where the wall turns back to form the bars. There are two types: the dry corn and the wet, or superating corn. In the dry corn, the underlying blood vessels have been crushed and haemorrhaging occurs. A wet corn is active and can sometimes be infected.

Causes: Commonly due to the shoes being left on too long, or the horse being shod too close at the heel. Bruising can also be the result of treading on a sharp object, e.g. a stone.

Signs: Lameness, which will be severe if infection is present. Pain on pressure, particularly when turning.

Treatment: Anti-inflammatories and pain-reducing drugs, along with rest. Antibiotics are needed if there is infection. Careful attention should be given to the balance of the feet and the use of bar shoes considered, to give maximum protection.

INFECTION IN THE FOOT (PUS IN THE FOOT, PRICKED SOLE)

Infection can enter the foot through any wound, commonly either from a nail mistakenly driven into the sensitive tissue, or through a puncture wound to the sole or frog by a sharp object. The position of the wound is significant, as a deep puncture may involve the pedal or navicular bone.

Signs: Inflammation leads to intense pain, as the hoof wall restricts swelling. The horse will be reluctant to bear weight on the foot, there will be a strong digital pulse and heat in the foot. The lower limb may fill. Hoof testers can pinpoint the site of the infection, although finger pressure is often sufficient.

Treatment: Left untreated, infection in the foot will take the line of least resistance, travelling between the horn and sensitive structures of the foot up to the coronet. It should therefore always be considered a potentially serious injury. Immediate attention is needed from the vet or farrier to remove the shoe, pare the sole to open the abscess and remove infected tissue. Hot poulticing (see Chapter Two) for two or three days followed by tubbing in warm water is usually successful in drawing out the remaining pus, if drainage is sufficient. The vet will check the horse is immunised against tetanus and may give antibiotics. If the heel is affected, antibiotics are unlikely to be effective as the underlying digital cushion has a very limited blood supply.

5 LIFE SUPPORT SYSTEMS

THE HEART AND CIRCULATION

The circulatory system delivers oxygen and nutrients to the organs of the body and removes waste products for elimination by the kidneys, liver and lungs. The important components are the heart, great arteries (aorta and pulmonary artery), arterioles (small arteries), capillaries, venules, great veins and lymphatics (which drain fluid that accumulates between cells). The system is divided into two circuits that work in series, one supplying the body and the other supplying the lungs.

Effective circulation depends on the cardiac structure, electrical activation and mechanical function of the heart all being normal, and the distribution network of the circulatory system being regulated in an appropriate way.

THE CARDIOVASCULAR SYSTEM

The peripheral cardiovascular system has an essential role in the distribution of blood to supply the requirements of tissues and to remove waste products. Oxygen is carried on haemoglobin molecules in red blood cells. The blood also contains

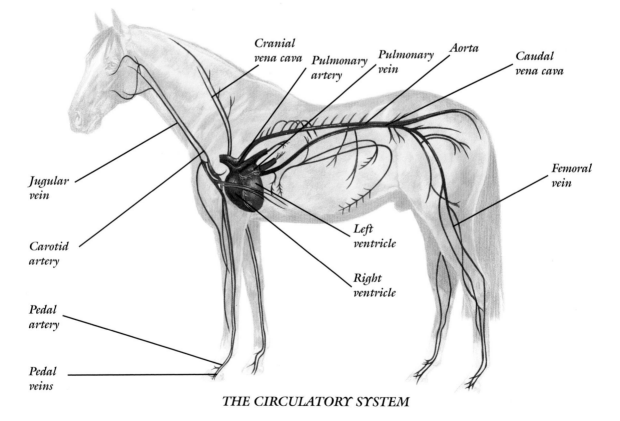

Cranial vena cava

Pulmonary artery

Pulmonary vein

Aorta

Caudal vena cava

Jugular vein

Femoral vein

Carotid artery

Left ventricle

Right ventricle

Pedal artery

Pedal veins

THE CIRCULATORY SYSTEM

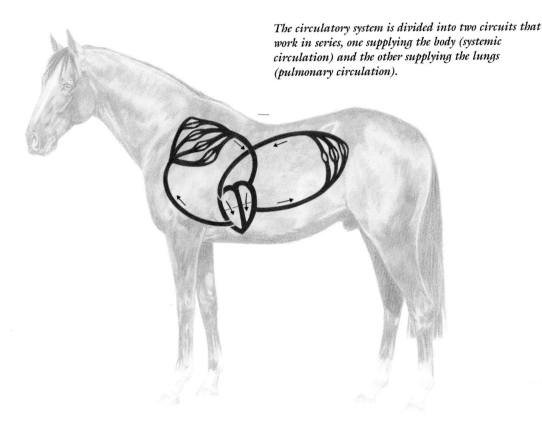

The circulatory system is divided into two circuits that work in series, one supplying the body (systemic circulation) and the other supplying the lungs (pulmonary circulation).

white blood cells to fight infection and platelets to help blood clot. Other waste products are carried on proteins, or dissolved in plasma.

The peripheral cardiovascular system is more than simple pipe-work; it controls the relative distribution of blood to different tissues in the body, according to demands.

The **aorta** is the main artery leading from the left ventricle (the main pump of the heart) to the body. It has a highly elastic wall, which stores the force of

contraction of the heart (systole) so that blood continues to be pumped around the circulation even when the heart is relaxing (diastole).

The **arterioles** are also elastic, but in addition they contain smooth muscle. Their diameter, and therefore the resistance they offer to blood flow, is controlled by the autonomic nervous system according to the demands of different organs (for example, to deliver blood to the gut for digestion or to muscles during exercise). The relative size of

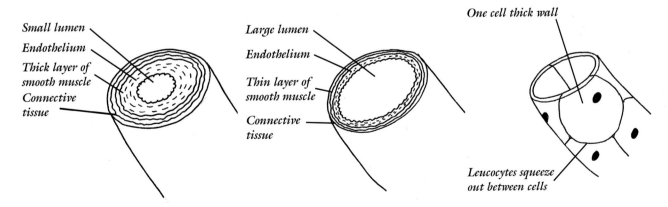

Section through an artery (left), a vein (centre) and a capillary (right)

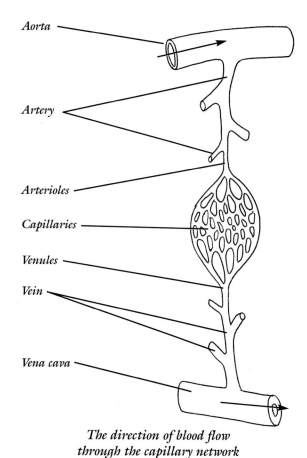

Aorta

Artery

Arterioles

Capillaries

Venules

Vein

Vena cava

The direction of blood flow
through the capillary network

circulation during exercise to increase oxygen-carrying capacity.

Blood pressure is maintained by heart output and the degree of contraction of the arteries and veins all co-ordinating in a regulated way.

The **lymphatic system** is responsible for returning excess fluid into the veins. This ensures that the fluid between and in the cells maintains the correct concentration of electrolytes and proteins.

THE HEART

The horse's heart is made up of three main structures: the *endocardium* (lining of the heart and the valves), *myocardium* (heart muscle) and *pericardium* (sac around the heart).

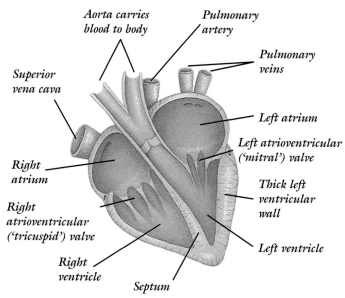

Aorta carries blood to body

Pulmonary artery

Pulmonary veins

Superior vena cava

Left atrium

Left atrioventricular ('mitral') valve

Right atrium

Thick left ventricular wall

Right atrioventricular ('tricuspid') valve

Left ventricle

Right ventricle

Septum

Vertical section through the heart

arterioles in different tissues controls the relative distribution of blood within the body.

The **capillaries** are where the exchange of nutrients and waste products takes place. A balance of pressures across the capillary wall controls the net flow of fluid and electrolytes (salts) into the space between the cells. Selective permeability of the capillary walls keeps some constituents of the blood in the circulation while allowing other molecules to pass through.

The **venules** collect blood from the capillaries and return it to the great veins. The majority of circulating blood volume is contained within the venules and veins; control of the tone of their walls plays an important role in maintaining blood pressure. When there is a demand for increased output from the heart, constriction of the venules maintains an adequate return of blood to allow cardiac output to increase.

The **veins** play a similar role to venules in control of blood pressure and circulating blood volume. The **spleen** also acts as a reservoir for blood, and can release a large number of red blood cells into the

MYOCARDIUM

The myocardium is surrounded by the epicardium and lined by endocardium. The bulk is made up of muscular fibres which contract when they are stimulated by an electrical signal. Some myocardial cells form a specialised electrical conduction system. When a heart cell is stimulated by an electrical impulse, a complex movement of ions, particularly calcium, results in contraction. A new electrical stimulation is required for each contraction so that the heart can relax between each contraction.

The heart is divided into four chambers: two atria which act as priming chambers, and two ventricles, which are the main pumps.

In the horse, the heart is positioned almost

vertically on the sternum, with the atria at the top. The cardiac chambers are adapted for maximum efficiency for the requirement of pumping blood through a high-pressure and a low-pressure circuit. The left ventricle drives blood around the body through the high-pressure, high-resistance 'systemic' circulation. It is constructed like a piston, forming a cylindrical chamber ideally suited to high-pressure pumping. The right ventricle has a large surface area in comparison to its volume and is more suited to low-pressure pumping. The right ventricle wraps around the front of the left ventricle and is responsible for pumping blood to the lungs.

The atria act as priming pumps, similar to a fuel injection-system for an engine. They store returning venous blood until it can empty into the ventricles, in early diastole. Blood returns to the right atrium from the caudal vena cava (which drains the rear half of the body), cranial vena cava (which drains the front half of the body), and the sinus venosus (which drains the heart).

Three pulmonary veins feed the left atrium with blood returning from the lungs. The atria have multiple folds, suiting them to their task of storing blood ready to fill the ventricles. They are relatively thin-walled because, in the normal heart, they pump against low pressure. The coronary arteries supply the heart muscle with blood.

ENDOCARDIUM

The chambers of the heart are lined with endocardium which is responsible for maintaining a smooth surface, free of blood clots. In addition, the endocardium forms the heart valves, which keep up one-way movement of blood through the heart chambers and prevent back-flow. Abnormalities of these valves may result in leaking (regurgitation) of blood, which reduces the efficiency of the heart. Such regurgitation is a very common abnormality in the horse. Valves can also be narrowed (stenosed), restricting outflow and increasing the workload on the chambers. However, this is very rare in horses.

Two types of valves are present in the heart. The atrioventricular (AV) valves divide the atria from the ventricles. They are supported by connective tissue fibres called the chordae tendineae and by the papillary muscles. The **chordae tendineae** act as guy ropes, anchored by papillary muscles, and these prevent the valve buckling backwards. Positioned between the ventricles and the great arteries, the semi-lunar valves have three leaflets.

PERICARDIUM

The pericardium is a fibrous sac which surrounds the heart and separates it from the lungs. Its function is mechanical; it acts as a barrier to infection and allows the heart to move freely within the thoracic cavity. It also limits the expansion of the ventricles, preventing expansion beyond their elastic limits.

HOW THE CARDIOVASCULAR SYSTEM WORKS

Movement of blood depends on pressure gradients between the chambers and the great vessels. These gradients are affected by disease, and changes in them are what cause signs of congestive heart failure. The speeding up and slowing down of blood during the cardiac cycle is responsible for the normal sounds we hear when listening to the heart (auscultation). Abnormal movement of the heart and blood within

Movement of blood through the circulatory system

1.
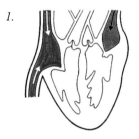

De-oxygenated blood flows via the vena cava into the right atrium from the head and body. The left atrium fills with oxygenated blood sent from the lungs via the pulmonary veins.

2.
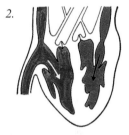

De-oxygenated blood is allowed through the tricuspid valve to fill the right ventricle. Oxygenated blood passes the mitral valve to fill the left ventricle.

3.
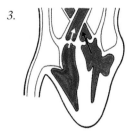

The de-oxygenated blood is pumped through the pulmonary valve (right semilunar valve) into the pulmonary artery.

4.
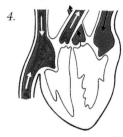

The de-oxygenated blood is sent to the lungs for re-oxygenation. The oxygenated blood is sent via the aorta to the head and body.

121

it can be detected as abnormal heart sounds and during examination, these may indicate the presence of cardiac disease.

THE CARDIAC CYCLE

Contraction and relaxation of the heart happens in a predictable cycle determined by electrical and mechanical events. The period during which the ventricles contract is known as systole. As pressure builds up, the semi-lunar valves open, and blood is ejected. Diastole is the period during which the filling of the ventricles occurs. At the end of systole, the semi-lunar valves shut, the ventricles relax, and the AV valves open allowing blood that has been stored in the atria to fill the ventricles.

In the resting horse, diastole is longer than systole. Late in diastole the atria contract and fill the ventricles as a 'pump-priming' action which increases the strength of ventricular contraction.

CONTROL OF THE CARDIOVASCULAR SYSTEM

Control of the working of the cardiovascular system is autonomic, that is, self-governing. The main aim is to maintain blood supply to vital organs, particularly the brain. This requires adequate blood pressure and all depends on adjusting the resistance of the arteries and veins and altering the output of the heart. In the longer term, blood pressure is controlled by adjusting blood volume, and this happens via a complex hormonal mechanism involving the brain, adrenal gland and kidney.

The rate and force of contraction of the heart is controlled by nerves from the cardiac centre in the medulla of the brain, and by the release of the hormones adrenaline and noradrenaline.

Information on blood pressure is fed to the brain from pressure receptors in the carotid arteries and heart, so that necessary adjustments can be made. For example, if a horse becomes excited or is exercised, the heart rate will increase so that more blood can be pumped to the muscles to allow activity. The horse has a remarkable capacity to increase the output of the heart by a factor of around six-fold from resting values. This is almost entirely due to an increase in heart rate from approximately 24-40 beats per minute, to a maximal heart rate of the order of 220-250 bpm.

Normal electrical activity, taking place via the specialised conduction pathway within the heart, results in co-ordinated contraction and relaxation. This is essential for the efficient working of the heart.

THE EFFECTS OF EXERCISE ON THE SYSTEM

In an athletic animal such as the horse, it is important to understand the effects of exercise on the cardiovascular system.

In humans and small animals, our main concerns with heart disease focus upon survival and quality of life. Signs are usually noticed only in those with moderate or severe disease. However, in the horse, clinical cardiology is principally concerned with how relatively minor cardiac disease can affect athletic performance.

Short-term effects of exercise

The short-term effects of exercise usually begin before the horse has even begun to trot. Excitement plays an important part in preparing the body to cope with the demands of exercise. The heart rate is raised and blood vessels to muscles dilate to deliver as much oxygen as possible. Blood is diverted from other organs, such as the gut, by constriction of local blood vessels.

Increased force of contraction of the heart and an increase in the amount of blood in the circulation allow the output of the heart for each beat (stroke volume) to increase. During exercise, skeletal muscle contraction, together with the marked negative pressure caused by the swinging of the huge bulk of the abdominal contents moving backwards and forwards during galloping, pump more blood back to the heart (see page 130).

The horse has a tremendous capacity to increase oxygen delivery to muscle, more than many other species, including man. The huge cardiac reserve is reflected by the low resting heart-rates in horses compared with animals of similar body size, such as cattle.

Long-term effects of fitness training and breeding

In the long term, exercise training leads to an increase in the heart muscle mass and the diameter of the ventricle, so that the heart pumps more blood per beat. The distribution of blood flow to skeletal muscles increases due to an increase in the number of blood vessels, and the skeletal muscle adapts to be able to extract more oxygen from blood.

Selective breeding has led to a difference in the oxygen-carrying capacity blood of the 'hot-blooded' breeds, which have a higher concentration of red blood cells (responsible for carrying oxygen) than ponies and heavy horses. Fit animals also appear to be able to move faster at the same maximal oxygen

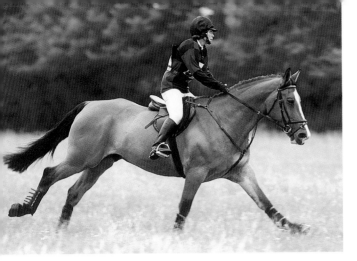

The force of the abdominal contents moving backwards and forwards as the horse gallops helps to pump more blood back into the heart, increasing the capacity to deliver more oxygen to the muscles.

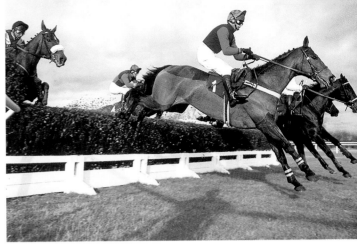

'Hot-blooded' breeds such as Thoroughbreds have a higher concentration of oxygen-carrying red blood cells than ponies and draft horses.

capacity. Athletic ability may also be related to an individual animal's capacity to tolerate increased levels of by-products such as lactic acid, which build up in the muscles during exercise and can affect anaerobic exercise capacity.

CLINICAL SIGNS OF HEART DISEASE

The first signs of heart disease largely depend on the use of the horse. In performance horses, poor performance is generally the first indication. These horses usually start work well but tire and take a longer time than normal to recover.

In general-purpose riding horses this phase may be missed and more profound signs may be the first to be noticed. In this case, the signs are those of congestive heart failure. Distension of the jugular veins, oedema fluid forming under the girth area, filling of the sheath in males and occasionally filling of the legs may be seen. Some horses will have an increased breathing rate, but coughing is very rarely associated with heart disease in horses.

The other circumstance in which heart disease is often first detected is when the horse is examined for some other reason, for example at a pre-purchase examination. This may come as a bolt from the blue for an owner, who may obviously be concerned by such a finding. Owners should rest assured that sudden death is a rare complication of heart disease in horses. Although a heart attack is often blamed for sudden death, this is usually unproven. No doubt some horses do die from a sudden, very irregular heart rhythm, but the vast majority of horses with heart murmurs will not suffer this fate. Only when they develop signs of heart failure is this a distinct possibility. The most commonly-proven cause of sudden death is rupture of a major internal artery.

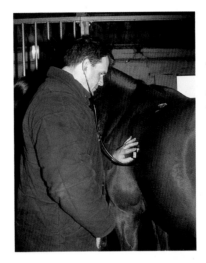

Auscultation (listening) with a stethoscope is the simplest form of investigation for heart problems, but one of the most difficult to interpret accurately.

INVESTIGATING HEART DISEASE IN HORSES

There are three main ways of investigating heart disease in horses.

The first and simplest in terms of equipment, but perhaps the most complicated in terms of potential findings, is **auscultation** (listening) using a stethoscope. At first sight this seems simple, and indeed, detection of heart rate and loud murmurs may be simple, but assigning significance to the findings can be difficult. Quiet murmurs can be difficult to hear, especially in a noisy environment. Murmurs are especially difficult to detect at high heart rates or in windy conditions, such as after exercise in a horse during a pre-purchase examination (see below).

An **ECG** (electrocardiogram) is a method of recording the rhythm of the heart and is invaluable in identifying irregularities in the heart rhythm which can be very significant. Unfortunately, ECGs tell us very little, if anything, about heart size in the horse, unlike the situation in humans and dogs. Over the years, a lot has been read into ECGs with little proven validity. The concept of 'heart score' was

123

pioneered in Australia and is still used in the southern hemisphere. It assumes a connection between the length of a complex on the ECG and heart size, and between heart size and athletic capacity and potential. It is now largely discredited. The diagnosis of heart strain from altered T-waves on the ECG in horses is also unreliable, and in fact there was never any evidence of what 'heart strain' was.

A useful form of ECG recording is radiotelemetry. With this technique the ECG is transmitted from a small box to a base unit, and the ECG can be recorded while the horse is lunged or ridden. For horses with intermittent irregularities, an ECG can be recorded over a 24-hour period to try to detect the irregularity.

Echocardiography (ultrasound of the heart) is a technique which has revolutionised our understanding of heart disease in horses and transformed the accuracy of judgements of its severity. It is particularly useful for assessing the clinical significance of cardiac murmurs.

Echocardiography allows the structure of the heart to be assessed, so that gross abnormalities, such as a ventricular septal defect, can be detected. Unfortunately, lesions seen are often subtle. Assessment of the motion of the valves and walls of the ventricles can also give useful information about valvular and myocardial function. An echocardiogram is particularly valuable for assessing the effects of the disease by measuring changes in the chamber size compared with normal animals. We therefore have to rely largely on accurate measurement and comparison of the results to a suitable normal range. Repeated measurements in the same individual are useful for monitoring the progression of disease and guiding the prognosis.

Doppler echocardiography is a technique which is used to measure the direction and velocity of blood flow. It can be used to detect abnormal jets of blood within the heart and great arteries, such as those associated with valvular disease or congenital defects such as holes in the heart.

CONDITIONS OF THE CARDIOVASCULAR SYSTEM

MURMURS

A 'murmur' is an abnormal sound caused by vibrations from turbulent blood flow. It is detected when listening to the heart with a stethoscope.

Murmurs are characterised by their intensity (loudness), which is usually graded from 1 to 6 over 6; their timing (part, or all, of systole or diastole); the change in intensity during the murmur (e.g. getting gradually louder or quieter); and by the place at which they are loudest.

NORMAL MURMURS

Around 60 per cent of normal horses have a heart murmur. In the vast majority this is quiet and may be missed without careful auscultation. Normal heart murmurs are called 'flow murmurs' and are present in horses because they have such a large volume of blood flowing rapidly into the large aorta and pulmonary artery. Most often they are heard at rest and are less apparent after exercise; however, they can be louder after exercise, so the commonly used rule of thumb that murmurs which disappear after exercise are insignificant is actually a poor guide.

ABNORMAL MURMURS

Abnormal murmurs can be caused by:

Valve disease: This is caused by a degenerative disease with no known cause. There is no evidence to suggest it is due to over-work or respiratory disease. Severe cases result in the leakage (regurgitation) of blood. Any valve may be affected, but in general either mitral, triscuspid or aortic regurgitation is involved – pulmonary regurgitation is rarely severe enough to be detected. Nothing can affect the rate of progression. In particular, it makes no difference whether the horse is worked hard or rested.

Anaemia: In the author's opinion this is over-diagnosed, as anaemia needs to be severe before there is a murmur (see page 126).

Congenital heart disease: Many foals have murmurs at birth, and in the vast majority this is not a cause for concern. In the first few hours of life the *ductus arteriosus*, which diverts blood away from the lung when the foal is in the uterus, closes off, but a murmur results from the limited flow through it until it seals off completely after a few hours or days.

A few horses are born with a deformed heart. The most common defect is a 'hole in the heart', which allows blood to flow from the high-pressure left ventricle into the low-pressure right ventricle, diverting it from going round the body. Although this is inefficient, often no signs are seen until the horse is two or three years old or more (holes have been detected for the first time in horses as old as 14 years). Horses with this condition are unlikely to be suitable for hard work and are unsuitable for breeding.

ASSESSING THE SIGNIFICANCE OF MURMURS

The significance of a leaking heart valve depends largely on the amount of blood that is leaking. The heart may have to pump an increased load to compensate, but up to a certain level copes well. However, there will come a point at which the output can no longer meet the demands put on it. This will be most marked during exercise, when up to six times the normal output may be required. Signs of heart disease are therefore most likely to be noticed during exercise, primarily as slowing down and tiring. Or the horse may take longer to recover from exercise.

For this reason it is important that when a murmur is detected it is thoroughly investigated to determine its significance.

However, heart murmurs seldom affect a horse's safety for riding. They do not cause sudden death or collapse unless they are very severe, or something suddenly occurs, such as the tearing of a diseased valve or the supporting structures, or a sudden irregularity in the heart rhythm.

Heart 'attacks' are in all probability nowhere near as common as we are led to believe. The owner of a horse with a heart murmur does not need to stop riding their horse, provided that the cause and severity has been examined by their vet or a qualified veterinary cardiologist.

ENDOCARDITIS

Endocarditis is an infection of a heart valve. It is a rare but life-threatening disease.

In some cases the horse is known to have had an infection of some sort, and subsequently develops weight loss, often a fever, and usually a murmur (commonly involving the aortic valve).

The infection proceeds both by destroying the valve, leading to reduced cardiac efficiency or heart failure, and by giving the horse a general illness that affects the whole body.

Endocarditis must be diagnosed early and treated aggressively if there is to be any chance of recovery. An ultrasound scan usually diagnoses the condition and gives an indication of the severity of the damage to the valves.

If this is very severe, the horse would be euthanased. If there is little damage, aggressive long-term treatment with antibiotics can bring about a cure. However, this may require extremely costly drugs over a long (4-8 week) period, without any guarantee of success, so treatment should not be undertaken lightly.

ABNORMAL HEART RHYTHMS (ARRHYTHMIAS)

Assessment of the rhythm of the heart is very important. As with murmurs, however, this is made difficult by the common presence in horses of irregularities which are normal. The crucial thing is, therefore, to distinguish the 'normal' from the 'abnormal'. Although the most significant types of irregularity can usually be diagnosed on auscultation, an ECG recording may be needed for confirmation. Common arrhythmias include:

- **Second degree atrio-ventricular block**
  Also known as a 'blocked', 'missed' or 'dropped' beat – a 'b-lub' sound only is heard, rather than a 'b-lub-dup'. This affects around 20 per cent of all horses and is of no clinical significance except in exceptional circumstances.

- **Atrial fibrillation (AF)**
  This is the most common arrhythmia affecting performance. The atria contract with a series of flutters and the ventricle contract irregulary, reducing the efficiency of the heart. Commonly found in horses without underlying heart disease, but can also occur with dilation of the atria due to valve disease. It is uncommon in horses under 15hh. Unlike most other heart conditions in horses, some cases where there is no underlying heart disease can be cured by drug treatment (quinidine sulphate), although this treatment is not without risk. Where AF is likely to have been present for some time and the horse is performing satisfactorily at a low work level, no action may be necessary and, in the author's opinion, there is no increased risk of collapse. It is when the condition is accompanied by significant heart disease and the horse is asked to work hard when it is tired, that a risk develops. The first sign of compromise due to the condition and/or the underlying disease is likely to be tiring.

Atrial fibrillation can occur for a short period before normal rhythm returns, without treatment, within 24 hours. Called 'paroxysmal' AF, this usually occurs during exercise and causes a significant reduction in performance. It can be difficult to diagnose because the horse is often normal by the time it is examined, but usually no treatment is needed.

- **Premature beats**
  Can originate from the atria and associated tissue or the ventricles themselves. Occur uncommonly in normal animals, but may indicate underlying

heart disease or other abnormality having a secondary effect on the heart (e.g. colic or electrolyte imbalance). If frequent, the horse should not be ridden, as performance may be reduced, and under some circumstances collapse would be possible. Often the cause is not found, although anecdotal evidence has suggested a link with recent respiratory disease. Rest usually resolves the premature beat within a few months, or steroid treatment may be successful. Where there is known disease outside the heart, the underlying condition should be treated. The long-term prognosis is very variable and usually impossible to predict at the outset.

Dangerously fast, irregular heart rhythms are fortunately relatively rare in horses compared to other species. Most often there will be a severe accompanying disease such as a surgical colic, when treatment is given to slow the heart rate and return it to a regular rhythm. A primary cardiac defect is only responsible in very few cases and the horse should be referred to a specialist cardiologist.

BREEDING AND HEART DISEASE
Animals with congenital heart disease should not be used for breeding purposes because it is possible that these conditions have a hereditary element. At present, there is no evidence that acquired valvular or myocardial disease has a hereditary basis in the horse. Horses with moderate or severe cardiac disease are often used for breeding and may continue to be useful for some years after the identification of the problem.

BLOOD TESTING
Disease, stress and electrolyte imbalances all cause changes to the normal parameters of the constituents of the blood. These can be identified and analysed from a blood sample. Performance horses are routinely blood-tested to monitor health and fitness. More generally, a blood sample may be taken as an aid to diagnosing a particular health problem.

ANAEMIA
Anaemia refers to reduced levels of the oxygen-carrying protein haemoglobin in the red blood cells. It is not a disease in itself, but a symptom of disease. A healthy horse has a red blood cell count of 7-8 million per cubic mm and a haemoglobin level of 14g per 100mls. If these levels drop to 3-6 million/8-12g, the horse is said to be anaemic.
Causes:
• Stress or over-work can depress production and increase fragility of red blood cells
• Excessive bleeding (internal or external) after traumatic injury, or rupturing of the wall of blood vessels due to parasitic damage
• Deficiency of iron, copper or cobalt in diet
• Increased destruction of red blood cells from infection by bacteria, virus or toxins.
Signs:
• Pale gums and mucous membranes
• Weakness and lethargy
• Loss of appetite and condition
• Poor, dull coat
• Increased rate and force of heart beat.
Treatment and prevention: Good nutrition (including a vitamin and mineral supplement for susceptible horses) and a correct worming programme should avoid anaemia. Blood-testing will give an accurate diagnosis. Iron and vitamin B12 supplements can be given, or iron injections if levels are very low. If internal blood loss is suspected, get immediate veterinary attention. External bleeding should be controlled as far as possible by direct pressure (see

HEART PROBLEMS & PRE-PURCHASE EXAMINATIONS
Cardiac murmurs and arrhythmias are frequently detected at a pre-purchase examination (PPE) and may be a cause of concern. The problem is that murmurs and arrhythmias may be due to normal or to pathological changes that commonly occur in normal horses, and may be of no clinical significance. As normal features it is perfectly acceptable to make no comment on them in a report.

The first task is therefore to distinguish physiological and functional murmurs and arrhythmias from those which indicate the presence of abnormality. If abnormalities are detected, the vet must give the owner some indication of the significance of the findings, not just at that time, but also in the foreseeable future for that horse, for the specific purpose for which it is intended.
Further diagnostic aids may be appropriate to help quantify the risk of disease.

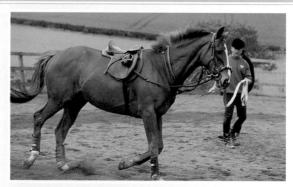

Energetic exercising that forms part of the pre-purchasing examination aims to expose any abnormalities in the functioning of the heart. Assessing the significance of irregularities is very difficult, however.

Chapter Two) and the vet called. Rest is crucial to recovery.

DISORDERS OF THE LYMPHATIC SYSTEM

FILLED LEGS/LYMPHANGITIS

If the water balance between the circulatory system and the tissue is upset, excess water can build up in the lymphatic system. This is particularly noticeable in the lower legs, where gravity creates the greatest pressure in the blood vessels.

Causes: Usually the result of a combination of too little exercise and too much feed, upsetting the delicate protein/blood salt balance. There may be a connection with a high-protein diet. Damage and inflammation of the vessel walls from toxins, allergy or infection may also be implicated.

Signs: Filled, swollen legs – particularly the hind limbs. May be warm to the touch. Swelling may subside with exercise, but in true lymphangitis this can be permanent, with the horse showing lameness. Hot abscesses may rupture the skin of the lower legs.

Treatment and prevention: Correct nutrition for the individual and its work-load, and sufficient regular exercise, should avoid problems. Massage and the application of stable bandages will help reduce swelling. Seek veterinary attention for lymphangitis.

THE RESPIRATORY SYSTEM

THE FUNCTION OF THE RESPIRATORY SYSTEM

A healthy and functional respiratory system is required by all horses. It is a necessity of life. The respiratory system brings air into close relationship with the mixed venous blood in the lungs, enabling gas exchange to take place. Gas exchange is the major function of the lung, which ensures the transport of oxygen (O_2) from the air into the blood and of carbon dioxide (CO_2) in the reverse direction. The intimate contact between inspired air, with the multiplicity of organisms, particles and gases it contains, and the internal lining of the lungs (with a surface area some three times that of the body) leads to efficient gas exchange. It also, however, creates

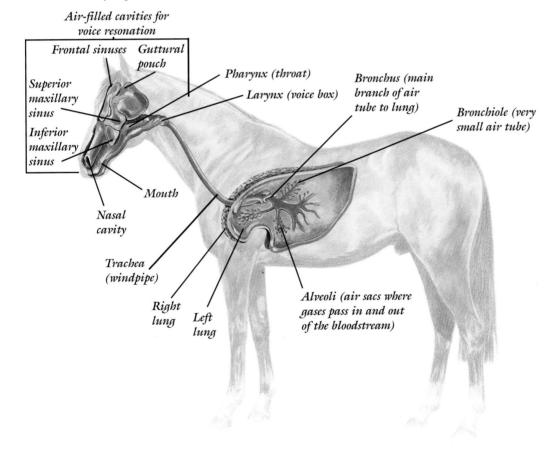

Air-filled cavities for voice resonation

Frontal sinuses   Guttural pouch

Superior maxillary sinus

Inferior maxillary sinus

Pharynx (throat)

Larynx (voice box)

Bronchus (main branch of air tube to lung)

Bronchiole (very small air tube)

Mouth

Nasal cavity

Trachea (windpipe)

Right lung   Left lung

Alveoli (air sacs where gases pass in and out of the bloodstream)

THE RESPIRATORY SYSTEM

repeated opportunities for damage to the lungs and for absorption into the body of harmful substances.

Virtually all processes in the body require O_2. Many of these processes produce a waste gas, CO_2, which needs to be removed from the body. A functional respiratory system is, therefore, essential for all horses, including those at rest. During exercise the demands for increased respiration rise dramatically. If the O_2 supply to the working muscles should reduce, then the muscles will be unable to burn sufficient sugar to provide the necessary energy, and fatigue or exercise intolerance results.

Research carried out over the last 20 years in exercising horses has provided strong evidence that the respiratory system is commonly a limiting factor for maximal performance, even in healthy animals. Therefore, any respiratory disease, even mild or sub-clinical, may significantly impair the exercise tolerance of the horse.

STRUCTURE OF THE EQUINE RESPIRATORY TRACT

The respiratory system may be divided into the upper and lower respiratory tracts. The upper respiratory tract includes the nostrils, nasal cavities, pharynx, larynx and trachea. The lower respiratory tract includes the bronchi and lungs. The lungs fill a cavity in the chest known as the pleural cavity or thoracic cavity.

Nostrils: The equine nostrils are large and mobile. Activation of muscles around the nostrils during exercise results in flaring (widening) of the nostrils which aids increased airflow.

Nasal cavities: The paired nasal cavities contain an intricately-folded surface (the turbinates) with a very rich blood supply. The large surface area within the nasal cavities is important for heat and water exchange.

Para-nasal sinuses: There are five paired para-nasal sinuses (frontal, sphenopalatine, ethmoidal, caudal maxillary and rostral maxillary). These are air spaces within the skull bones and all connect with the nasal cavities via small drainage holes.

Pharynx: The soft palate divides the pharynx into the naso-pharynx and oro-pharynx. The walls of the pharynx are soft and flexible and tend to collapse during inspiration due to negative pressures in the upper airways during this phase of respiration. This

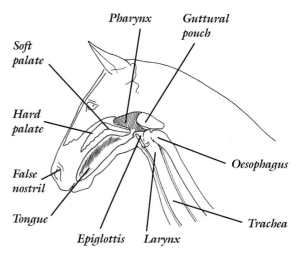

THE UPPER RESPIRATORY TRACT

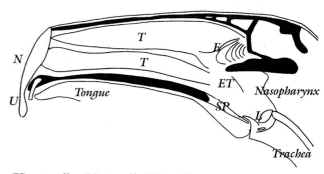

(U) upper lip, (N) nostrils, (T) turbinates, (E) ethoturbinates, (ET) opening to the Eustachian tube, (SP) soft palate, (L) larynx

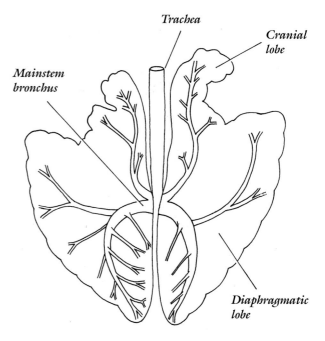

THE LUNGS AND LOWER RESPIRATORY TRACT

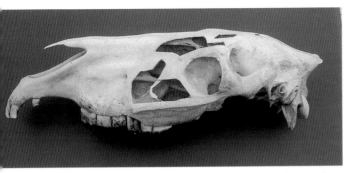

The skull with superficial bone removed to reveal the major paranasal sinuses.

tendency is limited by active muscular contraction in the walls.

The **Eustachian tubes** open into the naso-pharynx via slit-like openings on either side of the pharyngeal walls. The horse is unique in possessing a large out-pouching of each Eustachian tube, the **guttural pouches**. The function of the guttural pouches is unknown, but within their walls are some major blood vessels (including the internal carotid artery) and nerves. Diseases of the guttural pouches which result in damage to one or more of these structures may have severe, and sometimes life-threatening, consequences.

Another important structural peculiarity of the equine upper airway is the intra-pharyngeal ostium, an opening in the posterior part of the soft palate through which the larynx normally sits, rather like a button through a button-hole (see diagram, below). The larynx is thus fixed into the naso-pharynx by an airtight seal, which means that the horse can only breathe in and out through the nose. It is unable, under normal circumstances, to breathe through the mouth. The larynx normally only becomes 'unbuttoned' from the soft palate during swallowing;

when the horse has finished swallowing, the larynx normally returns immediately to its usual 'buttoned-up' position.

Larynx: The larynx is a valve-like structure that guards the opening to the trachea. It consists of several cartilage plates jointed together. The airway through the larynx (the glottis) can open or close by the action of various muscles attaching to these cartilages. During exercise the glottis will open widely to increase the diameter of the airway and help the large flow of air in and out of the lungs. During swallowing, on the other hand, the glottis will close, thereby preventing the accidental passage of food material into the trachea.

Trachea: The trachea, or windpipe, is a single tube, 70 to 80 cm long, that conducts air from the upper airways to the bronchi. The tube is supported by 50 to 60 cartilage rings in its wall.

Bronchi: At the end of the trachea, the airway divides into two (the right and left principal bronchi), which enter the right and left lungs. The bronchi continue to divide, rather like the branches of a tree, as they spread throughout the lungs. These airways become smaller and smaller at each division and the rigidity of their walls becomes less and less as they get smaller. The larger airways (bronchi) have cartilage plates in their walls, whereas the small airways (bronchioles) lack any cartilage support. The airways also have muscle in their walls, which controls their calibre, and which plays an important role in some diseases such as Chronic Obstructive Pulmonary Disease (COPD).

Mucus is constantly being produced in the bronchi and bronchioles. This is normally rapidly cleared and propelled back up the bronchial tree and trachea by

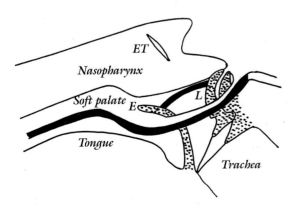

(E) epiglottis, (ET) Eustachian tube (L) opening of larynx
The normal arrangement of the larynx and soft palate. The larynx sits in the opening of the soft palate, like a button through a button-hole.

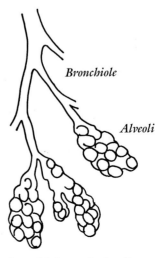

The bronchioles and alveoli

millions of tiny beating hair-like structures (cilia) on the surface cells lining these airways. When mucus is propelled as far back as the pharynx it is normally swallowed. This mucus blanket is an important defence mechanism in the airways, trapping and removing dust and other particles breathed in with the inspired air.

Lungs: From the final divisions of the bronchial tree (the bronchioles), tiny air sacs (alveoli) protrude, rather like a bunch of grapes on a stalk. The lining of these air sacs is extremely thin and a very rich network of blood capillaries passes through them. This is where gas exchange takes place. The ultra-fine membrane between the air and the blood allows for the rapid diffusion of O_2 from the inspired air to the blood, and of CO_2 from the blood to the air which is then exhaled.

The horse's lung is a large, well-developed organ. It weighs only about 1 per cent of the total body weight yet contains in the region of 10 million alveoli. The alveolar surface area is very large and the alveolar walls are thin compared with other mammals.

Thoracic cavity: The thoracic cavity, in which the lungs sit, is roughly pyramidal in shape. Its base is formed by the diaphragm, the roof by the thoracic vertebrae and muscles, and the walls by the ribs and intercostal muscles. The floor is formed by the sternum.

Respiratory muscles: In the resting animal, inspiration is an active process brought about by the action of various muscles (most importantly the diaphragm) which expand the size of the thoracic cavity, thereby forcing air to be drawn into the airways and lungs. Expiration is mainly a passive process, brought about by the elastic recoil of the lungs and thoracic wall, which reduces the size of the thoracic cavity thereby squeezing air out of the lungs. Various muscles (most importantly the abdominal muscles) may be recruited to aid expiration if needed (for example, during exercise or in some diseases).

RESPIRATION DURING EXERCISE

During exercise, the demand for oxygen by the muscles increases and the respiratory rate increases in order to supply this. The O_2 levels in the blood are thus maintained at a steady level. During strenuous exercise, however, the respiratory rate of the horse fails to increase sufficiently and the blood O_2 levels start to fall. This phenomenon seems to be unique to the horse and is not seen in other species such as man.

One reason why this phenomenon occurs in the horse is the locomotion-respiration coupling that occurs during galloping and limits how high the respiratory rate can reach. At the canter and gallop, respiration and locomotion are linked such that one inspiration-expiration cycle occurs for every locomotion cycle; the horse breathes out as the leading fore-leg hits the ground. The respiratory rate is therefore controlled and limited by the locomotion rate.

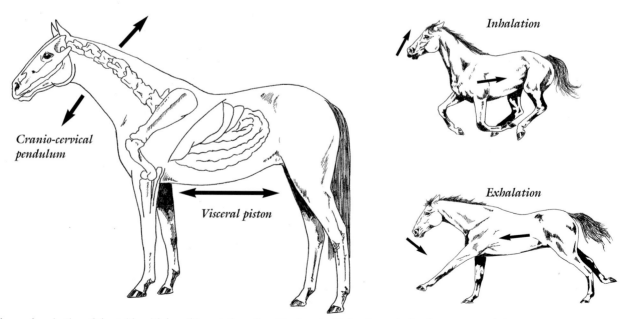

Cranio-cervical pendulum

Visceral piston

Inhalation

Exhalation

The synchronisation of the stride with breathing at the gallop. During the flight phase, the head comes up and the gut moves back, allowing the horse to inhale, filling its lungs. As the forelegs reach the ground the weight of the guts within the abdomen swings forward, and the horse exhales and empties its lungs.

DISEASES & DISORDERS OF THE RESPIRATORY SYSTEM

The horse can be affected by a diverse range of diseases affecting the respiratory system. These include infections, parasitic and allergic diseases. Neurological and structural disorders that result in functional obstruction of the airways are particularly important in performance horses, such as racehorses and eventers, because they can have a profound effect on exercise tolerance and athletic ability.

CLINICAL SIGNS OF RESPIRATORY DISEASE

Cough: Many diseases of the respiratory tract cause coughing. This is a reflex defence mechanism which is initiated by the presence of foreign material or excessive secretions in the larynx, trachea or bronchi. A cough consists of three phases: a deep inspiration, forced expiration against a closed glottis and then an explosive respiratory blast due to sudden opening of the glottis.

Coughing is seen in many infectious and allergic respiratory diseases. In upper airway infections, such as influenza, the cough often appears to be harsh, dry and painful, whereas in lower airway diseases, such as COPD, the cough tends to be moist and deeper.

Nasal discharge: A nasal discharge most commonly arises from excessive mucus production present in infectious and allergic diseases. When the discharge originates from the lower respiratory tract, it will usually be seen as a bilateral nasal discharge (that is, it is present at both nostrils). If it originates from a site in one nasal cavity or from the para-nasal sinuses, it will tend to appear at one nostril only (unilateral). Some diseases may result in other types of nasal discharge, such as pus (for example, in strangles), blood (in guttural pouch mycosis) or food (in diseases that impair swallowing).

Respiratory distress or difficult breathing (dyspnoea): Respiratory distress at rest may occur in cases of severe upper airway obstruction (e.g. strangles) or with widespread disease affecting the small airways in the lung (e.g. COPD and pneumonia). Upper airway obstruction generally results in inspiratory dyspnoea (difficulty breathing in), whereas small airway disease usually results in expiratory dyspnoea (difficulty breathing out). A number of upper airway obstructions may only manifest at fast exercise (e.g. recurrent laryngeal

neuropathy), and in such cases the airway obstruction may cause an abnormal inspiratory noise (e.g. roaring).

Exercise intolerance: Virtually any disease of the respiratory tract that interferes with air flow or gas exchange can cause exercise intolerance. Some upper airway obstructions occur suddenly during exercise and result in an abrupt onset of exercise intolerance. Many other diseases will affect exercise tolerance throughout the period of exercise resulting in a gradual onset of fatigue.

INFECTIOUS DISEASES

EQUINE INFLUENZA
There are two distinct subtypes of equine influenza virus: A/equine/1 and A/equine/2. Influenza is a major and economically important cause of acute respiratory disease throughout the world. In North America and some parts of Europe, the virus is constantly present. Horses of all ages are susceptible, but infection is commonest in young (2-3 years) unvaccinated horses. Infection may occur in vaccinated horses, although the severity of clinical disease and degree of viral shedding are reduced.
Cause: Viral infection.
Signs: Large amounts of virus are aerosolised from affected horses due to frequent coughing. The incubation period is short (one to three days) and horses are contagious for up to 10 days. Outbreaks

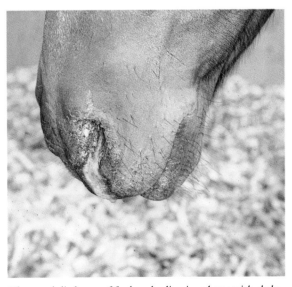

The nasal discharge of food and saliva in a horse with choke (obstruction of the oesophagus) differs from other types associated with the respiratory tract.

131

are most common when large numbers of young susceptible horses are brought together at sales and shows, or for weaning and training.

In individual horses the clinical signs include:
- cough (harsh and dry; sudden onset)
- fever (up to 107 F, 41.7 C)
- lethargy
- inappetence
- enlargement and tenderness of sub-mandibular lymph nodes
- watery bilateral nasal discharge (becoming thicker with secondary bacterial infections).

In uncomplicated cases, recovery occurs in one to three weeks. In some cases, secondary bacterial infection of the lower respiratory tract may lead to bronchopneumonia. In partially immune or vaccinated horses, the clinical signs are usually mild or the infection may be sub-clinical. Performance horses may demonstrate only exercise intolerance.

Treatment:
- Complete rest for minimum of 3-4 weeks in clean, dust-free environment
- General nursing care and provision of palatable food
- Antibiotic treatment is necessary only if there is significant secondary bacterial infection.
- Non-steroidal anti-inflammatory drugs such as phenylbutazone and banamine are helpful in horses with high fever, depression or muscle stiffness.

Prevention and control:
- Isolate new arrivals for three weeks
- Maintain adequate ventilation rates for all stabled horses, especially in barns
- Routine vaccination. Most vaccines require two primary doses three to six weeks apart, followed by a booster dose six months later, and thereafter annually (or more frequently for high-risk horses). See Chapter Two.
- Isolate infected horses as soon as possible (as soon as a temperature rise is identified).
- Provide adequate ventilation and dust-free conditions.
- Avoid all contact between healthy and sick horses.
- Cease exercise/training to minimise stress.
- Maintain separate feeding, cleaning and grooming equipment and personnel for sick horses.
- Quarantine the premises.
- Vaccinate healthy horses in the face of the outbreak.

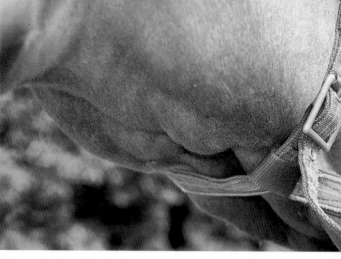

Enlarged submandibular lymph glands in a horse infected by flu.

EQUINE HERPES

Cause: Two viruses, EHV1 and 4, are associated with serious clinical disease in horses.

Signs: EHV1 infection is associated with respiratory disease, abortion, neonatal disease and neurological disease. The virus has a world-wide distribution.

The incubation period is 2 to 10 days. Respiratory disease is commonest in young horses (up to three years). Older horses usually show mild or sub-clinical respiratory disease. Immunity following infection or vaccination is short-lived and horses may become re-infected on numerous occasions throughout their lives.

Clinical signs include:
- fever (up to 106 F, 41.1C)
- watery nasal discharge (which becomes thicker later)
- coughing
- depression
- enlargement of sub-mandibular lymph nodes.

Uncomplicated cases recover in 8 to 10 days. Secondary bacterial infections may prolong the course of the disease. Older horses show milder or sub-clinical disease; this may be associated with exercise intolerance or low-grade lower airway inflammation.

Abortion, neurological disease and disease of new-born foals are rare complications of EHV1 infections. Abortion usually occurs in late gestation (7 to 11 months). The initial respiratory infection is often sub-clinical. Abortions may be sporadic or multiple (abortion 'storms'). Foals infected in the uterus may be affected by severe respiratory disease and are born ill and weak, dying within a few days. Alternatively, foals may appear normal at birth, but develop severe illness after a few days.

Neurological disease may occur in association with or in the absence of respiratory disease or abortion. Any age group may be affected. Single, isolated cases or outbreaks may occur. Clinical signs vary in severity, but usually include weakness and incoordination of the hind legs, which may progress to recumbency. Non-recumbent horses usually recover, but full neurological function may not return for several months.

EHV 4 causes respiratory disease indistinguishable from EHV 1. EHV 4 has also been linked with sporadic abortions but has not been associated with abortion 'storms'. It is not generally linked with neonatal disease or neurological disease.

Treatment:
Respiratory disease
• rest
• antibiotics as necessary to control secondary bacterial infections
Abortion
• none
Neonatal disease
• antibiotics
• general nursing and respiratory care
Neurological disease
• general nursing care
• treatment of recumbent horses is difficult and many cases require euthanasia due to complications of muscle damage, skin damage, pneumonia etc.

Prevention and control:
• Isolate incoming horses for two to three weeks.
• Age segregation of horses.
• Pregnant mares should be separated from young stock and ideally kept in small groups according to the gestational stage.
• Horses showing clinical respiratory disease should be isolated.
• Personnel handling infected horses should be isolated from healthy stock.
• Bedding of infected horses should be burned.
• Contaminated stable equipment/clothing should be disinfected.
• Aborting mares should be kept and managed in isolation. The foetus and membranes are potential sources of infection and must be handled and disposed of carefully.
• In cases of abortion, all mares due to foal in the same season should remain on the farm until they have foaled. Horses that leave the farm should not be allowed contact with pregnant mares.
• In cases of neurological disease, infected horses should be isolated, and all horses on the premises should be confined until three weeks after the identification of the last new case.
• Vaccination. EHV 1 and 4 vaccines are available but provide only partial and short-

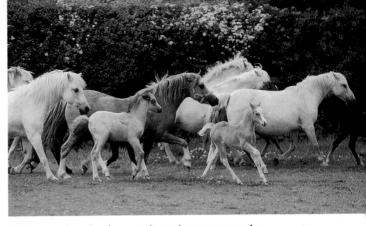

Studs must have in place a strict regime to prevent the outbreak of EHV.

lived immunity. However, repeated vaccination can reduce the severity of respiratory disease and reduce the incidence of abortions. Two initial doses given several weeks apart are followed by regular boosters at intervals varying between three months and one year (depending on vaccine).

EQUINE VIRAL ARTERITIS (EVA)

Cause: EVA is caused by Equine Arteritis Virus (EAV). EAV is widely distributed throughout the world and EVA has been reported in the UK. Transmission of the virus occurs via the respiratory tract (aerosolised particles). In addition, stallions can transmit the virus venereally in the acute stage of the disease and as long-term carriers.

Signs: The incubation period is 3 to 14 days. Infection may result in clinical disease or be sub-clinical. The clinical signs vary widely but may include:
• fever (up to 106 F, 41 C)
• depression and inappetence
• limb swelling (especially hind limbs)
• stiffness
• nasal discharge
• conjunctivitis
• swellings around the eyes, lower abdomen, sheath or udder
• abortion (any stage of gestation)
• coughing, respiratory distress.

Clinical disease tends to be most severe in young or old horses. Most infected horses make a full recovery and the mortality rate is low.

A carrier state is established in 30-60% of infected stallions. The duration of the carrier state varies from several weeks to lifetime. Carrier stallions shed the virus constantly in the semen but there is no effect on fertility.

Treatment:
• rest
• symptomatic treatments.

Prevention and control:
A vaccine is available and is safe and effective in stallions and non-pregnant mares.

Prevention and control depend on management practices (as described for influenza and EHV 1) and selective use of the vaccine, including vaccination of the at-risk stallion population. Stallions should be vaccinated annually at least 28 days before the onset of the next breeding season. Measures should be taken to prevent the spread of EAV in fresh or frozen semen used for artificial insemination.

BACTERIAL DISEASES

STRANGLES

Strangles is a common acute, contagious respiratory infection.

Cause: Infection by the bacterium *Streptococcus equi.*

Signs: Strangles is most commonly seen in young animals (foals and yearlings), although it can occur at any age. It is a highly contagious disease and spreads easily among stabled populations of susceptible horses, generally after being introduced into a yard by an animal incubating the disease or by a carrier horse. Spread is slower than that of respiratory viruses and requires direct contact or contact with contaminated equipment, tack, etc. However, copious discharges from infected horses result in rapid contamination of the environment, where the bacteria can survive for several months.

The incubation period is usually 4 to 10 days and clinical disease lasts about three weeks. The clinical signs include:

- fever (103-105F)
- inappetence
- dullness and lethargy
- nasal discharge; watery then thick pus
- enlargement of the lymph glands under the jaw, which eventually soften and burst yielding thick, creamy pus
- respiratory distress and noise
- difficulty swallowing
- conjunctivitis.

Complications of strangles occur in a small number of cases due to spread of the infection to other parts of the body (known as 'bastard strangles'). Some cases may develop a persistent nasal discharge due to chronic infection of the guttural pouches or sinusitis. Horses can carry the organism in the guttural pouches for prolonged periods (from weeks to years) and these carrier horses can be a source of infection of other horses.

Treatment: General nursing care with provision of soft food and poulticing of the lymph node abscesses is most important. Some abscesses may require surgical drainage (lancing). The use of antibiotics is controversial: if given once abscesses have already developed they may simply prolong the course of the disease.

Prevention and control:

- Isolate all confirmed and suspected cases.
- General hygiene is important to prevent the spread of the disease. Spread via handlers and equipment must be prevented. Thorough cleaning and disinfection of contaminated stables and the environment. The bacteria can remain viable within the grazing environment for several months.
- Restrict movement of horses from the premises for at least six weeks.
- Quarantine all new arrivals.
- On studs, maintain separate animal groups, especially foals.
- Vaccination is not available at present in the UK, but a new intra-nasal vaccine is now in use in North America and is proving very successful.

RHODOCOCCUS EQUI PNEUMONIA

Cause: Rhodococcus equi is responsible for pneumonia of foals, especially in the one to six months age group. The organism survives in the soil and the disease tends to become endemic (that is, it recurs year after year) on certain farms. The prevalence of disease increases with dusty environments and dry weather.

Signs: Two clinical forms of *R. equi* pneumonia are recognised. The sub-acute form is characterised by a severe pneumonia with a short clinical course usually resulting in death. The chronic form is characterised by solitary or multiple lung abscesses and has a prolonged clinical disease of weeks to months.

Sub-acute form:

Acute onset of fever, increased respiratory rate and dyspnoea. Coughing and nasal discharge are variable. Affected foals often die within a few days of onset of clinical signs.

Chronic form:

Fever, depression, dyspnoea, weight loss and unthriftiness. Coughing and nasal discharge are variable.

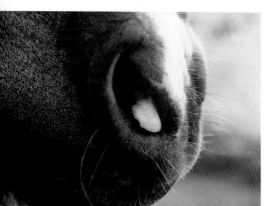

The nasal discharge of a horse with strangles is thick and creamy.

Treatment: The combination of two antibiotics, erythromycin and rifampicin, gives the best results. Treatment must be continued for 4 to 12 weeks. Approximately 80% of foals recover with this treatment, with good prognosis for future athletic soundness.

PLEUROPNEUMONIA

Cause: Pleuropneumonia is caused by a severe bacterial infection of the lungs and pleural cavity. The disease is not contagious and a number of different bacteria may be involved. The disease occurs most commonly following stress, e.g. long-distance travel ('transit fever', see Chapter Nine) or surgery.

The disease causes consolidation of some or all of the lungs, sometimes with abscess formation. Pus-like fluid fills the thoracic cavity.

Signs:
- Initially fever and pain (reluctance to move).
- Later, fever, inappetence, dyspnoea (inspiratory and expiratory), cough and weight loss.
- Nasal discharge is variable, occasionally blood-tinged. There may be malodorous breath.

Treatment:
- Appropriate antibiotics (preferably identified by bacteriological cultures) for prolonged periods.
- Anti-inflammatory drugs.
- Supportive nursing care.
- Drainage of pleural fluid.

LOWER-AIRWAY INFECTIONS

Cause: Lower airway infections can be associated with mild clinical signs but often cause exercise intolerance and poor performance in athletic horses (especially racehorses).

Some cases follow an initial viral infection ('chronic post-viral coughing'). The initial viral infection may be sub-clinical (especially EHV 1 and 4 infections). A variety of bacteria can cause these infections.

Signs:
- fever
- chronic cough (especially during exercise)
- mucopurulent nasal discharge (variable)
- exercise intolerance in performance horses.

Treatment:
- 'dust-free' management as for COPD
- bronchodilators
- mucolytics
- antibiotics.

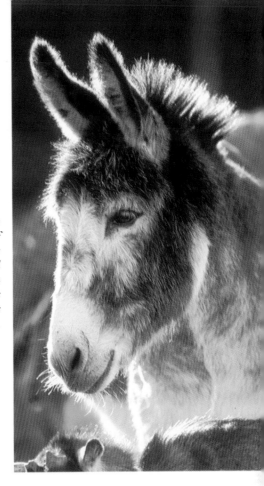

Donkeys, the natural hosts of lungworm, rarely show the clinical signs of infection that can debilitate horses that share their pasture.

PARASITIC DISEASES

LUNGWORM

Cause: Lungworm is caused by the parasite *Dictyocaulus arnfieldi*. Donkeys are the natural host of lungworms, and commonly carry infections without any clinical signs. Horses usually become infected by grazing pasture contaminated by donkeys. Eggs passed out in donkey faeces can develop rapidly into infective larvae which can survive six to seven weeks on pasture under suitable conditions (damp/shade). The larvae cannot over-winter.

Horses become infected by ingesting larvae, which migrate to the lungs. The disease is usually recognised in late summer/autumn.

Signs: Chronic coughing. Signs may be indistinguishable from COPD.

Treatment: Appropriate anthelmintics (wormers).

PARASCARIS EQUORUM INFECTION

Cause: Parascaris equorum is the ascarid (roundworm) that affects foals and weanlings. This is an unusual cause of coughing in foals, weanlings and yearlings, associated with the migration of larvae through the lungs.

Signs: Cough, watery nasal discharge, inappetence and weight loss.

Treatment: Appropriate anthelmintics (wormers).

ALLERGIC RESPIRATORY DISEASES

CHRONIC OBSTRUCTIVE PULMONARY DISEASE (COPD)

This disease is also known as chronic small airway disease (SAD), chronic pulmonary disease (CPD), broken wind, heaves or chronic alveolar emphysema. *Cause:* COPD is a common condition that results from obstruction of small airways (bronchioles) and cases may also have bronchitis. In the late stages of the disease some horses develop emphysema (structural destruction of the lung).

COPD occurs in all breeds of horses, ponies and donkeys. The incidence tends to increase with age, the disease usually occurring in horses older than four years. In performance horses, low-grade COPD may cause few overt clinical signs other than exercise intolerance and poor performance.

COPD is caused by a hypersensitivity (allergy) associated with the inhalation of organic dusts, primarily hay and straw dusts. An allergy to fungal and thermophilic actinomycete spores (the major component of hay and straw dust, especially from 'heated' bales) is involved in most cases. COPD is primarily a disease of the stabled horse, although some cases appear to be sensitive to pollens. The net results of the allergic reactions are:
• spasm and constriction of small airways
• excessive mucus secretion
• inflammation of the airways.

These reactions result in small airway obstruction; airflow is impeded, especially during expiration. Most of these reactions are totally reversible if exposure to the offending dust is eliminated. In severe cases, however, chronic airflow obstruction results in alveolar over-inflation and eventually areas of emphysema. In a minority of cases, secondary infection by opportunist bacteria may occur.

Signs: The disease may follow an acute respiratory infection, but most commonly the onset is insidious. The severity of the disease is extremely variable, ranging from sub-clinical to mild to severe. If left untreated, the severity tends to worsen. The clinical signs may be continuous or intermittent.

Sub-clinical disease:
This is most likely to be recognised in performance horses demonstrating exercise intolerance with no other overt clinical signs.

Mild clinical disease:
There is usually a chronic cough that is occasional

and sporadic; it is frequently noticed at the start of exercise or whilst feeding. There may be a slight watery/mucoid bilateral nasal discharge (especially after exercise) and exercise intolerance (performance horses).

Severe clinical disease:
Chronic cough that may occur at any time, but is most marked if the horse is exerted and during feeding. Increased respiratory effort with expiratory dyspnoea. Expiration becomes laboured with the use of the abdominal muscles. An 'abdominal lift' occurs at the end of expiration resulting in a double expiratory effort. The resting respiratory rate may be normal or mildly elevated (16-20/min). There is usually a bilateral nasal discharge, but this is not invariably present and may be worse after exercise or when the head is lowered. Exercise intolerance is marked in performance horses, and the recovery period after exercise is prolonged.

Treatment: Treatment can be divided into measures to relieve clinical signs and measures to prevent the recurrence of the disease.

To relieve clinical signs:
• 'Dust-free' management (see page 138)
• Bronchiodilators
  These drugs help by opening up constricted small airways.
• Mucolytics and expectorants
  These drugs loosen up the excessive mucus and help the horse to clear the discharges.
• Corticosteroids.
  These are anti-allergy drugs that can be used, usually for short-term use only.

To prevent recurrence of disease:
• Maintain strict 'dust-free' conditions
• Sodium cromoglycate
  This is another anti-allergy drug. It is administered by nebulisation through a face mask.

SUMMER PASTURE-ASSOCIATED OBSTRUCTIVE PULMONARY DISEASE (SPAOPD)

This is a syndrome with similar clinical signs as COPD, but occurring in horses at grass in the summer.
Cause: The precise cause is uncertain, but probably involves an allergy to pollens. Anecdotal reports in

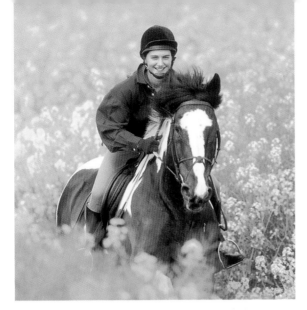

Pollen allergy is associated with symptoms of obstructive pulmonary disease that occur in the spring and summer months. Rape seed appears to be a culprit in many cases.

the UK suggest an association with oilseed rape (canola) pollen.

Signs: These are similar to COPD: expiratory dyspnoea and exercise intolerance. Coughing is not usually as marked as with COPD. There is sometimes inappetence and weight loss.

Treatment: Drug therapy is similar to COPD. In addition, the horse should be stabled and fed a diet of hay and nuts.

DISEASES OF THE NASAL CAVITIES AND PARA-NASAL SINUSES

SINUSITIS

Cause: Infection in one or more of the para-nasal sinuses may occur as a sequel to a viral upper respiratory tract infection or may occur secondary to dental disease. The roots of the last four upper cheek teeth on each side lie close to the maxillary sinuses and infection of the tooth roots often results in a secondary infection of the sinuses. Cysts sometimes arise within the sinuses that gradually enlarge and fill the sinus cavity.

Signs: The clinical signs of para-nasal sinus diseases almost invariably include a nasal discharge, which may be mucoid, purulent, haemorrhagic or a combination of these. There may also be facial swelling and obstructive dyspnoea (difficulty in breathing). The nasal discharge is usually unilateral (present on the same side as the diseased sinus). The nasal discharge may be foul-smelling, especially in sinusitis secondary to dental disease.

Treatment: Non-surgical treatments for sinusitis include antibiotics, mucolytics, steam inhalations, volatile inhalations and continued controlled exercise. The objective is the return of normal mucus clearance from the sinuses.

Surgical treatments include trephination (drilling a

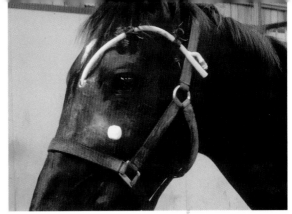

Trephination of the paranasal sinuses. A flushing catheter has been secured into the frontal sinus via a trephine hole to the side of the eye. Another trephine hole has been made into the maxillary sinus (the hole is plugged with a gauze bung).

hole through the side of the face into the sinus), which permits drainage as well as providing a route to flush and medicate the sinus. Facial flap surgery allows greater access to the sinuses to permit more extensive surgery to be performed.

PROGRESSIVE ETHMOIDAL HAEMATOMA (PEH)

Cause: The cause is unknown. The lesion is a non-cancerous mass containing blood which grows on the walls of the nasal cavity or sinuses.

Signs: Repeated low-grade haemorrhage from one nostril is the most common sign. The blood is not fresh and epistaxis is not related to exercise. Varying degrees of nasal obstruction will be present and in competition horses noisy breathing may be observed.

Treatment: Treatment is surgical.

DISEASES OF THE GUTTURAL POUCHES

The guttural pouches are balloon-like structures lying between the base of the skull and the pharynx. The volume of each pouch is approximately 300 ml, and medially the two pouches are in contact with one another, divided only by a thin layer of tissue.

GUTTURAL POUCH TYMPANY

Cause: In this condition the opening to one or both pouches acts as a non-return valve so that air can enter the pouch but cannot escape.

Signs: This is a condition of foals which is seen within a few days of birth. The disorder appears to be more common in fillies than colts. Air accumulates and produces a swelling on the side of the face.

Treatment: Treatment is surgical.

GUTTURAL POUCH EMPYEMA AND CHONDROIDS

Cause: Empyema of the guttural pouches occurs when mucus and/or pus accumulate within the

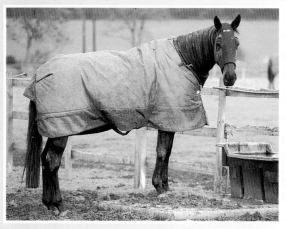

▲ *Affected horses should be managed from pasture or, where this is not an option, given as much turn-out time as possible with no access to hay or straw.*

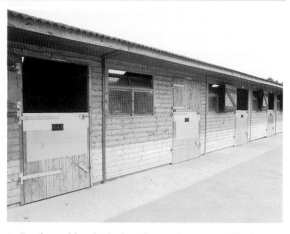

▲ *In the stable, check there is maximum ventilation without creating draughts. Always leave top doors open, using additional rugs to maintain warmth if necessary. The horse's air space should be completely separate from that of others not on a dust-free management regime. Avoid over-head lofts.*

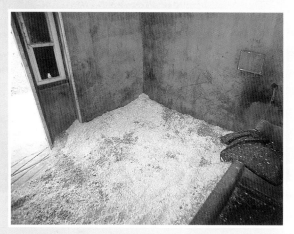

▲ *Use dust-free bedding such as shavings, shredded paper, hemp (e.g. Aubiose), synthetic bedding or rubber matting. Consider fitting a dust extractor in the stable. Maintain a clean, dry bed at all times. Deep litter should be avoided. Muck heaps must be positioned well away from the stable. Remove the horse from the stable during mucking out and for at least 30 minutes afterwards.*

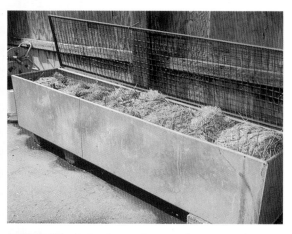

▲ *If possible, feed a hay replacer, such as a complete or high-fibre mix/nuts, chaff, silage or vacuum-packed haylage. If hay must be fed it should be good quality and be throughly soaked for approximately one hour and drained, prior to feeding. Dampen all concentrates and feed from ground level.*

pouches because they are failing to drain satisfactorily. Pus which is stagnant within the pouch eventually dries, leading to the formation of solid concretions (chondroids).
Signs: The clinical signs of empyema include a purulent nasal discharge (pus) and swelling of the side of face. The distension of the affected pouch into the pharynx may produce obstructive dyspnoea.
Treatment: Treatment is surgical.

GUTTURAL POUCH MYCOSIS

Cause: Guttural pouch mycosis is caused by a fungal infection in the pouch. Many of the fungal infections occur close to the internal carotid artery.
Signs: Clinical signs are variable. A nose bleed at rest is the most frequent sign and usually consists of a small quantity of fresh blood at one nostril in the first instance. A number of further minor haemorrhages may follow but, if untreated, a fatal haemorrhage may occur.

Some horses may suffer nerve damage as a consequence of the infection, resulting in difficulty or inability to swallow.
Treatment: The treatment is surgical.

UPPER AIRWAY OBSTRUCTIONS

RECURRENT LARYNGEAL NEUROPATHY (RLN)

Cause: RLN causes a permanent dysfunction of the muscles of the larynx. The result is partial obstruction of the airway evident during exercise and compromised athletic performance. The condition almost invariably involves the left side of the larynx. The resistance to normal airflow causes turbulence in the air stream which is the source of the characteristic abnormal inspiratory noises – 'whistling' or 'roaring'. Horses over 16 hands high are most susceptible.
Signs: Abnormal respiratory sounds are present at exercise, usually throughout the period of exertion at the canter and gallop. The noises range from a low grade musical 'whistle', to a harsh 'roaring' noise like sawing wood. The noise stops soon after the completion of exercise. There may or may not be obvious exercise intolerance. The diagnosis is confirmed by examination with an endoscope.
Treatment: A variety of surgical treatments are available including ventriculectomy (Hobday procedure), laryngeal prosthesis (tie-back procedure), nerve/muscle pedicle grafting and tracheotomy.

DORSAL DISPLACEMENT OF THE SOFT PALATE (DDSP)

Cause: The function of the intra-pharyngeal ostium is to provide an airtight seal that locks the larynx into the wall of the pharynx. This mechanism renders the horse at exercise an obligatory nose-breather. DDSP arises as an acute respiratory obstruction which

occurs while a horse is at fast exercise and when the free border of the soft palate becomes dislodged from its position and the unsupported soft palate is inhaled towards the larynx.

DDSP is frequently a symptom rather than a disease in its own right. Underlying causes include conditions causing fatigue (e.g. unfitness; heart and lung diseases; other obstructions of the conducting airways such as RLN), diseases of the larynx (e.g. epiglottic entrapment) and dental disorders.
Signs: The abrupt respiratory obstruction which accompanies DDSP not only causes a loud, vibrant noise but precipitates a serious interference with the progress of the horse. In most cases, the horse completely loses its stride rhythm as it makes gulping attempts to restore the larynx into the intra-narial position. As soon as the normal anatomical configuration is restored, the horse is able to resume galloping and will no longer appear distressed.
Treatment: Treatment involves identifying any underlying condition and treating that. Aids to prevent mouth-breathing, such as a dropped or crossed noseband, should be tried and a change of bit to a simple rubber snaffle or, if applicable, a bitless bridle may be recommended. The position of the bit in the mouth may be modified by an Australian noseband. Tongue straps or tongue-ties are used to discourage swallowing. A number of different surgical treatments can be used.

EPIGLOTTIC ENTRAPMENT (EE)

Cause: A fold of tissue becomes enveloped around the epiglottis (part of the larynx). The precise cause is unknown.
Signs: The signs associated with EE include exercise intolerance with inspiratory and/or expiratory noises at exercise, intermittent gurgling from secondary DDSP and coughing after eating.
Treatment: Treatment is surgical.

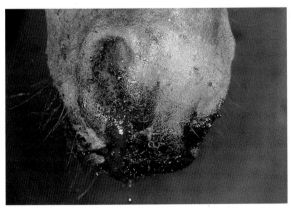

Uni-lateral nosebleed due to guttural pouch mycosis.

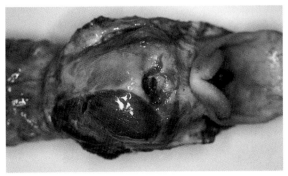

Recurrent laryngeal neuropathy. The post-mortem showed atrophy (shrinkage) of the muscles over the left side of the larynx (seen here on the upper half of the specimen – compare with the well developed muscle on the right side, lower half).

139

6 THE HORSE'S WORLD

Over many millions of years, horses evolved a physique and patterns of behaviour that were necessary for their survival in the wild. Like all animals, they have to respond appropriately to events occurring in the world around them. They need to be able to communicate socially with other members of their own species. With domestication, horses also had to adapt to the conditions and demands imposed on them by humans.

All the responses and activities which make up a horse's behaviour are directed by the nervous system. Sensory systems continuously feed information from the external environment (sight, sound, smell, taste, touch) and from within the body (position, temperature, pain) to the central nervous system, where they are filtered and processed in various ways.

As a result of this processing, messages are sent to the skeletal muscles. Nearly all behavioural activities are carried out by the contractions of skeletal muscle. Some responses, termed 'reflex', are automatic, immediate and fixed. Other 'voluntary' responses may involve a decision to act based on a number of factors such as motivation and previous experience.

As well as its outwardly-directed activities, the nervous system has the task of co-ordinating most of the body's internal functions. For example, it controls digestion, respiration, the contractions of the heart and of smooth muscles in blood vessels, and the release, by the endocrine system, of hormones which regulate metabolism and growth. Hormones themselves can influence behaviour by their effects on specific parts of the brain. For example, a stallion's aggressiveness and libido is affected by the male sex hormone, testosterone.

HOW THE NERVOUS SYSTEM FUNCTIONS

The basic units of the nervous system are nerve cells, or **neurones.**

An animal is born with its full complement of neurones (tens of billions!) and produces no more during its life. While their size and shape vary with location in the nervous system, most neurones contain the same parts: a cell body; a number of highly-branched outgrowths of the cell body called dendrites; a single, long nerve fibre (or axon) extending from the cell body; and branches at the end of the nerve fibre (axon terminals).

Wherever their location, the neurones also operate in the same way. In response to signals received at the cell body and dendrites, they generate electrical signals which travel rapidly to the ends of the cell. This process can be likened to what happens when a match is applied to one end of a line of gunpowder – once lit, the flame moves down the line to the other end. Depending on the type of neurone, the speed at which this signal can travel can range from about 1mph to over 250mph.

Neurones communicate with each other, and with other cells of the body (such as muscle or secretory cells). The junction between two neurones is called a synapse. Rather than there being a direct electrical connection between neurones, a chemical called a neurotransmitter is released into the gap between the cells. Depending on the neurotransmitter released, this can either tend to provoke the second cell to fire off its own electrical signal (excitatory) or put a damper on its activity and make it less likely to fire off (inhibitory).

A nerve cell in the brain may have contacts with many other nerve cells – some have more than 100,000 contacts. Whether a particular cell fires or not depends on the combined activity of the cells which contact it at any moment in time. Furthermore, the efficiency of a synapse may improve the more it is used, and new branches and synapses may be formed over a period of time. This provides a possible cellular basis for storing memories.

In addition to nerve cells, the nervous system also contains **glial** cells. Some of these serve to increase the speed at which signals can travel along axons. Others help sustain the nerve cells, providing nutrients, mopping up unwanted chemicals and stimulating the growth of axons and dendrites. They may even play a role in processing information.

THE STRUCTURE OF THE NERVOUS SYSTEM

The nervous system can be divided into two main parts: central and peripheral. The central nervous system (CNS) lies within a series of protective bones: the brain inside the skull, and the spinal cord in the vertebrae that make up the spine. The peripheral system comprises the nerves.

THE BRAIN

The brain is a very complex organ with many parts. A horse's brain is similar in shape and function to that of other mammals. Specific groups of nerve cells, or 'centres', in different parts of the brain, are specialised to perform different tasks.

The brain's shape conforms approximately to the cranial cavity of the skull. Between the delicate nervous tissue and the protective bones are three membranes, the **meninges**. The space between the two inner membranes is filled with clear, colourless, cerebro-spinal fluid which provides additional mechanical protection and a stable chemical environment for the brain.

An adult horse's brain weighs 400-700g, accounting for 0.1 per cent of body weight. This compares with 2 per cent for humans. This percentage difference has been used simplistically to compare intelligence amongst different animal species. As each animal has its own kind of intelligence, such comparisons are ultimately rather meaningless. IQ depends on how it is defined and tested. It is more useful to recognise that horses are good at being horses, and to study their particular strengths. Like the brains of all mammals, the horse's brain is divided anatomically into three sections: the hind-brain, the mid-brain and the fore-brain.

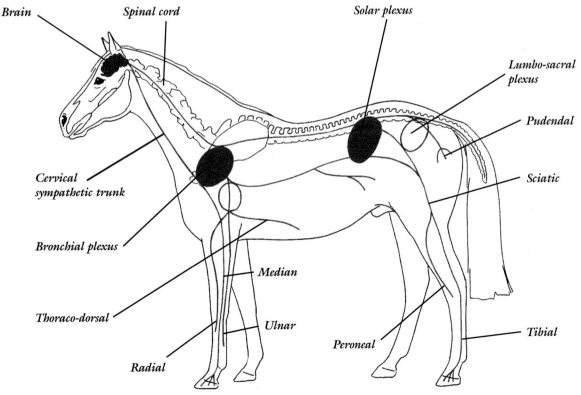

THE POSITION OF THE MAJOR NERVES OF THE HORSE

THE MAIN DIVISIONS OF THE EQUINE BRAIN AND THEIR FUNCTIONS

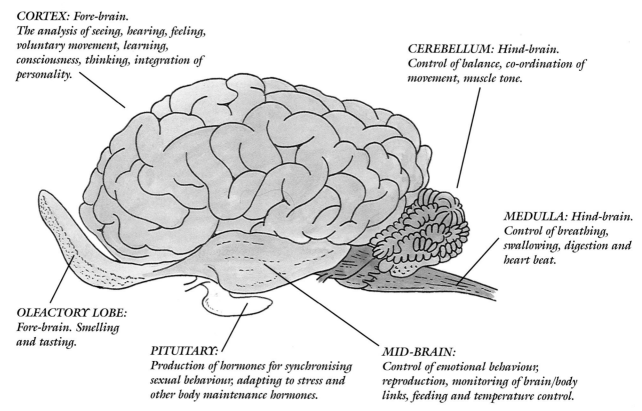

CORTEX: *Fore-brain.*
The analysis of seeing, hearing, feeling,
voluntary movement, learning,
consciousness, thinking, integration of
personality.

CEREBELLUM: *Hind-brain.*
Control of balance, co-ordination of
movement, muscle tone.

MEDULLA: *Hind-brain.*
Control of breathing,
swallowing, digestion and
heart beat.

OLFACTORY LOBE:
Fore-brain. Smelling
and tasting.

PITUITARY:
Production of hormones for synchronising
sexual behaviour, adapting to stress and
other body maintenance hormones.

MID-BRAIN:
Control of emotional behaviour,
reproduction, monitoring of brain/body
links, feeding and temperature control.

The hind-brain consists of the brainstem (literally the 'stalk' of the brain) through which pass all the nerve fibres that relay signals from the spinal cord. The **medulla** and **pons** of the brainstem contain neuronal 'centres' (groups of nerve cells) that control, automatically and without volition, breathing rhythm, coughing, blood pressure and heart rate. Other centres control posture and muscle tone and others promote sleep and wakefulness. The **cerebellum,** a globular structure at the back of the brain, is important for co-ordinating and learning movements and for controlling posture and balance.

Tucked underneath, the mid-brain is a short portion containing centres for visual and auditory reflexes and for voluntary movement. The mid-brain leads directly to the **diencephalon** (part of the fore-brain) consisting of various structures including the pituitary and pineal glands, hypothalamus and thalamus. Another fore-brain area, the **limbic system,** is involved with olfactory (smell) sensations, emotions, learning, endocrine functions, and (along with the hypothalamus) the expression of sexual behaviour, fear and rage. The remaining fore-brain structure is the **cerebrum,** which makes up the bulk of the brain. Its two separate left and right cerebral hemispheres are connected by bundles of nerve fibres, the largest being the **corpus callosum**.

The **cerebral cortex** is the rumpled grey outer layer of the brain. It is relatively thin but accounts for almost half of the volume of the cerebrum because it is so highly folded. Ascending pathways transmit information from touch-sensitive receptors in the skin, through the brainstem and thalamus, finally projecting a map of the whole body on to a discrete (somato-sensory) part of the cortex.

Neurones in another area, the motor cortex, contribute directly to movements involving the use of individual muscle groups. In these maps, the size of the projection is exaggerated according to how many nerves supply each part of the body. As the horse chiefly uses its lips and muzzle for tactile exploration, these areas are extensively represented in the brain. There are similar projections for the visual and auditory senses. Smells are not seen because the visual areas of the brain do not receive impulses from olfactory receptors! The cerebral cortex is also considered to be the part of the brain responsible for an animal's awareness of objects and situations, and for mental activities such as problem-solving.

While it is convenient to sub-divide the brain into

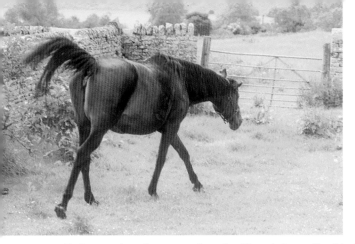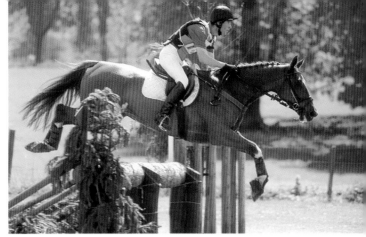

Reflex muscle action ranges from the skin twitch or tail swish that removes an irritating fly, to the complex co-ordination of muscles involved in maintaining balance throughout even the most demanding athletic activity.

parts on the basis of anatomy or function, all these parts are interlinked and influence each other in ways which we do not yet understand.

THE SPINAL CORD

The spinal cord, which is the thickness of a thumb, runs down the length of the vertebral canal, on average reaching a couple of metres from head to tail. Inside the cord is a butterfly-shaped core of nerve cells (grey matter) surrounded by the tracts of the nerve fibres (white matter) which carry impulses up and down the cord.

All the ascending and descending nerve tracts that link the trunk and limbs with the brain pass through the spinal cord in the white matter. Nerve bundles emerge from the spinal cord in pairs through holes between adjoining vertebrae: 7 cervical (neck), 18 thoracic (chest), 5 or 6 lumbar (loins), 5 fused sacral (croup) and 5 out of 20 or so caudal (tail) vertebrae.

The grey matter contains the large nerve cells, the motor neurones, that innervate the skeletal muscles. In part, they respond to impulses in pathways descending from the brain, but they are also involved in reflex loops within the spinal cord.

SPINAL CORD REFLEXES

Skeletal muscles are often called 'voluntary' muscles, because their actions are under conscious control. However, not all skeletal muscle activity is voluntary. Many reflex responses occur which involve specific sensory stimuli leading automatically to a fixed set of muscle contractions.

Many reflexes have a protective function. For example, an object moving close to the eye or a tap on the bone just below the eye will cause the horse to blink (the eyelid or palpebral reflex). Blinking also occurs when the surface of the eye starts to dry out or become irritated. Foreign matter in the eye also leads to the production of tears (lachrymal reflex). Bright light directed into one eye causes the pupil to narrow (pupillary light reflex), thereby preventing the light-sensitive cells in the eye from being

overwhelmed. One reflex horses possess that we lack is the skin twitch (panniculus) reflex which is particularly evident when a horse is being troubled by biting flies. Reflex muscle action also is important in the control of posture and muscle tone, providing a background level of muscle activity appropriate for effective voluntary actions. Vets use the absence of standard reflexes to diagnose neurological problems, or during surgery, to determine the depth of anaesthesia.

At the cellular level, reflexes involve a sensory detector and afferent neurones which are linked, within the central nervous system, to an efferent motor neurone. This pathway is known as the reflex arc. In a few reflexes there is a direct connection via a single synapse in the spinal cord between the afferent and efferent neurone. An example is the 'knee-jerk' reflex, which involves a sudden twitch of a limb muscle caused by tapping the tendon.

Most reflexes, however, are 'polysynaptic' as they involve one or more intermediate neurones. An unpleasant stimulus, such as a pin prick, applied to a limb will cause it to be promptly withdrawn. As the flexor muscle is made to contract, signals to the antagonistic extensor muscle, which acts in the opposite direction, are inhibited allowing it to relax. This stops the two muscles from working against each other. But if the horse simply pulled one leg up, it might lose balance and fall over. So the muscles in the other limbs are commanded to re-distribute the weight of the body to maintain balance.

Co-ordination of movement in this way occurs more or less automatically. Usually, higher brain centres, and not just the spinal cord, are involved in these more complex reflexes. Although the initial response to the pin prick is instantaneous and involuntary, the message is likely to filter up to a level where the horse becomes aware of a painful or unpleasant sensation. This may then provoke a voluntary reaction, such as running away or kicking out.

THE PERIPHERAL NERVOUS SYSTEM

The peripheral nervous system consists of nerve bundles extending out from the CNS to the body and limbs. Peripheral nerves may be classified by function into afferent nerves (bringing signals into the CNS) and efferent nerves (carrying signals out). The efferent nerves can be sub-divided into somatic and autonomic nerves.

Somatic nerves have cell bodies in the brainstem or spinal cord and run their axons directly to muscle cells. These are often called 'motor' neurones because their activity leads to contraction of the innervated muscle. Autonomic nerves make connections, via synapses in cell clusters called ganglia, to smooth muscle in blood vessels and to glands throughout the body.

THE ENDOCRINE (HORMONAL) SYSTEM

A hormone is a chemical messenger secreted into the circulation by an endocrine gland. It is carried by the blood stream to target cells which contain receptors for the particular message.

When hormone molecules bind to receptors, a response is initiated. For example, when blood pressure falls, perhaps as a result of haemorrhage and reduction in blood volume, the pituitary gland secretes a hormone called ADH (anti-diuretic hormone) which acts on the kidneys, its target organs. This causes them to reabsorb more water and produce a concentrated urine, thus limiting further fluid loss.

The endocrine and nervous systems are similar in that both involve the transmission of a message that is triggered by a stimulus and produces a response. But because nerve impulses can travel much faster than blood-borne substances, nervous system responses are more rapid.

On the other hand, hormonal responses are often long-lasting because it takes time (anything between minutes and days) for hormones to be broken down or excreted. In contrast, nervous responses are short-lived: for example, the twitch of a muscle is over in a fraction of a second.

One other difference between the two systems is that nerve impulses are transmitted to specific destinations, whereas hormones circulate throughout the body and may affect several target organs in different locations.

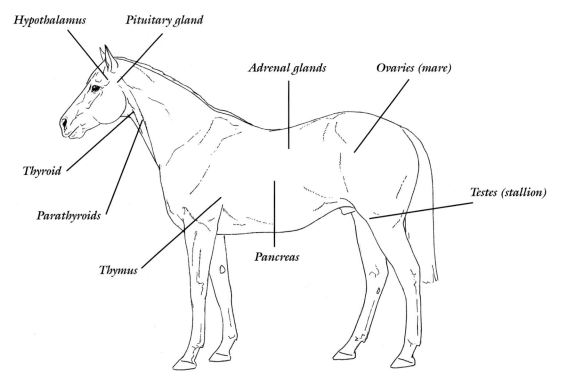

THE ENDOCRINE SYSTEM OF THE HORSE, SHOWING THE MAJOR GLANDS

ENDOCRINE TABLE

Endocrine gland/ source of hormone	Hormone	Target organ or tissue	Major function is control of:-
Hypothalamus	Numerous releasing factors	Pituitary gland	Hormones released by pituitary
Anterior pituitary (adenohypophysis)	ACTH (adrenocorticotrophic hormone)	Adrenal cortex	Cortisol secretion
	FSH (follicle stimulating hormone)	Ovaries / testes (tubules)	Ovarian follicle growth, oestrogen secretion/spermatogenesis
	LH (luteinising hormone)	Ovaries / testes (Leydig cells)	Ovulation, luteinisation of follicle/ testosterone secretion
	GH (growth hormone)	All tissues	Growth; carbohydrate, protein and fat metabolism
	TSH (thyroid stimulating hormone)	Thyroid gland	Thyroxine secretion
	Prolactin	Mammary gland	Milk secretion (stimulates)
Posterior pituitary (neurohypophysis)	ADH (antidiuretic hormone)	Kidney tubules Smooth muscle in arterioles	Water excretion Blood pressure
	Oxytocin	Uterine smooth muscle Mammary gland	Uterine contractions Milk 'let-down'
Pineal gland	Melatonin	Various tissues	Circadian rhythm; reproduction
Thyroid	Thyroxine (T4) Triiodothyronine (T3)	Most tissues	Metabolic rate; growth and development
	Calcitonin	Bone	Plasma calcium and phosphate (lowers)
Parathyroids	PTH (parathyroid hormone)	Bone, kidneys, intestine	Plasma calcium and phosphate (elevates)
Thymus (regresses in adulthood)	Thymopoetin	T-lymphocyte cells in blood	Immune responses
Pancreas (islet cells)	Insulin (from beta cells)	Most tissues, notably muscle and liver	Glucose utilisation; blood glucose (lowers)
	Glucagon (from alpha cells)	Primarily liver	Blood glucose (elevates)
Intestinal mucosa	Gastrin	Stomach	Acid secretion
	Secretin	Pancreas	Digestive secretions
	Cholecystokinin	Gallbladder	Release of bile
	Somatostatin	Intestine	Acid and intestinal secretions (inhibits)
Adrenal medulla	Adrenaline Noradrenaline	All tissues	Metabolism; heart rate and output; response to stress and exercise
Adrenal cortex	Cortisol Corticosterone	All tissues	Metabolism; response to stress and exercise
	Aldosterone	Primarily kidneys	Sodium, potassium and pH balance
Kidneys	Renin (converted to Angiotensin-II)	Blood vessel smooth muscle Adrenal cortex	Blood pressure Aldosterone secretion
Ovaries	Oestrogens	Reproductive organs	Reproductive development; also has effects on oestrus behaviour
	Progesterone (from corpus luteum)	Uterus	Uterine condition
Uterus	Prostaglandin (PGF2u)	Corpus luteum	Breakdown of corpus luteum (luteolysis)
Placenta (in pregnant mare)	Progesterone and oestrogens	Corpus luteum	Maintenance of pregnancy
	eCG (Equine chorionic gonadotrophin, PMSG)	Ovaries	Maintenance of pregnancy
	Relaxin	Uterus Cervix, pelvic ligaments	Uterine contraction (inhibits) Increase in distensibility
Testes	Testosterone	Reproductive organs	Reproductive development; also has effects on behaviour

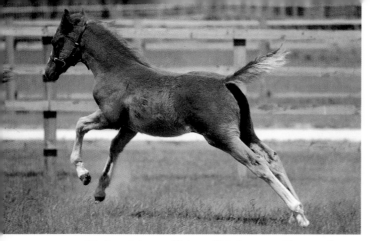

The horse's innate 'fight or flight' response illustrates how closely, and rapidly, the endrocrine and nervous systems work together for survival.

The table on page 145 illustrates the great diversity of endocrine glands and hormones. Some glands secrete hormones in response to a simple change in the level of a substance (e.g. calcium) in the surrounding fluid. Others respond to nervous system signals. For example, when a foal suckles its dam, receptors in the teat are activated and impulses conveyed to the pituitary gland by way of the spinal cord. This results in the prompt release of oxytocin into the blood. When this reaches the mammary gland, 20 seconds or so later, it diffuses out of the capillaries and causes contraction of the cells surrounding the alveolar ducts, leading to milk ejection or 'let-down'. Finally, a number of endocrine organs respond to hormones from other glands.

Organs may be primarily endocrine in nature: the pituitary, the pineal, and the thyroid, parathyroid and adrenal glands. Other organs combine endocrine with other important related functions: the pancreas, testes, ovaries and placenta. A third group comprises organs with quite different primary function, but which are also capable of producing hormones: the kidneys, liver, thymus, heart and gastro-intestinal tract.

The pituitary gland is sometimes called the 'master gland' because many of its hormones function chiefly to regulate the activity of other endocrine glands. It is an appendage of the brain, suspended below the hypothalamus by a thin stalk containing nerve fibres and small blood vessels.

The close connection between the endocrine and nervous systems is illustrated by the combined activities of the sympathetic nervous system and adrenal glands. In stressful situations, when an animal is forced to challenge an attacker or run from it (the 'fight or flight' response), there is widespread stimulation of the sympathetic system of the body. This results in a rapid pulse and rise in blood pressure. The output of the heart is increased and the flow of blood directed primarily to the skeletal muscles, at the expense of that to the skin and abdominal organs.

The middle part of the adrenal glands, the adrenal medulla, secretes the hormone adrenaline, which is chemically very similar to the substance noradrenaline produced at the endings of sympathetic nerves. Adrenaline evokes the same responses as impulses in the sympathetic nerves. It also produces a marked increase in metabolic rate.

Thus the combined effect of the endocrine and nervous systems is to prepare the body for emergency.

THE SENSES

Horses perceive the world around them using the same senses that we do. Broadly speaking, a horse's senses work in the same ways as ours, but differ in their capabilities and in *how* they are used. We will never know what it is really like to see or hear like a horse. Still, some appreciation of horses' unique perceptivity is crucial to understanding why they behave in the way they do.

The central nervous system is supplied with input from an extensive array of sensory receptor cells.

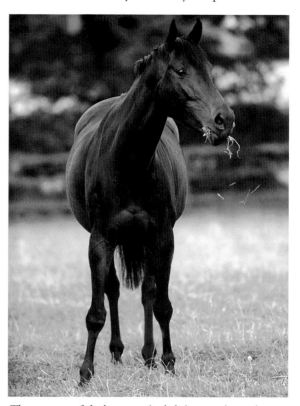

The ancestors of the horse survived their precarious existence as prey animals by fleeing first and thinking later. Every sense works as part of a sophisticated 'early warning system'.

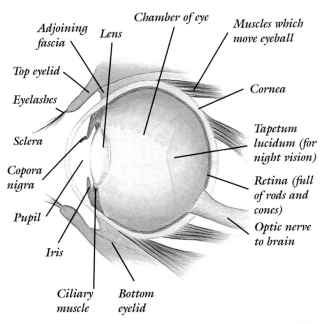

THE STRUCTURE OF THE HORSE'S EYE

Labels: Adjoining fascia, Lens, Chamber of eye, Muscles which move eyeball, Top eyelid, Cornea, Eyelashes, Sclera, Tapetum lucidum (for night vision), Copora nigra, Retina (full of rods and cones), Pupil, Optic nerve to brain, Iris, Ciliary muscle, Bottom eyelid

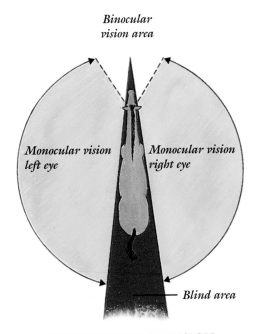

EQUINE FIELD OF VISION

Labels: Binocular vision area, Monocular vision left eye, Monocular vision right eye, Blind area

Some are scattered throughout the body, in every muscle, tendon, ligament and joint capsule. These pick up changes in mechanical strain, and keep the brain updated from moment to moment about the relative positions of the limbs, neck and head. The skin contains a great variety of receptors too, which make possible a range of cutaneous sensations.

All these receptors are modified nerve endings, whose shape and type of encapsulation determines the kind of stimulus to which they respond. They occur singly or in small groups. In contrast, large numbers of receptors are gathered together within the eyes, ears and nose, highly-specialised sense organs which enable features of the outside world to be discerned in considerable detail.

SIGHT

The ancestors of modern horses avoided being eaten by fleeing first and evaluating the situation later. Vision is the primary danger detector for a horse, as well as influencing almost every other aspect of his behaviour. The size of the eyes (the largest of any land mammal), the area of the cerebrum devoted to processing visual information, and the fact that a third of all sensory input to the brain comes from the eyes, indicate the relative importance of sight.

HOW THE EYES WORK

Eyes work by focusing rays of light from external objects to form an upside-down image on a layer at

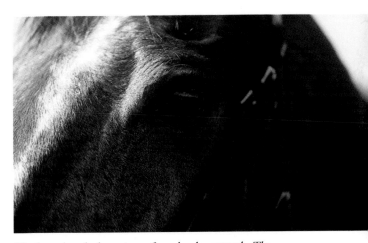

The horse has the largest eye of any land mammal. The perspective on his world that his vision provides, however, is quite different to that of the human eye.

the back of the eye called the **retina**. There photoreceptors (light-sensitive cells) transform the image into a pattern of nerve impulses which are conveyed, via the optic nerve, to the brain.

Two types of photoreceptors are present in both horse and human retina: rods and cones. Rod cells are more sensitive to light of low intensity, but provide no information about its wavelength (colour). Thus they are more suited to night vision. Cone cells need more light to be activated, so come into play more during daylight hours. They also respond differently to different colours, depending

147

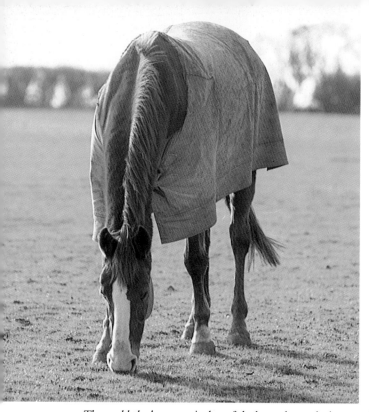
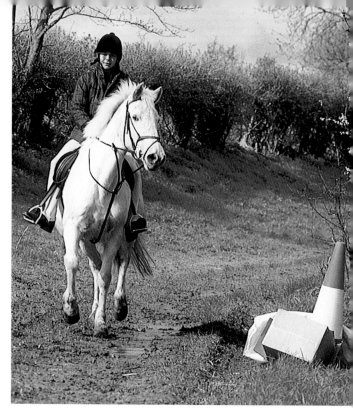

The world the horse sees is that of the hunted, not the hunter. Prominent and set to the side, his eyes have a huge range of vision. The grazing horse can see 340 degrees around him. The speciality of his eyes, however, is to detect movement. Detail and depth perception is only possible with accuracy in the narrow field of binocular vision in front. An unfamiliar object to one side causes this pony to shy – by swinging his body round to face the object head on, he can get a better look.

on the photo-pigment present in the cell. Humans have three cone types (red, green and blue); stimulation of these by varying amounts allows us to discriminate many subtly different shades.

The extent to which horses are able to distinguish colours is still the subject of inquiry. What is clear, however, is that horses have at least some colour vision, contrary to the old belief. Recent research indicates that they can discriminate between grey and four individual colours (red, yellow, green and blue), though some horses seem to have a more difficult time telling yellow or green apart from grey. This suggests that horses have only two cone types, in common with some other mammals including dogs, pigs and squirrels.

In the human retina, there is a central spot where photoreceptors and connecting neurones are packed together more tightly. Images focused at this point are seen with the greatest detail and visual acuity is at its highest. Because we cannot see equally well in all parts of the visual field, we use eye movements to shift attention from one feature to another. The equine retina also has a high-acuity spot, called the **area centralis**. When horses look face-on at an object, this is where the image falls. But there is also a second area of high-density photoreceptors and acute perception, which extends in a horizontal band across the equine retina. The location of this so-called 'visual streak' allows the horse to scan the horizon while grazing. Most of the time, the eyeball

is reflexively rotated by two (of seven) attached muscles to keep the eye aligned with the horizon.

Although horses have an extended field of gaze, they are not quite as able to make out fine detail as a person with average eyesight. However, they are extremely sensitive to variation in all parts of the visual field. This accounts for their tendency to become alarmed at the slightest unfamiliar movement and their ability to notice subtle body-language cues.

FIELD OF VISION
Equine eyes are set to the side of the head, and forward. The field of vision is obstructed only by the body and the shape of the head. Apart from a narrow blind area behind, in an arc of 10 degrees or so, a horse can see almost all of the 360 degrees around him in the horizontal plane. In the vertical plane, the retinal field of view is almost 180 degrees.

While grazing, a horse has only to turn his head slightly to check for signs of danger behind him. Although horses have laterally-placed eyes, there is a region in front of 60-70 degrees (depending on the breed) in which the two eyes can focus on objects - roughly half that of man and typical predators.

An advantage of this binocular mode of vision is that the brain can combine two slightly different images to judge the distance of an object, a process called stereopsis. In the horse, the binocular area is limited by the nose, which obscures anything

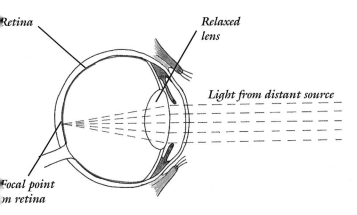

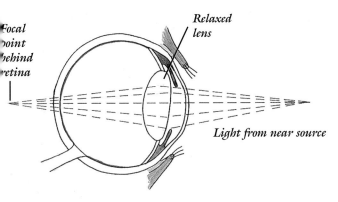

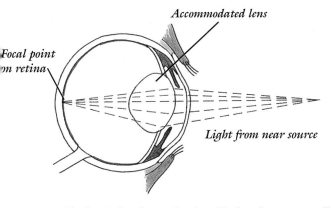

The horse's focusing mechanism. The lens focuses naturally on more distant objects. There is only a limited ability to 'accommodate' to bring objects at a closer range into sharp focus.

directly underneath and up to four foot in front of it. Therefore, a horse must be able to turn or lower his head in order to see where he is treading and to navigate obstacles safely. It is worth bearing this in mind whilst riding and particularly when jumping. Your horse needs a degree of freedom to move his head to obtain a good view of the jump in the approach phase and also to see where his front feet will land.

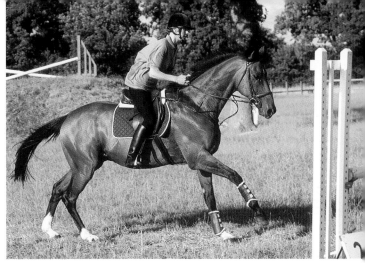

Awareness of the way the horse's vision works is essential for riders and trainers. The horse must be free to use its head to help focus and to judge distance and depth, particularly at close range. Too tight a rein contact, or the over-use of schooling gadgets, is not only counter-productive, but extremely unfair and stressful for the horse.

FOCUSING

For an object to appear sharp and not blurred, its image must be focused precisely on to the retina. The ability of the eye to focus on near and far objects is called accommodation. Much of the necessary bending of light rays is done by the curved surface of the transparent cornea. Changes in focus are brought about by the contraction of ciliary muscles which pull on the elastic lens located towards the front of the eye. When these muscles are relaxed and the lens is more spherical, the eye focuses on distant objects – thus horses are naturally 'long-sighted'. However, horses are subject to the same kinds of visual defect and deterioration with age as we are. It has even been suggested that domestication and in-breeding of the horse has introduced a degree of myopia, or near-sightedness.

According to the 'ramp retina' theory, it was assumed that the equine lens is inflexible and that a horse must raise and lower its head to bring objects at different distances into focus on upper and lower parts of the retina. This has now been disproved by optical measurements. Any head movements probably have more to do with bringing things out of blind spots and into binocular view. Nevertheless, it is likely that horses are unable to bring about changes in focus as rapidly as we can, so sudden moves nearby may be all the more startling.

Horses are vigilant for virtually 24 hours a day, so good vision is required both in daylight and in darkness. The **iris**, a flat ring of tissue containing smooth muscles between the cornea and lens, limits the amount of light entering the eye through the pupil. Under reflex control, the pupil closes to a narrow horizontal slit in bright light, matching the orientation of the visual streak. Extra shading is provided by irregular lumps, the **corpora nigra**, on the top edge of the pupil.

149

In dim conditions, the pupil enlarges and becomes more circular, admitting the maximum amount of light. Horses' eyes contain an additional shiny layer behind the retina called the **tapetum lucidum**, a feature shared by nocturnal animals. This is responsible for 'eyeshine', when the eyes are illuminated at night. Light that has passed through the retina without being absorbed, and hence not registered, is reflected by the tapetum back through the photoreceptor layer, giving it a second chance to be detected. As a result of these adaptations, horses have much better night vision than humans and are quite able to find their way around in the dark.

SELF-PROTECTION

The eyeball itself is quite tough, given shape and stiffness by the outer, fibrous **sclera**. However, the eye has delicate parts, injury to which is always a serious matter as it could spell disaster for a wild horse.

The eye has a blood supply to sustain its tissues. A dense network of blood vessels forms the **uvea**, comprising choroid, ciliary body and the iris. Several structures protect the eye. The eyelid, with its lining of conjunctiva, is perhaps the most obvious. The orbit has a strong ridge of bone, and fat in the cavity

behind the eyeball acts as a cushion. Lachrymal glands produce fluid secretion which passes through ducts to the surface of the eye, where it prevents abrasion and damage to the cornea. Tears also contain lysosyme which has an anti-bacterial effect.

Finally, horses are born with protective reflex responses (see above), although it may take several days for a neonate foal to acquire a 'menace response' to sudden movement.

HEARING AND BALANCE

Sound carries messages in a different way to light – as vibrations in the air. Sound can go around corners and carry over large distances. Horses have a well-developed sense of hearing, using it both to detect predators and in communicating with other members of the herd. Horses also readily learn to respond to vocal cues from their human handlers and riders.

HOW THE EARS WORK

The ear converts sound waves in the environment into action potentials in the auditory nerves by finely-tuned structures located inside the temporal bone of the skull.

The part of the ear we can see is the external ear, or **pinna**, which collects sound and funnels it down on to the eardrum. Within the middle ear, sound is transmitted through a series of three tiny bones (**ossicles**) – the hammer (malleus), anvil (incus) and stirrup (stapes) – to the oval window where it sets up vibrations in the cochlea.

The **cochlea** consists of a spiral canal, set in bone and filled with a fluid called endolymph. Running up the spiral is row of exquisitely sensitive 'hair cells' which synapse with the neurones of the cochlear nerve. High-pitched sounds are picked up towards the near end of the row; low-pitched sounds towards the far end. Very loud sounds initiate the tympanic reflex: the contraction of two small muscles in the middle ear which dampen sound transmission and protect the fragile cochlear mechanism.

In another part of the fluid-filled bony labyrinth of the inner ear are three semi-circular canals and a pair of sacs, the **utricle** and **saccule**. These serve the second major sensory function of the ear, which is to provide the brain with information about head movements and position, which it then uses to maintain balance.

USE OF THE EARS

Each ear can be swivelled independently through 180 degrees, or laid back, shutting it off. Such

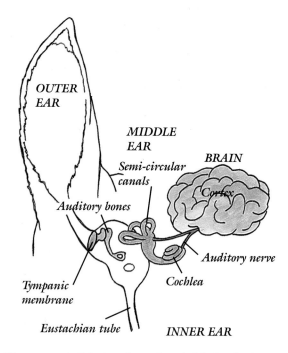

The structure of the horse's ear. Sound picked up by the tympanic membrane is transferred through vibration of the bones of the middle ear to the inner ear and cochlea and then via the auditory nerve to the brain.

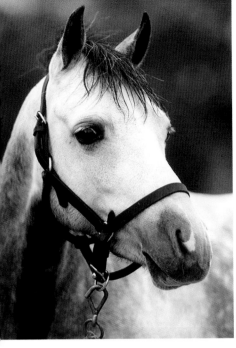

The 'Pryer reflex' enables the horse to instinctively direct his ears -either together or separately – towards the source of an interesting sound.

mobility is achieved with 16 auricular muscles attached to the base of the pinna. Humans have only three such muscles, all of which are vestigial.

Easily visible at the top of the head, a horse's ears are used to signal emotional state and intent. Laid-back ears may indicate aggression, or may simply be protection against a loud noise.

In response to directional sounds, a horse flicks an ear towards the source, or, if the sound is coming from the front, pricks both ears forward. This so-called 'Pryer reflex' improves the acuity of hearing and gives us an indication of what the horse is listening to. It also provides a way to test a horse's hearing abilities. In this way we find that their sense of hearing is somewhat better than ours. Horses can hear high-pitched tones with frequencies of 25kHz or above – almost an octave higher than we can. However, the frequencies at which sensitivity is best are much lower in horses and humans: around 2kHz and 4kHz respectively. In this middle range, horses have been shown to be capable of discriminating very small differences in tone and loudness. Yet, like us, their hearing does decline with age.

Some horses have been reported to become agitated before earthquakes. They may indeed be responding to low-frequency sound waves, but through feel rather than hearing.

Despite their evident sensitivity, horses do not react to all sounds in their environment. Clearly, a considerable amount of filtering takes place in the brain to ensure that, in general, only relevant sounds are acted upon.

What makes a sound interesting to a horse? That will depend on factors such as novelty, biological relevance and motivation. Instinctively, horses attend to vocalisations of other horses. But they may also learn to distinguish sounds which are not part of their natural repertoire. For example, horses kept next to a main road have been known to whinny in anticipation of feeding on hearing the approach of their owner's car, while totally ignoring all the other passing cars. Anything, such as wind, which hampers detection and pinpointing of sounds, can make a horse nervous and 'spooky'.

SMELL

As a horse approaches a strange object to investigate, not only are his eyes and ears directed towards it, but he also extends his head and neck to sniff with open nostrils. The equine skull evolved to be its present shape due to the need for a large set of grinding molar teeth. Having an elongated nose, however, also means there is a large surface area within the nasal cavity for detecting odours.

Smell is used to locate water, select food, and avoid predators. It is involved in aspects of social behaviour too: mares and foals recognise each other partly by smell, horses exchange breath on meeting, stallions assess the sexual status of mares and leave aromatic messages in their dung piles.

HOW THE SENSE OF SMELL WORKS

Air containing volatile substances enters the nasal passages when the horse inspires. Closer to the nostrils, the surface tissue (epithelial mucosa) contains few sensory cells and is more concerned with cleaning, warming and humidifying the air before it comes into contact with the olfactory areas. Further up, the air flows through tightly-rolled 'turbinate' bones which are over-laid with yellow-brown mucosal tissue. This is a mixture of chemo-receptor cells and supporting cells which secrete a layer of mucus, covering the epithelium.

Projecting from the peripheral end of each receptor cell are microscopic filaments which further increase the area of surface membrane available for reception of chemical stimuli. The axon of the receptor neurone join others to form the olfactory nerves, which pass through tiny holes in the ethmoid bone, converging finally on the olfactory bulbs of the brain.

In man, the olfactory epithelium is only 3-4 square cm in area; in a horse, it may be a hundred times or more larger than this. Imagine, then, the richness and importance to horses of their sense of smell!

Opening into the floor of the nasal cavity is a pair of accessory ducts that are also involved in scent sampling in horses and other domestic animals, though not in humans – the vomero-nasal organ (also called the Organ of Jacobsen). This screens the air for pheromones, chemical signals linked to specific behavioural reactions.

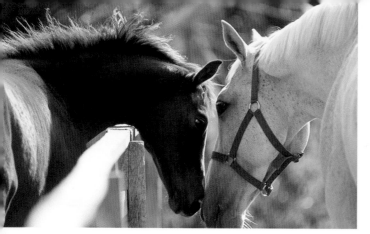

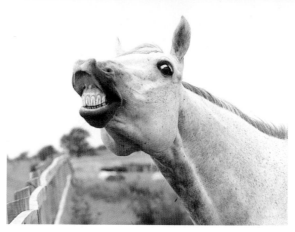

Far more sensitive than in human beings, the horse's sense of smell plays a pivotal role in feeding, reproduction and socialising. The exchange of breath on meeting is an opportunity to identify and assess the other horse.

The Flehmen response is a way of channelling intriguing smells up into the super-sensitive areas of the Jacobsen's organ, deep within the nasal passages.

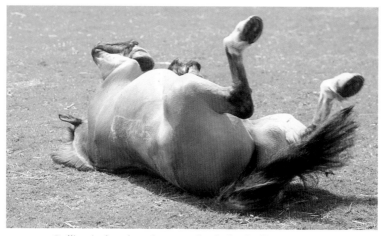

Rolling is thought to be a way for the herd's distinctive smell to be thoroughly 'ground into' the coat.a

A stallion will often curl his upper lip in the 'Flehmen' response after sniffing the urine of a mare. This is thought to facilitate the transfer of pheromones, dissolved in nasal secretion, into the vomero-nasal organ. Pungent or unusual smells may also provoke Flehmen, not only in stallions.

TASTE

Taste, also referred to as the gustatory sense, plays a significant role in survival by allowing horses to avoid ingesting unpalatable and potentially harmful food (or tainted water). Horses have to be particularly cautious about what they eat because, unlike many other animals, they are unable to vomit. How something tastes also depends on its smell, so the two senses are closely related.

HOW TASTE WORKS

In the epithelium of the mouth, chemo-receptors and supporting cells are grouped together in onion-shaped taste buds, about 0.2mm across. These occur on the soft palate and epiglottis as well as in papillae on the tongue. To stimulate the receptor cells, substances dissolved in oral fluids must reach the tiny pore of the taste bud, through which hair-like microvilli project. There they interact with the cell membrane, where they generate action potentials in sensory neurones. Relatively slow-conducting axons from the taste buds are routed via cranial nerves to unite in the medulla of the brain.

In man there are four basic taste 'modalities': sweet, sour (or acid), bitter and salty. It would be wrong to assume that the same tastes are experienced by animals: what is sweet to us may be perceived entirely differently by a horse. One can, however, find out whether horses can tell the difference between, for example, pure water and water with something added to it. Thus we know that horses can detect the above modalities, though there are variations between individuals.

It is not surprising that salt is tasted, as a deficit of sodium in the body stimulates an appetite for salt. In one study with foals, sugar solutions were preferred to tap water, supporting the notion that horses have a natural 'sweet tooth'. One notable difference between horses and humans is that horses seem to tolerate things which would taste extremely bitter to us.

VICE PREVENTION: LOWERING STRESS LEVELS

Horses are designed by evolution to spend two-thirds of their day eating, constantly on the move and in the company of others of their own kind. Unsympathetic modern management methods prevent a horse being able to fulfil his natural repertoire of behaviour and in-built urges. The abnormal and obsessive behaviours (*stereotypes*) frequently seen in stabled horses have traditionally been described as 'vices', although they in no way indicate maliciousness.

Such repetitive actions appear to provide a mechanism for the horse to cope with a situation he finds intolerably stressful yet cannot escape. Once established, these habits are difficult or impossible to eradicate even once the primary cause has been removed, and can affect the horse's ability to eat and rest properly. Prevention is clearly a better option.

Stereotyped behaviours are unknown amongst wild and free-living horses. In domestication they can readily be prevented by making greater efforts to occupy and enrich the lives of stabled horses, reducing stress levels, particularly among more nervy or anxious personalities that have low 'stress tolerance' thresholds. A relaxed horse will be both psychologically and physically healthier and easier to keep and handle.

TABLE OF STEREOTYPES & THEIR ORIGIN

Stereotypes related to:

Eating	Movement	Irritation	Social interaction
Chewing	Pacing	Box kicking	Head extension
Licking lips	Weaving	Rubbing	(nodding, with ears back)
Licking environment	Pawing	Self-mutilation	Box kicking
Crib-biting	Tail swishing	Head-tossing	
Wind-sucking	Kicking door	Head-circling	
Wind-sucking		Head-shaking	
		Head-nodding	

EATING

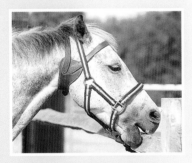

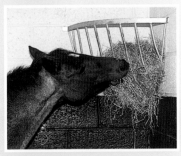

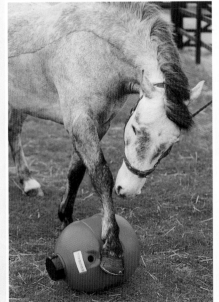

Modern high-energy feed provides a domesticated horse's nutritional requirements in a rapidly consumed and easily processed, concentrated form, leaving a stabled horse with the majority of his day with nothing to occupy his mind or digestive system. The nature of many stereotyped actions, such as wind-sucking, crib-biting (top left) and rug-tearing, reflects the horse's unfulfilled urge to chew.

A stabled horse should have access to ad lib forage (bottom left). Small-holed haynets increase eating time. Stable 'toys' such as the horseball (right), that make the horse 'work' for his concentrate ration, are useful boredom-busters. Ensuring all horses in a yard are fed at the same times each day reduces anxiety.

SOCIAL INTERACTION

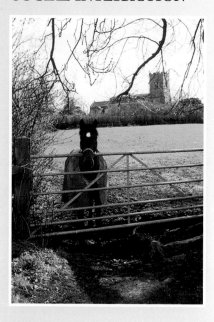

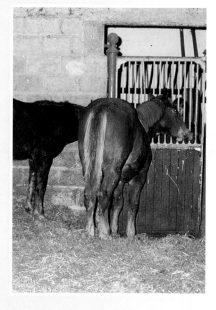

Stereotypes frequently become a habit after originating at times of trauma. Weaning that is too early, abrupt, or leaves the foal in unnecessary isolation is a typical precursor to cribbiting in later life.

Grazing companions should always be provided, ideally another equine, although any livestock is preferable to none. Stabling should be arranged so that horses in a yard are within sight of others and, preferably, are able to touch each other in safety, e.g. through dividing grilles.

Despite being a herd animal that feels intensely vulnerable when isolated, social contact is denied to many stabled horses, or those kept alone in fields. Settled friends can live together in large stables without problems. However, it should be remembered that over-crowding can also be a source of stress.

EXERCISE AND ACTIVITY

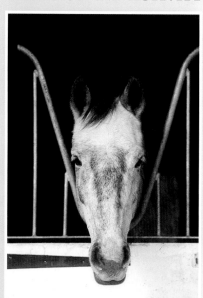

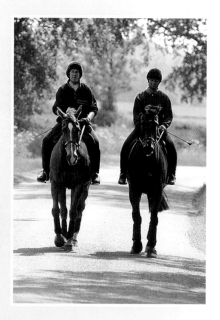

All horses should be provided with as much activity, whether ridden exercise, loose schooling or turn-out, as possible. Split exercise into several short spells a day if possible. Consider a daily total of two hours per day a minimum for a fully-stabled horse, with no days off. Stables should be as large as possible, with a high ceiling, and providing at least one accessible, interesting outlook.

A horse is psychologically programmed for continuous steady movement punctuated by bursts of energetic activity. He is naturally claustrophobic and would not freely choose to be in any enclosed space. Many domesticated horses spend 23 or more hours a day in small stables in which they can barely turn around and that allows for no 'escape options'. Exercise is strictly controlled and there is little or no opportunity for natural relaxation or play. Weaving and box-walking are typical symptoms of activity-related stress intolerance.

MEASURES OF CONTROL

Although established stereotyped behaviour can often be reduced by stress and boredom reduction, habitual 'vices' generally have to be managed rather than cured. Remove as many opportunities as possible for the horse to perform the behaviour. Weaving grilles and cribbing straps (see above and previous page) are examples of mechanical deterrents that can be used whilst addressing the background causes of the animal's distress.

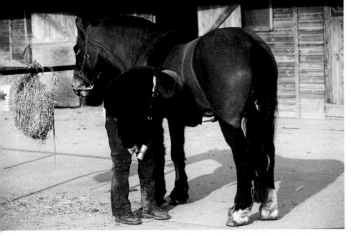

Touch plays a central role in equine social life. Most horses enjoy the sensation of sympathetic touch, although care must be taken with sensitive areas.

SKIN AND TOUCH

The skin, which will be covered in detail in the next chapter, covers the body, protecting it against injury, invasion by micro-organisms and dehydration. It participates in the control of body temperature through the cooling effect of sweating. The skin has a sensory function too: the immediate environment is felt through this medium, with sensations of touch, pressure, vibration, cold, heat and pain.

Some parts of the body surface are more sensitive than others. This is partly due to differences in thickness of coat and skin. The latter ranges from 1-6mm and is thickest where the mane grows from the neck crest and on the upper surface of the tail. Skin thickness also varies with age, sex and breed and from one individual to another. Thoroughbreds tend to have a rather thin and delicate skin, whereas draught horses have a thicker, coarser skin.

In addition, the number of sensory receptors varies from hundreds to thousands per square inch of skin on different parts of the body. Many of these receptors are simple nerve endings, while some, looking like tiny bulbs or discs, are specifically sensitive to either light or sustained touch. Tactile sensitivity is particularly great around the lips, nose and eyes, due to a higher concentration of receptors and the presence of long, stiff hairs whose follicles are surrounded by nerve endings. Whiskers are important to horses because they indicate when the nose is close to an object. They may also be used while feeding to judge textures. Shaving a horse's whiskers off just for cosmetic purposes should therefore be discouraged.

Touching plays a vital role in communication between horses, particularly between mare and foal, and in courtship. Mutual grooming helps to cement friendships within the herd. We also rely on the horse's keen tactile sense in riding, through the use of legs, seat, hands and whip. A responsive horse remains sensitive to subtle signals. On the other hand, repeated and indiscriminate use of harsh aids is likely to result in a 'hard' mouth and/or 'dead' sides, as the sense of touch becomes de-sensitised.

Horses prefer to be stroked rather than patted. Gentle stroking of certain areas of the body, such as the withers, may be used both to calm and to reward. Touching is the basis of massage therapies such as Tellington Touch and Shiatsu.

In conclusion, all the hormonal, nervous and sensory adaptations discussed in this chapter are genetically programmed and, to some extent, fixed. While a horse may learn new behaviours and skills, training can never completely overcome his innate instincts and drives. Knowledge of these systems and how they affect behaviour help us work with, rather than against, the horse.

LEARNING AND MEMORY

Throughout its life, a horse's innate abilities and instinctive responses are shaped, refined and extended by learning. Experiences perceived, using the senses described, lead to the formation of memories and lasting changes in behaviour. Sometimes, the fact that a horse has learned something is not immediately apparent, although the information may be used later (so-called 'latent learning').

Horses naturally learn best those things which are biologically relevant to them: what is dangerous and what is not, the smell and texture of good food, where to find water and shelter, who's who in the herd, sureness of foot, how to mate, or fight, or scratch those itchy spots. However, we also expect them to learn specific athletic skills, 'good manners', and how to live within the unnatural constraints we impose upon them.

Horses learn in various ways. One simple type of learning is 'habituation', in which the response to a particular stimulus becomes less and eventually ceases with repetition. Thus a horse becomes quickly de-sensitised to frequent sights and sounds which are initially alarming but turn out to be harmless. The horse may react again to the same stimulus after a long time without exposure ('spontaneous recovery'), but typically re-habituates more rapidly. Habituation may be used to get a horse accustomed to unfamiliar objects or procedures (e.g. clippers).

In 'flooding', a horse is confined or restrained so that it cannot escape while being exposed repeatedly to the stimulus, until the horse ignores the stimulus and becomes calm again. A gentler alternative is called 'progressive de-sensitisation'. Here exposure to the stimulus is carefully controlled so that the horse never becomes fearful enough to precipitate the flight reaction. This approach takes longer, but is less likely to have secondary effects on the horse's attitude to people.

Other kinds of learning involve associating between two events. In 'classical conditioning', a horse learns that a signal or cue, initially of no significance, is followed by an event or stimulus which is significant (and which produces a response). For example, in the wild, the appearance of a predator may be preceded by the alarm call of a bird. By learning this natural signal, a horse's ability to survive may be increased. In the domestic setting, a horse may similarly learn to associate the sound of buckets with feeding.

In 'operant conditioning', also known as trial and error learning, the performance of a behaviour is changed by the consequences of that behaviour, which may be pleasant or unpleasant. When a newborn foal discovers where its mother's teats are located, it is immediately rewarded with its first drink. The foal's tendency to head for a dark under-surface may be instinctive, but the most efficient ways to obtain milk are learned through trial and error. In this example, suckling behaviour is learned through 'positive reinforcement': something pleasant occurs after the initial action of sucking which makes the action more likely to occur again on future occasions. The 'something' here is the ingestion of milk, which satisfies a physiological need.

'Negative reinforcement' also increases the likelihood of an action. However, in this case the action is performed in order to escape or avoid an unpleasant or aversive stimulus. Thus a horse learns to yield to pressure applied through a halter. By moving his head in the direction of pull, he is rewarded by an instant release of pressure and regaining of comfort. With good timing, lighter and lighter contact can be learned.

In contrast, punishment is an aversive stimulus given after an action with the intention of decreasing its likelihood. It may succeed in stopping an unwanted behaviour, but in general it is an antiquated approach not well-suited to horses. It may make a fearful horse more afraid or an aggressive horse more aggressive. These emotional states are not conducive to learning.

Alternatively, a horse might habituate to repeated, ineffectual aversive stimuli. Some 'punishments', such as shouting at a horse that kicks its stable door, may actually reward the behaviour because the horse has succeeded in getting your attention. In such cases it is better to ignore the offending behaviour completely until it extinguishes itself.

In training which relies on associative learning, timing is crucial. The reward or release should be delivered as soon after the desired action as possible. If it is delayed more than a second or two, it may be useless, or worse - you may be rewarding the wrong thing. For this reason, verbal praise, stroking or some other signal (such as a click) may be used as 'secondary reinforcers' which can be given in a more precisely timed way. They may bridge the delay between the action and the primary reward (usually a treat), or may substitute for food if perceived as pleasant. Rewarding every time ('continuous reinforcement') is useful in the early stages of training. However, if the rewards stop so does the trained behaviour, a process called 'extinction'. By rewarding only once every few successful attempts ('intermittent reinforcement') extinction is reduced and the lesson retained for longer.

Teaching a horse a complex skill, such as jumping, is made easier by 'shaping'. This involves reinforcing successive approximations, a step at a time, towards the final goal. Sequences of actions can be taught by 'chaining' simpler actions together.

Horses may learn through imitation, though convincing scientific evidence for this is lacking. However, some learning, such as the location of water, may be facilitated by following and watching other horses. It is no longer thought that vices such as cribbing and weaving are acquired through imitation.

Studies of learning in horses have revealed aspects of memory, as well as sensory and other cognitive abilities. For example, one horse learned to obtain a food reward by picking the correct choice in each of 20 pairs of patterns. At the end of the training period, the horse's performance with four of the pairs was perfect, and even the 'hardest' pair was discriminated correctly 73 per cent of the time. A year later, the horse showed hardly any memory loss. Not all horses do equally well at such tests, though a poorer performance might indicate an individual was simply less motivated, rather than a lack of innate ability. Despite all the research done to date, we still have much to learn about the horse's mind.

DISORDERS OF THE NERVOUS AND ENDOCRINE SYSTEMS

Neurological disease in the horse may show in a variety of ways including alterations in behaviour, seizures and fits, facial abnormalities, locomotory difficulties and paralyses. Often financial constraints and welfare considerations will dictate a gloomy outlook. Despite this, many conditions can now be diagnosed and treated and in some cases spectacular and rewarding outcomes result.

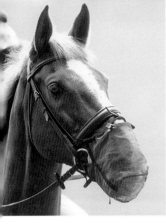

Head-shaking is a notoriously difficult condition to treat. Some horses find relief through the use of a fine mesh nose net.

CHANGES IN BEHAVIOUR
STABLE 'VICES'

So-called 'stable vices', such as weaving, crib-biting, head-nodding etc., are discussed in the section on stereotypic behaviour on pages 153-154.

HEAD-SHAKING

This may be involuntary or voluntary, causing the horse to shake its whole head or its nose or to sneeze repeatedly.

Cause: Causes can include flies, poorly-fitting tack, ear mites, harvest mites, sensitivity to ultra-violet light, rhinitis, sinusitis, skin and dental problems. Head-shaking is notoriously difficult to diagnose and most often no cause is identified.

Treatment: Ecto-parasiticides, fly control measures, nose nets and ear drops. Surgery to de-sensitise the facial nerves may help some cases.

SELF-MUTILATION SYNDROME

Cause: This generally occurs in stallions and is thought to be associated with confinement and isolation.

Treatment: Suggested treatments include increasing exercise, minimising stress and providing suitable animal companions, preferably equine.

NARCOLEPSY/CATAPLEXY

A rare syndrome where sleep occurs at inappropriate times. The animal falls to the ground and loses all tone and reflexes. No abnormalities can be detected between episodes.

Cause: Narcolepsy may be associated with restraint, feeding and change in environment.

Treatment: The condition is generally treated with the administration of stimulants.

TRAUMA

Cause: Injury to the brain and spinal cord occurs during accidental falls, collisions, falling over backward and direct blows (e.g. kicks). These may result in fractures with swelling and compression of nervous tissue.

Signs: Signs exhibited are dependent upon the neuro-anatomic location and the severity and extent of damage, but may include wandering, depression,

head tilt, circling, blindness, in-coordination and sudden death.

Treatment: The principles are to reduce swelling with the use of anti-inflammatory and diuretic drugs. Sedation is important for seizures, and supportive care such as deep-litter bedding and providing small moist feeds will aid recovery. If no or little response is observed, euthanasia may be needed.

HEPATIC ENCEPHALOPATHY

Cause: Hepatic encephalopathy is associated with liver failure, most commonly due to ragwort poisoning, although other causes have included fungal toxins, congenital diseases and liver infections.

Signs: Weight loss, depression, anorexia, yawning, sunburn over white and thinly-haired areas, weakness, laryngeal paralysis causing a rasping respiration, head pressing and in-coordination, progressing to recumbency and coma.

Treatment: The outlook is often hopeless if signs are advanced. Treatment should be directed at the underlying disease and at reducing the neurological signs.

SEIZURES AND FITS

NEONATAL MALADJUSTMENT SYNDROME

See Chapter Ten.

MENINGITIS

Cause: Common clinical signs include fever and loss of appetite, a stiff neck, convulsions, facial tremors, blindness, oscillating pupils, behavioural changes, weakness and recumbency, leading to coma.

Signs: Common in neo-natal foals receiving an inadequate intake of colostrum, or poor-quality colostrum if the mare suffered from a systemic disease or metritis whilst pregnant.

Treatment: Intensive antibiotic therapy and plasma transfusion. Sedation if patient is fitting, and supportive therapy including heat lamps and feeding by hand.

EPILEPSY

This condition is very rare and is poorly-documented in the horse, but may occur in some ponies and Arabians.

Cause: Metabolic disorders (Cushing's Disease, liver and kidney disease), trauma, inflammation, infection (e.g. parasite migration), vascular disorders (e.g. following an intra-carotid injection),

toxicity (e.g. poisoning from snail bait or organophosphates) or drug reaction.
Treatment: Treatment should be aimed at the underlying causes. Sedation may be required if seizures are severe.

HEAD TILT AND FACIAL ABNORMALITIES

HORNER'S SYNDROME
Cause: This is due to damage to a specific nerve known as the cervical sympathetic trunk. Damage may occur at any point along its pathway from the thorax, shoulder, neck and skull. More common causes include guttural pouch infections, abscesses in the neck, tumours in the thorax and injection damage.
Signs: Signs are usually one-sided and include a constricted pupil, protrusion of the third eyelid, a drooping eyelid and patchy sweating on the head and neck.
Treatment: Treatment is dependent upon cause.

FACIAL NERVE PARALYSIS
Cause: Guttural pouch infections, trauma to face and skull or inner-ear infection.
Signs: Asymmetry of the face, with an inability to close the eyelids or to move the lip or ear, and the drooling of saliva.
Treatment: Dependent upon cause, but if keratitis is present eye-drops will be required.

TRIGEMINAL NERVE TRAUMA
Cause: Trauma (dislocated jaw), parasitic migration, polyneuritis equi.
Signs: 'Dropped jaw' appearance (if bilateral), quidding, atrophy of the cheek muscles.
Treatment: The horse may need assistance in feeding, soft feeds and feeding from a height.

VESTIBULAR LESIONS
Vestibular disease can be divided into central or peripheral conditions, depending upon the site of the damage – in the brain or in the inner-ear respectively.
Cause: Extension of infection from guttural pouch, polyneuritis equi, traumatic fractures of the skull or septic meningitis (only with central vestibular disease).
Signs: Damage to these areas will result in in-coordination, head tilt, oscillating pupils, circling and falling over. A horse with central vestibular disease will also show depression, fever and loss of

appetite, ataxia and weakness and, eventually, recumbency. Symptoms of peripheral vestibular disease include ataxia (but without depression), facial nerve paralysis, and possible deafness.
Treatment: Dependent on cause.

WEAKNESS AND INCO-ORDINATION (ATAXIA)

CEREBELLAR HYPOPLASIA/ABIOTROPHY
Cause: A lack of brain tissue, generally affecting Arabian and Arabian-cross horses. A hereditary/familial relationship is suggested.
Signs: Signs generally begin at a few weeks or months of age and are progressive. Ataxia may vary from slight incoordination to complete dysfunction. There may be a stiff gait (but without weakness), hyperflexion of limbs, and head tremors. Clinical signs are accentuated by stimulation.
Treatment: None is available, although many foals will accommodate the problem.

BOTULISM
Cause: Usually associated with feeding poor-quality silage contaminated by toxins produced by *Clostridium botulinum*.
Signs: Difficulty eating due to paralysis of the muscles of chewing and swallowing. Flaccid muzzle and lips, pharyngeal paralysis and progressive muscle paralysis leading to trembling and recumbency, respiratory arrest and death.
Treatment: Remove the horse from suspected feed. Administer botulism antitoxin. Careful nursing (feeding by stomach tube, fluids etc.) will be required. Avoid excessive stimulation.

SPINAL CORD TRAUMA
Cause: A common neurological condition, particularly in horses that can attain high speeds. In adults the most frequent sites of damage are the head-neck joints, the base of the neck and the mid-back. In foals, mid-neck and mid-back fractures are commonly associated with falls.
Signs: Usually has a sudden onset with possible wounds, swellings and pain on palpation. The precise signs shown depend upon the site of the trauma. See Chapter Nine.
Treatment: Some cases will recover spontaneously. In those acutely affected, anti-inflammatories may be given. If the animal is unable to stand after several days or shows obvious distress, euthanasia may be the best option.

VERTEBRAL BODY ABSCESS/ OSTEOMYELITIS

Cause: Most cases appear in young animals and are associated with spread of infection from a site distant from the vertebrae via the bloodstream. Others are linked with wounds, injection abscesses, etc.

Signs: Two syndromes may present, either where there is direct compression of the spinal cord or where erosion of the bone and meninges occurs. In spinal cord compression the neurological signs mimic spinal trauma. Cases only occasionally have fever, depression, pain, heat and swelling over the site. With bone and meningeal cases there is hyper-sensitivity, spastic muscle contractions and recurrent sweating.

Treatment: Long-term (two to three month) antibiotic therapy. Surgical removal of necrotic bone and drainage of abscesses has been recommended, although this is difficult owing to the inaccessibility of the vertebral column.

CERVICAL VERTEBRAL MALFORMATION AND INSTABILITY ('WOBBLER' SYNDROME)

Cause: 'Wobbler syndrome' is commonly seen in young, fast-growing horses, especially Thoroughbreds and warmbloods. The clinical signs seen are due to stenosis (narrowing) of the cervical vertebral canal. Two types of stenosis may occur: static or dynamic. Static stenosis occurs where bony changes result in narrowing of the vertebral canal. In dynamic stenosis, narrowing results from flexion or extension of the neck. In addition, further developmental abnormalities of the bone and cartilage in the axial and appendicular skeleton may be found.

Signs: The most obvious sign is a clumsy ('tin soldier') walk, involving primarily hind-limb in-coordination and weakness although the fore-limbs may be involved. Knuckling, stumbling, scuffing of toes, crossing over of limbs, excessive sway of the pelvis can also be shown. The forelimbs often appear stiff.

Treatment: No treatment is universally regarded as successful. Rare recovery has been noted with short-term corticosteroid therapy and prolonged box rest. Successful surgical intervention has been used on a limited number of cases with mild signs. This might best be considered only in those required as breeding animals.

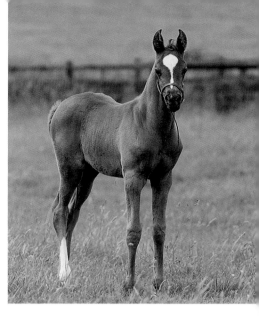

'Wobbler syndrome' is most commonly seen in fast-growing Thoroughbred and warm-blood youngsters.

EQUINE DEGENERATIVE MYELOENCEPHALOPATHY

Cause: A progressive degenerative disease of the spinal cord. A familial predisposition has been reported, although a lack of access to green forage (vitamin E) is necessary to produce the disease. The exact cause is unknown.

Signs: This condition primarily results in ataxia in young horses (three months to two years old). Signs affect all four limbs, with the hind limbs often being the worst affected. Ataxia and weakness, knuckling, stumbling and stiffness are frequently found.

Treatment: Supplementing vitamin E has been tried, although signs generally are irreversible and euthanasia is the usual outcome. Prevention is through supplying plenty of fresh, green forage.

GRASS SICKNESS/EQUINE DYSAUTONOMIA

A devastating disease with mortality rates of over 90 per cent. The clinical signs are related to dysfunction of the gastro-intestinal tract. See Chapter Three.

STRINGHALT

An involuntary, exaggerated flexion of one or both hind limbs.

Cause: The exact cause of stringhalt symptoms is unknown. Signs are usually sporadic, although outbreaks in Australia have been associated with grazing dandelion. Possible fungal toxin.

Signs: Flexion may be mild to marked and signs can be exaggerated by turning and backing.

Treatment: Mild cases still perform quite well. If severe, surgical muscle resection may result in variable degrees of improvement.

SHIVERING

Involuntary muscular movement (shivering) of hind limbs and tail. Occasionally the fore-limbs and face are affected.

Signs: The horse has great difficulty backing and may

not be able to. The hind limbs may flex, be held out to the side, then tremble and relax back to the ground.

Sometimes the early history indicates difficulty in lifting a hind limb for shoeing.

Cause: The cause is unknown, but may be due to a muscle disorder. There is a possible relationship between shivering and stringhalt.

Treatment: None is available.

TUMOURS

CUSHING'S DISEASE
Ponies seem most susceptible to this condition, which commonly affects older animals.

Cause: Usually a benign tumour affecting the pituitary gland at the base of the brain, which produces extra chemical messengers that confuse the rest of the body - in particular the adrenal gland. In Cushing's Syndrome, the adrenal glands themselves are affected.

Signs: Early stages are easily overlooked or attributed to general old age, as the disease often comes on gradually.

- excessive thirst
- excessive urination
- weight loss and muscle wastage, despite increased appetite
- pot-bellied/sway-backed appearance
- abnormally long and 'curly' coat, which may not be shed in summer
- abnormal sweating
- persistent infections, often involving the skin, feet or respiration
- lethargy/dullness
- laminitis
- mares not in-foal producing milk.

Treatment: The typical signs usually lead to diagnosis, though blood and urine tests will rule out other possibilities such as kidney disease or diabetes. Careful management can reduce the impact, e.g. clipping, appropriate feeding, rigorous hygiene and good foot care. There is no cure and surgery is rarely an option due to age. Drugs to control the pituitary gland problem are expensive but often bring rapid improvement.

PARALYSIS

TETANUS
A toxaemia (poisoning) produced by the anaerobic bacterium *Clostridium tetani* that attacks the nervous system, tetanus is a major threat to domesticated animals world-wide. Most cases prove fatal. Horses are particularly vulnerable due to their susceptibility to cuts, nail pricks etc. Tetanus is totally avoidable through preventative vaccination.

Cause: Clostriduim tetani bacteria live in the soil and manure where they are long-lived and highly-resistant to disinfectant. The bacteria enters a wound (frequently a puncture wound to the foot) and may lie dormant for up to four months until conditions are suitable for spores to multiply and produce toxin. New-born foals are particularly at risk from infection through the umbilicus.

Signs: Characterised by spasmodic muscle contractions over the whole body. The third eyelid comes partially across the eyes, the horse typically has a forward-thrust neck and raised tail. It has difficulty taking in food and chewing and getting up once down. Stiffness generally leads to convulsions and death in over 80 percent of cases.

Treatment and prevention: Seek immediate veterinary attention. Stable horse in darkened stable with deep bed, give soft, moist food and handle as little as possible. Spasms can be lessened with drugs. If an unvaccinated horse suffers a wound vulnerable to infection, an anti-toxin can be given to give temporary protection for two weeks. Regular vaccination with tetanus anti-serum (see Chapter Two) gives permanent protection and should be considered essential for all horses (foals can be vaccinated at 3-4 months of age).

SUPRA-SCAPULAR NERVE PARALYSIS ('SWEENEY')
See Chapter Four.

RADIAL NERVE PARALYSIS
Cause: Trauma to the shoulder region. Radial nerve paralysis can be associated with recumbency, first rib and humeral fractures. Multiple nerves to the fore-limb, in the brachial plexus, are usually damaged but signs of radial nerve paralysis predominate.

Signs: The horse is unable to extend the limb and flex the shoulder. The elbow is dropped and unable to bear weight.

Treatment: As for Sweeney.

PERONEAL NERVE PARALYSIS
Cause: Trauma to the lateral femur and stifle.

Signs: Knuckling at fetlock and pastern, hyper-extension of the hock and tripping.

Treatment: As above.

FOALING PARESIS

Cause: Femur fractures, dislocated hip or difficult foalings.

Signs: The foal sinks or is unable to stand on its hind limbs.

Treatment: As above. Provide deep bedding with firm footing.

POLYNEURITIS EQUI/CAUDA EQUINE NEURITIS

Cause: The cause is unknown, but is thought to be an allergic response, possibly associated with EHV. The condition occurs mainly in mature horses.

Signs: Signs are variable, dependent upon which nerve roots are involved.

There is usually a sudden observation of insensitivity around the perineum and progressive numbing, leading to paralysis of tail, bladder, rectum and anal sphincter. This leads to faecal incontinence, constipation, urinary incontinence, and in males, a protruded, relaxed penis. There can also be cranial nerve involvement, leading to signs dependent upon the nerves involved, but which may include atrophy of cheek muscles, facial paralysis, keratitis and corneal ulcers.

Treatment: Corticosteroids and supportive care (fluid therapy, manual evacuation of bladder and rectum) may be tried since progression is slow, but eventually all cases need to be euthanased.

SACRAL TRAUMA

Cause: Most cases follow an accident where the horse has reared up and fallen onto its rump, causing a mid-sacrum fracture (see Chapter Ten).

Signs: Symptoms involve the tail, anus, rectum and bladder as for polyneuritis equi but without any cranial nerve involvement.

Treatment: As for polyneuritis equi, above.

DISORDERS OF THE EYE

Eye disease is relatively common in horses, with traumatic and infectious problems being found most frequently. Disorders of the eye are understandably of great concern to the owner, for both aesthetic and functional reasons. More importantly, and more so, than in any other domesticated animal, devastating complications can occur.

ENTROPION

Signs: Inversion of the lower eyelid(s) margins. This is a relatively common and usually self-correcting disorder in foals and may be bilateral or unilateral.

Entropion produces signs of ocular irritation, excessive tears and photophobia (aversion to light) within a few days of birth.

Treatment: Most cases resolve with therapy, which may be as simple as eversion (turning out) of the lower eyelid. In more severe cases, surgical correction is required.

EYELID LACERATIONS

Cause: Tears and lacerations to the eyelids are very common and are generally caused by the horse rubbing its eyes on objects.

Treatment: Precise surgical repair is required. If left to heal on their own, the margins may distort, causing chronic corneal irritation.

CONJUNCTIVITIS

Cause: Wind and dust, fly irritation, trauma, invasion by a foreign body, bacterial infection and respiratory virus infection are common causes.

Signs: Pain, excessive tear production, redness and/or swelling of the conjunctiva and discharge from the eye.

Treatment: Regular topical application of antibiotics.

CORNEAL ABRASIONS AND ULCERS

Causes: Traumatic damage to the cornea, followed by bacterial infection. Infected corneal ulcers should be considered a medical emergency owing to their rapid progression and serious prognosis.

Signs: Pain, tear production, photophobia, ulceration (white/yellowish opacity), loss of ocular transparency and redness.

Treatment: Immediate antibiotic therapy must be repeated at hourly intervals. Attempts to prevent progression of the ulcer should be made using either topical or anti-collagenase treatments. Surgery is usually indicated. Anti-inflammatory and mydriatic (pupillary dilating) drugs should be used to alleviate pain and prevent the progression to uveitis (see below).

KERATITIS

This describes inflammation of the cornea.

Causes: Keratitis is usually due to superficial bacterial or fungal infections.

Signs: Pain, photophobia and excessive tear production.

Treatment: Topical antibiotic or anti-fungal therapy is effective for superficial infections. Pain should be managed by use of pupillary dilators together with anti-inflammatory drugs. Anti-collagenase therapy is essential if there is serious ulceration.

UVEAL DISORDERS

This describes inflammation of the uveal tract (iris, ciliary body and choroid).

Cause: This may occur as a primary or secondary disorder. Secondary disorders causing uveitis include keratitis, corneal ulceration or corneal trauma. Primary causes are more common although the exact causes are often unknown. Most are thought to be immune mediated, possibly a hypersensative reaction to bacteria (e.g. leptospira) or worms *(Onchocerca cervicalis)*.

Signs: This is the most common uveal disease of horses. It may affect one or both eyes, and may have quiet periods interspersed with periods of acute inflammation, resulting in progressive loss of vision. Pain, eyelids closed in discomfort, photophobia, excessive tear production, cloudy eye, redness ('ciliary flush') at the junction between the transparent cornea and white sclera, pupillary constriction, adhesions (synechiae) between the iris and cornea or between the iris and lens are commonly found abnormalities. Inflammation usually lasts 7-10 days and intervals between attacks are extremely variable (days, months or years). Over time, the retina degenerates, cataracts form and shrinkage of the eyeball occurs.

Treatment: Uveitis should be considered a medical emergency and intensive anti-inflammatory and pupillary dilator therapy should be initiated. Hospitalisation should be considered due to the need for concentrated treatments. Treatments should be continued at least three weeks beyond the remission of clinical signs. Recurrence is highly likely and anti-inflammatory therapy should be re-started as soon as clinical signs appear.

CATARACTS

Cataracts are an opacity (scarring) of the lens or its capsule. Congenital forms are more common than those acquired as a result of injury, uveitis or old age. The size can vary from a tiny pinpoint, to coverage of the entire lens.

Signs: Generally, if the cataract is local and small, no adverse signs are found. If large, vision can be reduced.

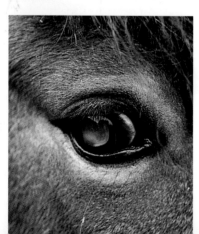

Corneal ulcers or uveitis will produce progressive clouding of the eye.

Treatment: Cataract surgery is usually only attempted in foals. In acquired cases, surgery is often difficult and has unsatisfactory results.

RETINAL DISEASE

Causes and signs: Disorders of the retina are rare in the horse, although a number of congenital and acquired (usually viral) conditions can affect vision. Most show little abnormality in the external appearance of the eye, but the animal has problems with night vision or displays true blindness.

Treatment: There is no effective treatment, but an accurate diagnosis is necessary for a prognosis to be given.

OPTIC NERVE DISEASE

Causes and signs: Problems with the optic nerve are rare, with no external signs of ocular disease, but various degrees of disturbance to vision are found. The most common cause of blindness due to optic nerve disease is head trauma.

Treatment: There is no treatment aside from treatment for head trauma.

SARCOIDS

Although not strictly ocular, these can affect the upper eyelid and their physical presence may cause problems. See Chapter Seven.

SQUAMOUS CELL CARCINOMA

Causes and signs: These common tumours of the horse may be found in a number of regions, but in the eye occur on the conjunctiva, the third eyelid and the limbus (the junction between cornea and sclera). Affected eyes usually discharge pus, due to irritation.

Treatment: Numerous treatments have been tried including surgery, cryosurgery and radiation therapy.

LYMPHOSARCOMA

Causes and signs: Usually associated with other systemic disease, owing to widespread invasion of further tissues by the tumour.

Treatment: Treatment is usually hopeless.

PSEUDO-TUMOURS

Causes and signs: Any space-occupying lesion behind the eye can cause the eye to protrude. In fat horses and ponies, ocular fat can herniate around the eye producing a smooth swelling.

Treatment: Surgical removal is successful.

7 THE SKIN

THE STRUCTURE AND FUNCTION OF THE SKIN

The skin is the largest and one of the most fascinating organs in the horse's body. For a start, it is the only organ we can actually see! Skin has over a dozen vital roles to play. Its most critical role is in maintaining a barrier separating horse from outside world, thus preventing loss of water and salts on the one hand and excluding harmful chemical, physical and microbial agents on the other.

GENERAL FUNCTIONS OF THE SKIN

Protective barrier
Hair and hoof production
Temperature regulation
Vitamin D production
Storage of essential nutrients
Production of glandular secretions
Elimination of waste products
Immune system regulation
Anti-microbial action
Pigment production and protection from the sun
Provision of shape and form
Perception of touch, pressure, pain, itch and heat.

The skin broadly contains two layers: the outer **epidermis**, itself consisting of five or six layers, and an inner **dermis** made up of fibres, cells, hair follicles, glands, blood and lymph vessels and nerves. A chemical gel, known as 'ground substance', binds the dermis together, allowing passage of salts, nutrients and cells from dermal blood vessels into the epidermis. The epidermis has no blood supply itself and is therefore dependent on the dermis for delivery of essential items. Cells in the dermis are involved in processes such as inflammation, immune system regulation and production of various pigments and fibres.

Skin contains the follicles which produce hair; production and the maintenance of a healthy coat is, of course, very important to horses and their owners. Hair does not grow constantly but in phases. A hair is produced in the growing (anagen) phase. The follicle then passes into a resting (telogen) phase and all growth stops. With time, the follicle reverts back again to the anagen phase and a new hair is formed. As new hair emerges, old ones are lost.

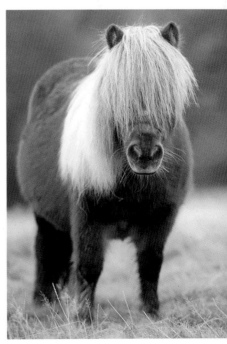

In the spring and autumn the coat is shed and new hair growth takes place. In preparation for winter conditions, longer temporary hair grows to cover the finer, shorter and denser under-coat. Differences between breeds reflect their environmental origins: draft and pony breeds are capable of growing remarkably effective protection against the most extreme weather.

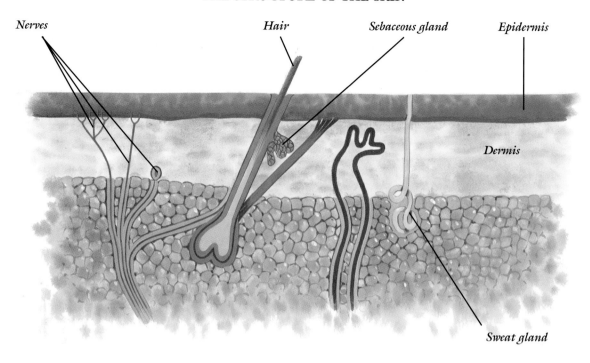

A horse has two patterns of hair growth: body hair growth which is periodically synchronised resulting in seasonal shedding, and mane and tail hair growth which is not synchronised and consequently does not produce seasonal shedding.

DISORDERS OF THE SKIN

This section is problem-oriented, with conditions discussed according to what owners see, e.g. irritation, weals, crusting and scaling, nodules. There are many mechanisms of disease production but most skin diseases are believed to arise through one or more of the following mechanisms:

- development of allergic reactions (to foods and food additives, medications or to substances in the external environment such as dust and forage mites, pollens and moulds)
- infection by micro-organisms such as bacteria, fungi and viruses
- infestation by parasites
- cancer formation
- auto-immune reactions which result in the horse's immune system turning on itself and destroying its own tissues
- irritant reactions (to toxic or caustic substances in the environment)
- dietary deficiency
- internal metabolic upset.

Like all animals, horses can react differently to the same disease process. This means that precise clinical signs may differ from one horse to another, so identical signs may well not be seen in horses given the same diagnosis. Equally, two horses which appear to have the same signs may have very different disorders.

PRURITUS (ITCHING OR IRRITATION)

Horses usually show pruritus by biting or rubbing themselves. Many pruritic conditions are caused by allergies or parasitic infestations.

INSECT-BITE HYPERSENSITIVITY (SWEET ITCH)

Incidence of sweet itch is seasonal, occurring between March and October depending on geographical location. The condition typically starts from horse's second summer onwards and may worsen with age. It is non-contagious – only one or a few out of a group of horses are normally affected.

Cause: Allergy to bites of midges and other insects.

Signs: There is mild to severe irritation resulting in rubbing of mane, tail and elsewhere. Self-trauma leads to crusting, scaling, hair loss, bleeding, skin-thickening and ridging. The horse or pony is understandably very restless.

Treatment: Diagnosis is usually based on the horse or pony's history and clinical signs, but intra-dermal allergy testing may be necessary to identify specific reactions. Treatment with steroids is cheap and very effective at reducing or even eliminating irritation, at least in the earlier years of the condition. However, these carry risks of short and long-term side-effects, including laminitis, increased thirst and urination, altered hormonal balance, increased susceptibility to infection, liver and kidney abnormalities, mood changes and many others, and so are best avoided if possible.

Alternative therapies include antihistamines (less effective and more expensive than steroids but less likely to cause serious side-effects), avoidance of insect-infested areas (draining ditches and ponds and moving an affected horse away from forests, rivers and streams) and protective stabling at certain times of the day (midges are most active around dusk) combined with insect repellents, hoods and all-over body sheets, mane and tail guards and sand-fly netting. Evening primrose and fish-oil supplements have helped some horses and regular use of shampoos may be soothing. Some people advocate homoeopathy, black box radionics and acupuncture.

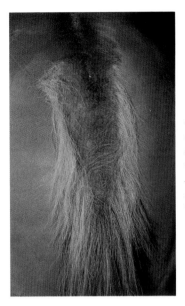

The intense irritation caused by sweet itch can result in large areas of hair being rubbed off and the skin broken. The crest and dock are usually worst affected.

PREVENTION AND MANAGEMENT OF SWEET ITCH

Precautions should be taken from early spring to help prevent problems becoming established in at-risk animals.

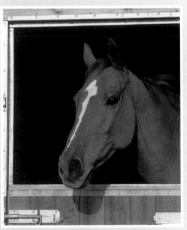

◀ *Stable horse at high-risk times of day when midges are most active, i.e. early morning and evening (until dark). Risk is reduced around mid-day. Stable away from muck heap. Windows and doors can be fitted with mosquito netting or an electric fan used to increase air movement.*

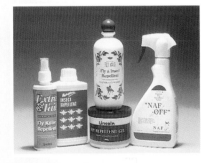

▲ *Apply an effective insecticide to kill midges on the horse before the feed. Treat the whole horse, as bites can occur anywhere. Follow manufacturer's instructions regarding frequency of application. Fly repellent measures, e.g. sprays, lotions or tags, should also be used daily as a deterrent. Supplements with insect repellent properties added to the feed e.g. garlic, can help.*

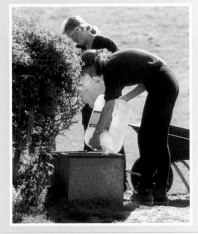

◀ *Use an open, breezy field for turning out. Avoid pasture containing ditches, ponds or rivers. Keep troughs scrupulously clean.*

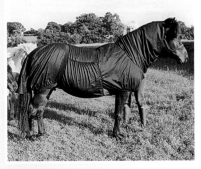

◀ *All-over clothing like this Boett blanket, can prevent midges getting to the skin, allowing affected horses and ponies to enjoy spring and summer at grass.*

FOOD ALLERGY

When an allergic reaction to a food is suspected, typically only one out of a group of horses will be affected. This may occur all year round unless a particular item is fed seasonally, and may start at any age. Reactions can develop to foods that have been eaten for years without problems.

Cause: Abnormal reaction to any food or food additive.

Signs: Irritation (either localised or generalised) and urticaria may occur either together or alone. Any type of skin lesion may develop.

Treatment: Involves identifying and avoiding the incriminated food substances. Diagnosis can be helped by an elimination diet of hay, silage or haylage only for at least three to six weeks, followed by challenge with full previous diet.

CONTACT DERMATITIS

Contact dermatitis can occur anywhere on the body. It may involve allergy (allergic contact dermatitis typically affects only one horse in a group) or straight irritation (irritant contact dermatitis often affects more than one horse exposed to the irritant substance). Dyes, preservatives, soaps, medications, insect repellents, plants, bedding, blankets and even excretory products may be incriminated. Moisture (e.g. rain, sweat, mud) may promote contact dermatitis as it decreases the efficacy of the normal skin barrier and increases the intimacy of contact between the agent and skin surface. Horses kept in wet or muddy environment, often develop contact dermatitis on the lower limbs.

Cause: Contact with irritant substances on horse or in its environment.

Signs: Irritation occurs in localised areas, e.g. lower limbs, backs of hind limbs, under tack. There may

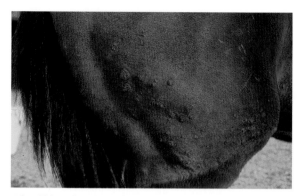

Identifying the trigger factor in a case of urticaria may or may not be easy!

be rubbing, crusting, scaling, bleeding, hair loss, skin-thickening and white hair formation.

Treatment: The cause needs to be identified and avoided and the area shampooed regularly with a medicated product. Steroid administration (creams, tablets, injections) may be indicated.

PARASITIC INFESTATIONS

PEDICULOSIS (LOUSE INFESTATION)

Lice are obligatory host-specific parasites. This means that they can only live and breed on their one host species. Horse lice cannot live on people or species other than horses or donkeys. The most common variety is *Werneckiella*, which prefers the neck, withers and tail head but may also be seen over the entire trunk. It feeds on surface scale and general skin debris. *Haematopinus asini* is less common but may be found all over the head, neck, trunk, axillae, groin and tail, and feeds on tissue fluids. Transmission of lice is by direct and indirect contact. Indirect contact may arise through a horse brushing against a post or tree (or person!) on

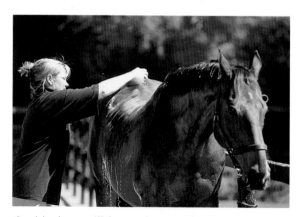

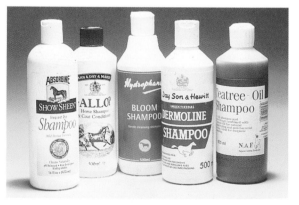

Sensitive horses will frequently react adversely to chemicals within shampoos and other coat preparations. Use only products specifically designed for horses.

which lice have previously been deposited by an infested horse. Typically, lice can survive off the horse for about seven days. Horses are affected mostly in winter, when skin and hair temperature is lower, and animals are housed indoors. High temperatures are fatal to lice.

Cause: Infestation with *Werneckiella, Damalinia equi* (biting louse) or *Haematopinus asini* (sucking louse).

Signs: Severe irritation, self-inflicted skin damage, shaggy coat, crusting, scaling and hair loss. Anaemia (see Chapter Five) may accompany heavy infestations of sucking lice.

Treatment: Diagnosis of louse infestation is based on clinical signs and demonstration of the lice or eggs (known as nits). Adult lice have six legs and are about 2 mm long. Nits are about 1-2 mm long and attach to hairs by a sticky substance secreted by the female. Good lighting and a magnifying glass are useful!

Insecticidal sprays, washes and powders are available. Therapy may need to be repeated weekly for at least three to four weeks to kill off lice from hatching eggs. Owners must follow the manufacturers' recommendations and instructions.

CHORIOPTIC MANGE

Chorioptes is a very superficial parasitic mite that feeds on surface debris. The mange infestation is usually easy to demonstrate. It can be transferred directly or indirectly, and heavily-feathered horses are particularly susceptible. Groups of horses are often affected.

Cause: Chorioptes equi infestation.

Signs: Severe irritation, self-trauma, crusting, scaling and hair loss especially on the fetlocks and lower limbs.

Treatment: Multiple skin scrapings taken from affected areas and examined microscopically will confirm the diagnosis. The hair must be clipped away and skin washed or sprayed with suitable preparation. All in-contact horses must be treated until several weeks after regression of the lesions. Bedding should be burnt and stables and tack thoroughly disinfected.

WEALS

Weals are well-defined fluid swellings that pit with pressure. No change in the overlying skin or hair coat is usually produced by a weal.

URTICARIA (NETTLE RASH, HIVES)

Of all the domestic species, the horse has the greatest prevalence of urticaria. Although it is often discussed as such, this is not a specific disease but a reaction pattern with many different causes. There is no age, breed or sex predisposition.

Cause: Foods, food additives, drugs, medications, pollens, moulds, mites, bites and stings, vaccinations, illnesses, stress, heat, cold, pressure, exercise, saddle soaps, leather conditioners, tack cleaners, preservatives, and just about anything else!

Signs: Localised or generalised weals that pit with pressure. There is variable irritation – many affected horses are not at all itchy and seem completely unconcerned. The condition may develop within minutes or hours of the eliciting factor, or days later. Weals may occur anywhere on the body but especially on face, neck and trunk. The legs and lower abdomen may swell. In severe cases, the horse may go into shock or respiratory distress.

Treatment: The trigger factor must be identified and avoided. Steroids or antihistamines will help signs subside. Whereas mild cases may last for several hours and resolve without treatment, chronic episodes may last for months. It is often difficult to identify the trigger, and recurrence is common. In North America, antigen injections are sometimes given after testing. This is useful in horses where the trigger cannot be found and removed.

CRUSTING AND SCALING

A scale is an accumulation of loose fragments or flakes of the outer layer of skin. A crust can be described as a mixture of scale, blood, cells, pus and sometimes medication at the skin surface. All conditions that cause itch and irritation can produce crusting and scaling.

FUNGAL DISEASES

DERMATOPHYTOSIS (RINGWORM)

Dermatophytosis is a more accurate term than the more commonly used 'ringworm', which leads to frequent misinterpretation by owners believing the condition to be caused by a worm and always to involve circular lesions.

The fungus is highly contagious to horses, to other animals and to people. Young horses under four years, fed a poor diet and living in dirty surroundings with little or no exposure to ultraviolet light, are perhaps most at risk. Adult horses are less likely to become infected and may recover more quickly.

The condition may affect only one or many animals in an exposed group and usually resolves without treatment within one to four months.

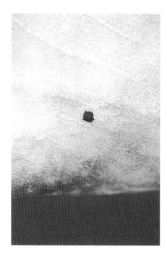

A typical ringworm lesion, here in the girth area.

Cause: Infection by dermatophyte fungi. Transmission is by direct contact with infected animals and also from contact with hair and scale or fungal elements in the environment. Fence posts, soil, trees, shoes, hands, tack, cleaning brushes, clippers and bedding and other items may become contaminated. Poor grooming, leaving sweat on the skin, gives the fungus a good food source.
Signs: Lesions may occur anywhere but especially in sweat areas (girth and saddle). There is a variable clinical appearance. Typically, small spots progress to thick crusts and hair loss. Nodular lesions are sometimes seen. Lesions not normally itchy.
Treatment: Isolation of the fungus confirms the diagnosis and good husbandry is the key to treatment. Each horse should have its own tack and grooming equipment and infected horses should be isolated.

Clip and wash affected horses repeatedly with an anti-fungal preparation until after the infection has

resolved. Dispose of all hair and crust that has been removed and disinfect stables and tack. Many therapies are probably ineffective but take the credit for spontaneous remission. Most horses get better on their own within 4 months.

BACTERIAL DISEASES
Equine skin is highly resistant to invasion by bacteria. When bacterial skin infection does become established, a horse's defence mechanisms are commonly impaired.

DERMATOPHILOSIS
Dermatophilosis occurs world-wide but is especially prevalent in tropical countries. It can be seen during or following periods of prolonged rainfall.
Cause: Infection by *Dermatophilus congolensis* bacteria. Moisture and trauma to skin is needed for infection to occur, as normal, healthy skin is very resistant to infection. The infective agents, called zoospores, are highly-resistant to drying and may remain dormant in crusts for many months until reactivated by adequate wetting. Chronically affected horses are the primary source of infection. Crusts on a horse, or those that have fallen or been rubbed off into bedding or around the environment, may harbour many infective organisms. The bacteria can also be transferred by biting and non-biting insects.
Signs: Signs are extremely variable but typically one of two areas of the body are affected:
1) back and flanks (commonly called rain scald),
2) lower limbs especially fetlocks (commonly called mud fever or greasy heel).

The muzzle and eyes may also be affected. Areas of skin lacking pigment are particularly susceptible. The terms 'rain scald' and 'mud fever' are commonly

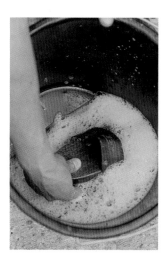

Ringworm is highly infectious. Affected horses must be isolated and their equipment kept separately and thoroughly disinfected after use.

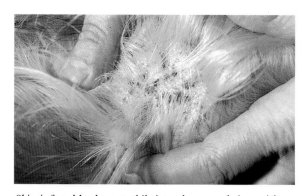

Skin infected by dermatophilosis produces sore lesions with the tufty 'paint-brush' owners associate with 'mud fever'. Areas of skin without pigment seem particularly susceptible.

used, rather vaguely, by horse owners and vets when a precise diagnosis has not been made. The term 'dermatophilosis' is preferable when the causal organism of this specific condition has been isolated.

Many horses develop crusting and scaling. In horses with long winter coats, groups of hairs may be seen matted together producing the so-called 'paint-brush' effect. In short-haired horses, lesions are smaller and occur as multiple spots covered with crusts or scale. Horses are rarely itchy but may show pronounced discomfort or pain. Severely affected horses may show depression, lethargy, weight loss, fever and enlarged lymph glands.

Treatment and prevention: Veterinary laboratory techniques are available to isolate the bacteria and rule out similar conditions. In temperate climates, the infection will often resolve spontaneously, but to treat the condition (and prevent it developing) the horse should be kept out of the rain and wet or muddy pastures. Avoid excessive moisture or sweating. Clipping of the affected areas may be required. Anti-bacterial solutions, shampoos, creams and ointments can be applied. Remove and carefully dispose of crusts.

No long-term immunity is acquired and if crust removal is incomplete, recurrence is likely.

PREVENTION AND MANAGEMENT OF MUD FEVER/GREASY HEEL

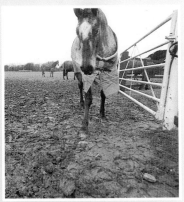

▲ *Avoid prolonged exposure to wet, muddy conditions. Regularly give the skin of the lower legs opportunity to dry out completely, if necessary by bringing the horse in. Keep an eye on the condition of the skin and legs in the vulnerable areas and take prompt action to control any signs of mud fever developing.*

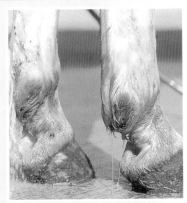

▲ *Clip away heavy feathering, which prevents air from getting to the skin. Mud can be washed off as necessary using warm water, but the heels and lower legs must be dried thoroughly afterwards. Dry mud can be removed with the fingers or a soft brush. Wet skin in this area is easily damaged.*

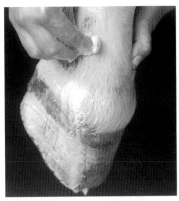

▲ *After exercise in muddy conditions, wash and dry the legs or allow mud to dry and carefully brush off before inspecting the legs. Any broken skin will allow in infection and needs to heal before the horse can be turned out again.*

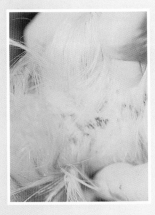

◀ *If signs of mud fever occur, stable the horse, clean and dry the legs. If it is possible to do so easily, remove scabs from affected areas to expose to the air. Dispose of scabs by burning or immersing in disinfectant. Apply medicated wash or other preparation recommended by vet to affected areas.*

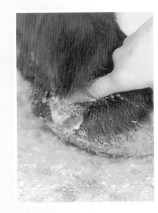

◀ *The legs must be kept as dry as possible until healing is complete. A barrier can be created between the dry skin and the wet environment using a suitable medicated ointment or cream. However, this should be regularly cleansed off and replaced, with the legs being allowed to dry again thoroughly before re-application.*

FOLLICULITIS AND FURUNCULOSIS (ACNE)

Folliculitis is an inflammation of the hair follicle. With time, inflammation can break through the follicle into the surrounding dermis and is then known as furunculosis.

Cause: Infection by *Staphylococcus aureus* and other bacteria, associated with trauma, pressure and increased environmental temperature and humidity. Most cases begin in spring and early summer and may be seen with increased work-loads, heavy riding and shedding of the coat. There is no age, breed or sex predilection.

Signs: Infection is often seen in areas subjected to repeated rubbing such as under the saddle but can also occur around the pastern and fetlock. Initially, small spots appear which last from weeks to months. These may spontaneously regress or enlarge but eventually flatten out to give gradually expanding areas of hair loss and scaling. Some continue to enlarge, resulting in large swollen areas which can ulcerate and scar, leading to white hair and skin formation. Spots are sometimes painful and may render the horse unfit for work.

Treatment: Mild cases may resolve spontaneously or with topical therapy. Antibiotics may be needed for more severe cases. The owner must improve general hygiene, feeding and other management procedures, ensure girths are correctly fitted and grooming is adequate. Washing a susceptible horse daily with an anti-bacterial solution before and after heavy work can help prevent a recurrence.

PHOTOSENSITISATION

Increased and abnormal response to sunlight.

Cause: Ingestion of or direct contact with certain plants (e.g. St. John's wort, clover, lucerne, rape, rye grass and wild carrots) or drugs that contain photo-dynamic agents. These agents exert toxic effects or induce allergic reactions when sunlight is absorbed through the skin. Liver disease can lead to an accumulation of a photo-dynamic agent within the skin.

Signs: Unpigmented and hairless areas most often affected. Signs can be variable but include redness, oedema, crusting and scaling, skin cracks, skin thickening, ulceration and skin death. Pain and irritation are sometimes present. In severe cases, clumsiness, blindness and shock can be seen.

Treatment: Reduce or prevent exposure to sunlight. Change the feed or pasture. Apply sun blocks or steroids. Any liver disease must be treated with urgency, although the prognosis is poor where liver disease is diagnosed.

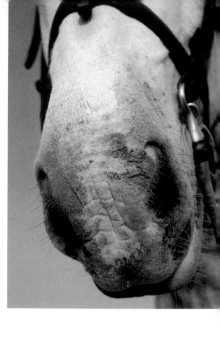

Unpigmented and hairless areas of the body are the most photo-sensitive. Severe cases can be extremely sore and painful.

NODULES

Nodules are firm, raised lesions that often extend into the deeper layers of the skin. Nodules typically result from massive infiltration of either inflammatory or cancer cells. They include granulomas (infectious or non-infectious swellings in the skin), abscesses, tumours (cancers) and cysts (cavities containing fluid or solid material).

COLLAGEN GRANULOMA

Cause: The cause is unknown, but there may be many causes including allergy to insect bites and reactions to foods and drugs. This is a very common condition seen throughout the world. More prevalent in warmer months, it usually causes no pain or irritation. No particular age, breed or sex is more predisposed to the condition, which has no effect on the health of the horse.

Signs: There are one or more lumps on the trunk that vary in size from around 0.5 to 5 cm ($^1/_4$ – 2 $^1/_2$ ins). The skin surface and hair coat are typically normal and there is no ulceration unless traumatised. With time, the lesions may become calcified and harden.

Treatment: The lumps are best left alone. Either steroid creams or ointments (if one or few lumps) or tablets (if multiple) can be given. Some vets inject steroid into or around larger lesions, or lesions can be removed surgically. Signs do often resolve themselves without therapy but recurrence is frequent. Calcified lesions are often non-responsive to steroids and will need to be surgically removed if treatment is required.

ABSCESSES

Cause: Bacterial contamination of wounds resulting from surgery, foreign bodies, insect or mite attack or other forms of trauma.

Signs: Well-defined accumulations of pus which form and enlarge under the skin.

Treatment and prevention: Surgical drainage and

flushing or packing with topical anti-microbial agents.

Antibiotics based on sensitivity testing may be necessary but should not be given before the abscess matures or points.

SARCOIDS

Sarcoids are the most common equine cancer. Although not malignant, they may invade local tissue causing loss of use depending on location. There is no definite age, sex, breed or colour incidence. Growths may occur anywhere on the body and many horses have multiple sarcoids.
Cause: Research suggests a hereditary predisposition to a specific viral infection.
Signs: Tumours are variable in appearance and may be warty, fleshy, flat or a mix of all of these. They may be static for long periods but will often become locally aggressive.
Treatment: Ligatures, creams, radiotherapy, chemotherapy, immunotherapy, surgery, freezing, electrocautery and lasers are used. No one treatment is always effective and multiple treatments are often needed.

Combination therapy gives maximum chance of successful resolution, and therapy needs to be tailored to each individual. Static sarcoids are probably best left alone as surgery or biopsy may lead to enlargement and local spread.

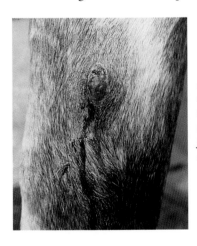

Sarcoid growths can appear anywhere on the body and are the most common form of cancer in horses.

MELANOMA

Some lines of grey- and white-coated horses are more susceptible to melanoma. Many cases are benign, although some are malignant. Depending on location, the growth may interfere with defaecation, urination and mating. Horses under six years old are rarely affected.
Signs: Small firm tumours in subcutaneous tissue

which slowly increase in size but are rapidly fatal once vital organs are involved. The anus, vulva and tail are commonly involved. Less commonly, the male genitalia, limbs, ears, eyelids and neck. Tumours sometimes ulcerate and produce a black discharge.
Treatment: Skin biopsies will confirm diagnosis. Radical surgical excision or cryotherapy (freezing) is then required. Cimetidine, a powerful antihistamine, has sometimes been helpful in treating actively-growing melanomas. Unfortunately the prognosis for severely-affected horses is poor, especially if the growths are malignant.

PAPILLOMATOSIS (WARTS)

Warts most commonly affect foals and yearlings, with no breed or sex predilection.
Cause: Viral infection.
Signs: Warts, usually found on the muzzle, lips, nostrils and eyes but also on external genitalia and lower limbs. May easily be confused with some types of sarcoid.
Treatment: Allow the warts to regress naturally. Spontaneous remission usually ensues within six months and immunity is lifelong.

AURAL PLAQUES

Cause: Viral infection, possibly transmitted by insects.
Signs: White, warty plaques on inner surface of one or both ears. Other possible sites include the anus and vulva.
Treatment: There is no known treatment or spontaneous remission. However, the lesions are not typically painful or itchy.

EPIDERMOID CYST (ATHEROMA, EPITHELIAL INCLUSION CYST)

A subcutaneous nodule found in, or over, the false nostril. Such cysts are uncommon and congenital cysts may not be noticed until horse is three to six months old. There is no breathing noise or obstruction. Cysts may also occur around base of the ear and produce mucus (dentigerous cyst).
Cause: Congenital, or acquired through blocked hair follicle or penetration of epidermis by a foreign body.
Signs: Nodules may be single or multiple. They are well-defined and firm but there is no pain or irritation, hair loss or damage to the skin surface.
Treatment: The cysts are unlikely to resolve without therapy and can be removed by surgical excision, although they are as well left alone.

8 THE HORSE IN WORK

FITTING SADDLERY

LISTEN TO YOUR HORSE

Given the opportunity to express himself fully, your horse will 'tell' you what he needs in almost every aspect of his care. This definitely applies to finding the 'right' saddle. A horse could not care less how much its saddle costs, what colour it is or whether it is made of the finest doeskin or a lump of moulded plastic. The saddle either allows the horse to use its body as nature intended, or it does not. It is either comfortable or gives varying degrees of discomfort right up to the downright painful.

So how does this help you to determine what saddle to go for? What really helps horse owners to choose a saddle, or at least what to eliminate as unsuitable, is a clear understanding of how the horse's body needs to move and how any saddle needs to interact with this movement.

MOVEMENT AS NATURE INTENDED
In trying to understand how nature intended the horse to move in order to be athletic, healthy, sound and comfortable, we can design and use equipment that interferes with this as little as possible. The further the horse's body and locomotion is taken away from nature, the more stresses are placed on the structures. Owners who are willing to give their horses the opportunity to try a variety of saddling systems, enable the horse to provide them the feedback they need to determine which is most appropriate.

Although there is not space to go into a great deal of detail in this chapter regarding the biomechanics of natural equine movement, when you look at the amount of activity in the saddle area of the horse's

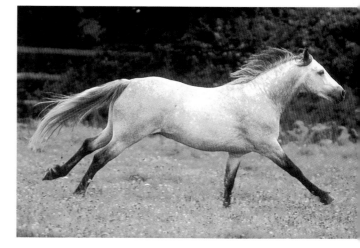

A horse should be expected to be able to move as freely under saddle as he is able to naturally, loose in the field.

body and the fact that when in motion, the horse's back is not the same shape as when static, it is immediately possible to appreciate the pitfalls of trying to make saddles that fit the static shape of the horse. Nevertheless, this has been done for years. Unfortunately, the horse is such a master at compensating when part of its body is restricted or damaged, that it often manages amazing feats of athleticism despite wearing a saddle that is creating a problem.

The conventional method of fitting saddles to horses has created a situation where the majority of ridden horses no longer have a natural body shape. A saddle that has been fitted to match the static contours of the body effectively 'locks' the horse into its static posture whilst in motion. This changes the entire biomechanics of the horse, which has to discover ways of accommodating the rider's commands whilst his natural patterns of movement

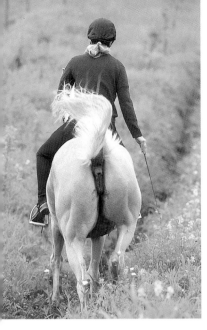

A horse with a poorly fitting saddle will be working in constant pain or discomfort. The correct fit of all tack should always be a primary concern of all owners and one of the first considerations when trying to find the cause of any behavioural problem.

are disabled. Over time, these compensations create a range of unnatural body postures and/or muscle development, which can include:

- A lack, or even loss, of muscle mass along the back, top of the neck and quarters of the horse, creating a more angular body shape
- Unnatural amount of definition of the thoracic spineous processes (withers) and scapula due to lack of healthy muscle mass around them
- Over-development of certain muscle groups
- Shortened stride
- Contraction of the tendons, caused by loss of elasticity in muscle groups at the top of the foreleg and shoulders
- A dropped back posture caused by constant contraction of the long back muscles into dorsi-flexion
- A protruding sternum
- Tendency toward overloading the heels of the front feet
- Tendency to overload the outside edges of the front feet.

It is often understandably assumed that if a horse can get around a Badminton three-day event, complete the Golden Horseshoe endurance ride or win a Grand Prix dressage test, that it cannot possibly have a problem with its saddle. But discomfort and stress are often part of a competition horse's existence. Look at any top human athlete or dancer and you will see that discomfort and even pain is often an accepted part of their lives.

The human athlete may choose to 'abuse' his body in order to get the performance he desires. But what of the horse? The horses that make it to the top may not necessarily be the most talented athletes, but are rather able to cope with physical and psychological stress better than others. As long as the horse is able to perform to a sufficiently good standard, the trainers are happy and look no further

than their current management methods and equipment. If the horse is not able to perform well enough, it is easy enough to discard it and get another. In an environment where comfort and ease is not a priority, it is easy to see that seeking the horse's opinion about a saddle is not going to be a priority!

For many humans entrenched in the need for competitive horse owning and riding, a new, more enlightened approach toward working with the saddle may be too challenging because it places the horse's needs as at least equal to our own.

NEW APPROACHES TO SADDLE DESIGN AND FIT

The issue of how to fit saddles to horses is currently creating a great deal of controversy and confusion amongst horse owners and the many professionals who are involved within the horse industry, such as vets, chiropractors, trainers and judges.

In the early 1990s and before, the story would have been very different. Saddle fitting had been done the same way for many years, often by people who knew little or nothing about horses. No-one questioned the validity of the conventional 'rules' of saddle 'fitting' and horse owners would not have dreamt of questioning the advice provided by their saddle retailer/fitter.

The English saddle industry was then working in the main with three standard widths of tree: narrow, medium and wide, to accommodate the needs of every horse. At the same time, it was busy creating many different variations to accommodate the needs and desires of the rider. A 'custom-made' saddle was generally considered to be the best kind to buy for your horse if you had the money. The old chestnut, "if the saddle fits, you dont need pads under it," abounded. No-one talked much about saddles in relation to the horse's needs or comfort.

In the late 1980's, a British group named BALANCE began researching the effects of saddles on the performance, health and soundness of the ridden horse. The information gathered has resulted in a massive increase in interest in this important topic. Highlighted was the far-reaching impact saddles have on the horse.

In terms of performance, the restrictive saddle can cause, or contribute to, any of the following:

- Inability or apparent reluctance to engage the hind legs
- Hollow outline
- Reluctance to bend
- Shortened stride

- Hanging legs when jumping
- Respiration affected adversely
- Apparent nervousness or 'spookiness'
- Reluctance to go forward
- Tension.

All of the above create difficulties for riders and trainers and can result in further abuse for the horse, when gadgets and riding techniques are employed to over-ride the horse's instinct to protect itself from discomfort. Unfortunately, whilst there are so many horses still being ridden in uncomfortable saddles, we will continue see the unnatural movement, postures and body shapes these create as 'normal'.

Although a variety of opinions on the subject is a healthy stimulation for improvements, it can also prove to be confusing for the poor horse owner who is simply trying to do the best for theis horse. For this reason, we don't feel that it is appropriate to give you a 'recipe' for the perfect saddle here by providing yet another set of saddle fitting rules. Rather, we want to give you some of the thinking behind the BALANCE Saddling System and invite you to consider them alongside some of the other saddle fitting theories that exist. Having considered the different approaches, you simply have to go with the one that feels most appropriate for you and your horse right now.

There can be no guarantees: the whole concept of using a saddle between horse and rider is doomed to create more problems than it solves and the only way to ensure that you will never ever have a saddle-related 'problem' or dilemma is to never use one.

A NEW PERSPECTIVE: PRINCIPLES OF THE BALANCE SADDLING SYSTEM

- The BALANCE Saddling System provides the horse owner with the means to protect their horses' natural patterns of movement, health and soundness, or to help recover it once lost as a result of previous poor saddle fit.
- The system consists of several different kinds of saddle in a variety of styles for the rider, used in conjunction with a specially-designed padding system.
- The saddles themselves have been created to incorporate the design features that horses consistently demonstrate that they prefer. The saddles are 'fitted' slightly wider than the horse's static posture to allow for the natural and desired increased width of the horse's back when moving. The padding system provides the comfort and

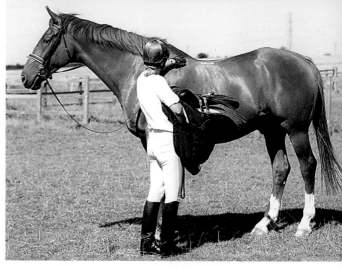

The horse provides us with feedback about everything he is exposed to – saddles, riding techniques, boots, bits or stables/turnout routine etc. The key is to be willing to offer our horses choices rather than always imposing our own rigid ideas about what is appropriate for them. Regular, monitoring of the on-going comfort of the horse in his saddle needs to be part of every rider's routine. Here, the rider checks for any 'tender' areas before putting her saddle on. In this way, she can detect tension or bruising which could be saddle-related and need investigating.

balance in the saddle and allows fine-tuning of both to ensure continued comfort for horse and rider.
- The exact combination of saddle and pads is 'chosen' by horse and rider by trying a variety, but with the horse's opinion being considered most important and also most reliable. Finding the saddle/pad combination that allows the horse to move most naturally and easily is the aim.
- The widths of BALANCE saddles are, by necessity, considerably wider than conventional narrow, medium and wide, because healthy, well-developed horses are considerably wider than these widths.

TIME FOR RE-EVALUATION
- If your horse is still being ridden in a conventional width of saddle.
- If your horse's saddle was made or fitted to his static shape.
- If your horse's comfort and long-term health and soundness are important to you.
- If you are aware that your horse moves beautifully when loose in the field but loses it when under saddle, it is time to take another look at this vital issue.

When one is willing to provide the horse with a choice, and be respectful of the feedback he provides, it is possible to get to the truth. This applies to any piece of equipment you want to put on his body, the training methods you employ, and the riding aims you invite him to participate in with you.

CONVENTIONAL RULES FOR CORRECT FIT: SADDLE

A saddle needs to suit the rider, but most importantly it must be comfortable and a correct fit for the individual horse. Owners should always bear in mind that each horse will be a different shape and that body contours can change with age, condition or fitness level. Regular checks by qualified professionals up-to-date with enlightened thinking in the fitting of saddlery are needed to ensure that the fit and condition of the saddle remain good. Fit should be considered both with and without a rider, standing still and on the move.

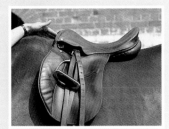

◀ *The saddle should sit level on the back with the lowest part of the seat midway between the pommel and cantle. There should be no twisting and no rocking backward and forward when the rider is doing rising trot (posting).*

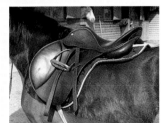

◀ *No part of the saddle must impede the horse's movement, even when the shoulders are at full stretch. The back of the saddle should not extend beyond the last rib or reach the weak and sensitive loin area.*

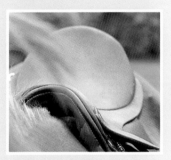

◀ *Plenty of daylight should be seen all the way down the gullet, even with the rider leaning forwards or back. Four fingers should fit easily between the withers and the pommel at all times.*

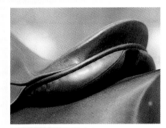

◀ *The panels are the saddle's shock absorbers and should spread the rider's weight over as wide an area as possible. Stuffing must be sufficient to provide protection – avoid thin panels or hard, over-stuffed panels which stand up off the horse's back.*

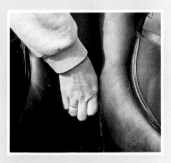

◀ *The gullet must be wide enough for the panels to rest well clear of the spine on either side.*

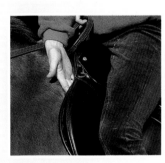

◀ *The fitting is too wide around the withers if the thin panels or saddle sits down low or is spacey at the sides, allowing movement. An over-narrow fitting will make the saddle sit up too high at the front and cause pinching. It should be possible to slide your fingers between the saddle and the sides of the withers.*

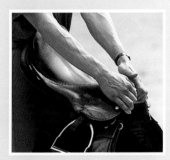

◀ *Take particular care when buying second-hand saddlery, checking for both condition and fit. This saddle is being tested to listen for the tell-tale creaking and excessive movement that are signs of a damaged tree. Keep a constant eye on saddle fit – all horses will change body shape according to their condition and fitness. Also, bear in mind that a saddle 'inherited' with a new horse does not necessarily fit him.*

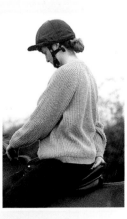

◀ *The saddle must also fit the rider, to help them to sit in an optimum position over the horse's centre of gravity.*

FITTING GUIDELINES: MARTINGALES

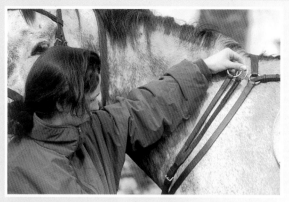 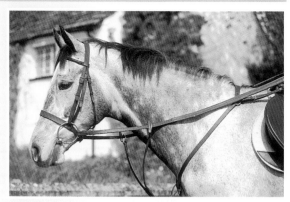

▲ *Whatever type of martingale is used, it should take effect only when the horse raises its head beyond the point of control. A martingale fitted too loosely is ineffectual. The restriction of too tight a fit will only cause further resistance, tension and evasion. All neckstraps should allow the width of a hand to be inserted easily underneath.*

▲ *The straps of a running martingale should reach to within a hand's width of the withers. Fitted too short, the martingale interferes with the correct use of the rein aids by altering the angle of the bit in the mouth.*

CORRECT FIT: BRIDLE AND BIT

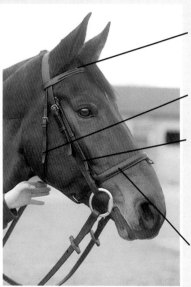

Browband should not pinch the base of the ears.

Throatlash should allow a hand's width between it and the cheek.

Adjust cheek pieces so the bit slightly wrinkles the corners of the lips. Bits fastened too low or too high cause great discomfort.

Noseband sits midway between the corner of the lips and the projecting cheekbone, fastened to allow two fingers to be easily inserted underneath.

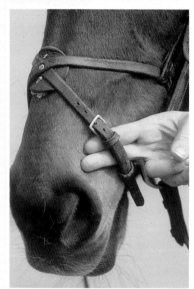

◀ *A drop-type noseband (e.g. dropped, Flash, Grakle) fastens below the bit. Care must be taken to ensure the upper strap sits well up the nose so there is no interference with the horse's breathing. Drop nosebands fit snugly but not too tightly. Two fingers should be able to fit underneath.*

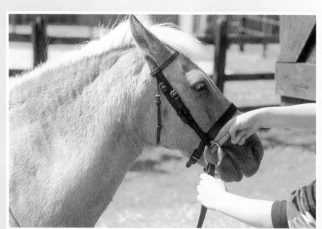

◀ *The correct width of bit allows a quarter-inch (0.5cm) of the mouthpiece to be seen. A bit too large for the horse will lose effectiveness, knocking against the teeth and injuring the roof of the mouth. Too small a bit is likely to pinch and cause sores on the lips.*

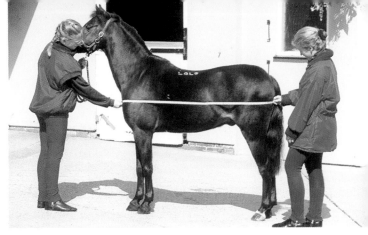

RUGS/BLANKETS

Depending on the type of horse and what you intend to do with him, a selection of rugs/blankets may be needed throughout the year.

During winter, a hardy, unclipped native type or a youngster in good condition given ad lib forage and provided with adequate shelter, will grow a thick protective coat of far more use to him than a rug. Finer-bred horses managed with a part-in, part-out system will benefit from the help of a turnout rug to keep off the worst of the wet and wind while they are outside. Any clipped horse, particularly of the Thoroughbred type, however, does need to be well wrapped up in much warmer attire from autumn onwards, if he is to keep condition until the spring, as will an old horse who feels the cold.

In summer, cotton sheets help to keep a horse clean and protect him against flies. A modern 'wicking' cooler rug is also indispensable to the busy horse owner, as it keeps a sweaty or wet horse comfortable and prevents chilling while he dries off.

Measuring for the correct length of rug. Sufficient depth and a close, but not tight, fit around the shoulder are also important for any rug to work effectively.

MATERIALS & FASTENINGS
Of the variety of materials now used to manufacture horse clothing, traditional canvas and jute are probably still the cheapest and seen in the most basic, inexpensive designs. At the top end of the price scale are lightweight, high-performance synthetics which aim to keep a horse at a comfortable temperature all winter, whatever the weather, by their use of 'breathable' fabrics.

As a general rule, quality has to be paid for and a tough, well-designed rug that is easy to use, does its job well and lasts, is worth the extra initial cost.

Rugs are held in place with breast clips or velcro fastenings at the front of the chest. Surcingles, attached to the lower edge, crossing under the belly and clipping to the opposite side, have now virtually replaced the traditional padded leather roller and they ease spine pressure considerably. Some designs of turnout rug have leg straps which loop around the hind legs to hold the back of the rug in place and prevent it blowing up. Alternatively, a fillet string simply passes from one side to the other under the tail.

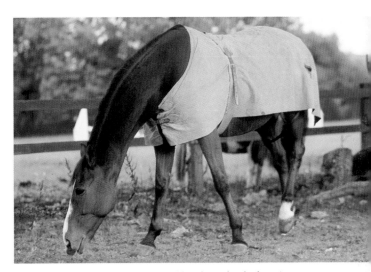

Modern designs and fabrics have at last brought the horse's comfort to the fore, making sights such as this poorly fitted canvas rug, secured with a tight surcingle, a thing of the past.

GETTING A GOOD FIT
Rugs are sized according to their length, from the smallest pony rugs at around 5 feet to the largest horse rugs at over 7 feet. Sizes traditionally go up in 3-inch increments, although some modern rugs are now in metres.

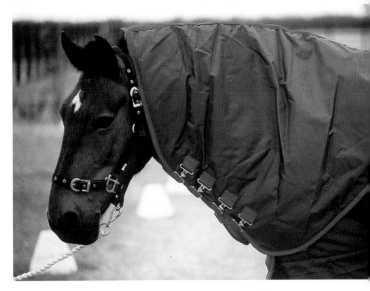

Neck covers may be separate, or an integral feature of modern stable and turn-out rugs.

To size a horse for a rug, measure from the centre of the chest all the way around the shoulder and along the barrel to the point of the buttock. In addition to the length, it is important to make sure depth is sufficient to cover the horse's belly. The rug should also be cut high across the neck to cover as much of the horse as possible and prevent it pulling round the shoulders and withers. The most recent designs extend right up the neck, adding extra warmth and eliminating the need for a neck cover on a clipped horse.

RUG ACCESSORIES

- Shaped thermal liners fit under the normal rug for extra warmth.
- 'Shoulder savers' are designed to fit under the rug around the chest and shoulders as a kind of collar to prevent rubbing.
- Hoods cover the neck and sometimes the head also, protecting the horse from mud, rain and cold. Usually attached to D-rings on the rug, these can be padded for stable use or waterproofed for turnout.

RUGGING TIPS

- Sew simulated sheepskin or silk on the inside of the rug, around the withers and shoulders, to prevent rubbing.
- Search markets for cheap duvets or blankets to use as an extra lining in very cold weather.
- Make basic alterations and repairs yourself. Extra D-rings, webbing straps, velcro, strong plastic fastenings, dog clips and extra-strong thread can be found in outdoor-leisure shops and department stores.
- Every rug, no matter how expensive, will begin to leak if it is not properly cared for. Clean all clothing after use (and re-proof turnout rugs) before storage. There are a number of products which are designed for this and rug manufacturers will advise on which is most suitable.
- A cotton sheet worn under a rug can be regularly washed, keeping the lining clean and hygienic.

TYPES OF RUG

The items of clothing a horse requires will depend on how he is managed and the type of work done. The numerous styles available for all purposes fall into the following main categories.

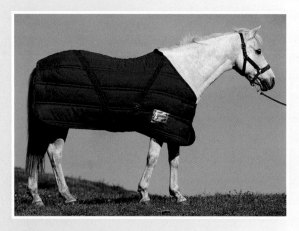

▲ *Stable rug: Old-style jute and woollen rugs and blankets, fastened around the girth with a roller, are now rarely seen. Today's indoor wear comes in the form of a well-insulated 'duvet-type' stable rug, again using modern synthetic fibres to produce warm yet 'breathable' clothing, fastened by broad surcingles or leg straps designed for comfort and security. With their movement restricted, all stabled horses will require rugging during cold weather.*

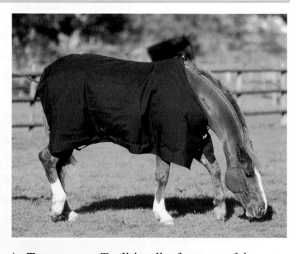

▲ *Turnout rug: Traditionally of waterproofed canvas (known as a New Zealand rug) most turnout rugs are now made from synthetic fabrics that combine warmth and water resistance with the ability to 'breathe', so allowing moisture to be 'wicked' away from the skin back to the air. Such rugs are often suitable for indoor use too. Differing weights are available for various weather conditions, temperature, etc. The rug is designed to stay in place, however active the horse. Whilst unclipped, hardy animals with adequate shelter and forage can winter outside quite happily without a turnout rug, finer-bred or older horses will appreciate the added warmth and protection. Clipped animals should always be rugged up when turned out.*

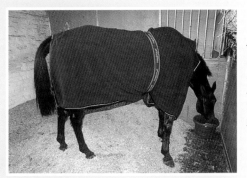

◀ Cooler: A lightweight sheet, which may extend to cover the neck and is designed to allow a horse to cool off without chilling. Moisture is drawn through the fabric to evaporate at the surface. Again, these advances in technology mean the cooler has largely replaced the old 'string-vest' style anti-sweat sheet. These rugs are particularly useful for travelling.

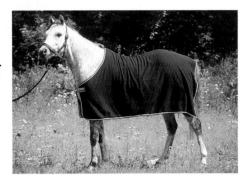

Summer sheet: A general-purpose lightweight sheet for spring ▶ and summer. Useful for travelling and protection from dust and flies.

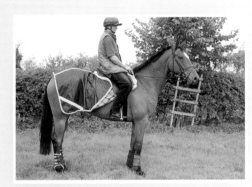

◀ Exercise sheet: If a clipped horse needs to be exercised in cold conditions, particularly if the going or the horse's state of fitness mean work must be slow, an exercise sheet provides warmth and weather protection for the quarters. Usually either a waterproof sheet or woollen half-blanket, this is a useful addition to most equine owners' wardrobes, allowing a horse to be kept largely dry during rides in the rain, so the stable or turnout rug can be replaced immediately on the return home without further drying off.

RUG FITTING

Correct fitting is essential to get the most from a rug. Too small or tight a fit creates constant discomfort to the horse and will soon cause rubs or even sores. A baggy, over-large rug lets in draughts or wet, with drooping straps likely to cause an accident.

1. Adequate length from withers to covering the dock
2. Shaping along the back will help rug stay in place
3. Plenty of depth to protect belly from draughts
4. Secure fastenings, fitted snugly but allowing a hand to be inserted easily
5. Shoulder and quarter darts mould rug to horse's shape and help prevent rubs
6. Adequate coverage at the chest
7. Room at the shoulders to allow movement but not let in wet/cold

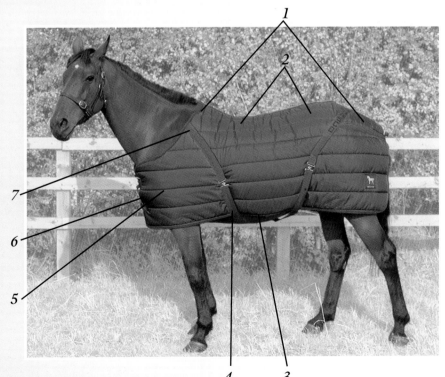

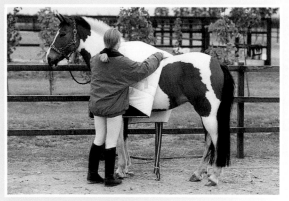

▲ *Fold the rug in half and put it over the neck, well forward. Fasten chest straps.*

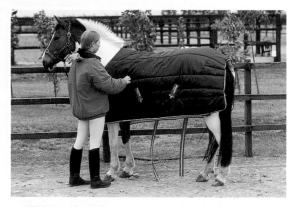

▲ *Slide rug back into position and fold other half down to cover quarters. Fasten belly surcingles or roller, if used. Now fasten any hind-leg straps.*

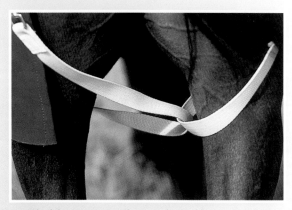

▲ *Hind-leg straps are frequently used instead of, or in addition to, cross-surcingles. These should be looped through each other before fastening to help keep the rug stable and prevent chafing. Avoid fastening too tightly. A 'spider' strap is seen in some turnout rugs. This reaches from the chest between the forelegs, then divides into two straps that thread through each side of the rug and then between the hind legs to fasten at the back.*

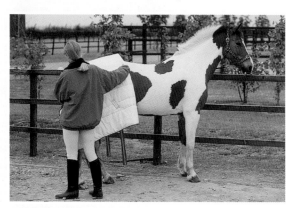

▲ *To remove a rug, unfasten the straps furthest back first and work forwards. When all are undone, knot any cross-surcingles loosely together and re-fasten any leg straps to prevent them knocking against the horse. Folding the front half of the rug back, pull it off carefully in one backward sweep. Avoid standing directly behind the horse.*

LEG PROTECTION

WHY USE LEG PROTECTION?
There are various types of boots and bandages which will protect your horse's most valuable assets – his legs. By asking the domestic horse to deal with the unbalancing effect of a rider and to perform movements on a daily basis which he would rarely use in the wild (such as working in small circles, side-stepping in lateral work, or jumping combinations of fences), we considerably increase the chances of him knocking or stepping on himself. A horse can inflict severe damage to his own legs, especially if he is shod. It makes safety sense to take the precaution of spending a few minutes fitting leg protection before you start riding, whatever your intended activity.

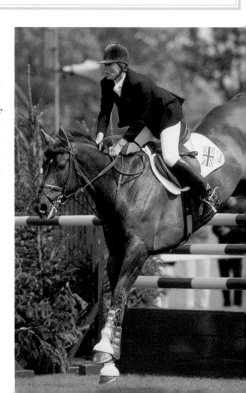

A horse's legs are its most valuable asset, but easily at risk of damage during the athletic activities we ask of him. Leg protection minimises that risk.

BOOTS OR BANDAGES?

While bandages may be the perfectionist's choice, offering greater support and conforming to the leg, these do require a great deal of practice to put on correctly and can easily do more harm than good when wrongly applied. For daily exercise, boots are quicker and easier to fit and keep clean.

Some owners even choose to turn their horses out in the field wearing boots if they are inclined to play rough games, but this can cause skin problems if mud and grit get beneath them. Generally, a horse at liberty is quite good at balancing and looking after himself without the need for boots.

Whilst some types of boot offer general, all-round protection, others are designed to give maximum protection to a particular area or during specific risk situations (see page 182).

WHICH MATERIALS?

Once solely made of leather, boots now more commonly use a variety of synthetic materials including plastic and high-impact neoprene, which have high shock-absorbency yet are comfortable to wear and easy to care for. Manufacturers might use a range of shock-absorbing linings such as rubber or sheepskin. Fastenings are generally velcro (with or without elastic inserts), straps with buckles, or 'hook-and-eye' type fixtures. Clearly a leather boot with sheepskin lining will be more time-consuming to clean and maintain than, say, a neoprene boot, which can be scrubbed off under the tap or put in the washing machine, but leather is generally the most expensive.

HOW DO I CHOOSE?

When choosing boots to buy, a balance has to be struck between the need for maximum protection (such as when taking a stiff cross-country course, for example), and what you feel are reasonable precautions to take for your particular horse when exercising on a daily basis.

The rider of a sensible, well-schooled horse with straight movement may decide their horse can manage without any leg protection at all except when jumping. An argument does suggest that it is more beneficial for a horse to be able to feel where his legs and feet are, particularly youngsters, and that 'wrapping them up in cotton wool' is counter-productive. This is the thinking behind the open-fronted tendon boot described below. Used by show jumpers, these boots protect the tendon behind the knee, but are open at the front so exposing the cannon bone and allowing the horse to feel it should he hit a pole.

The type of leg protection which suits you and your horse, and how often you intend to use it, is a matter of personal preference. Be warned, however. The nature of the beast is that the day you decide not to put boots on is the day the horse will knock himself!

FITTING BOOTS

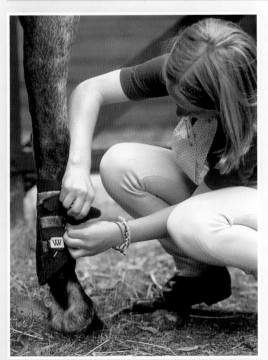

Boots provide protection to the lower legs from self-inflicted injuries (see Chapter Four, Interference) and other knocks or wounds, such as during competition or schooling.

Fitting points to watch include:

- *Boots are always fastened on the outside of the leg.*
- *Straps always point backwards.*
- *Front and hind pairs are usually shaped differently, with hinds generally having more straps.*
- *Fasten snugly but not tightly – a finger should fit down inside.*
- *Ensure the boot does not impede movement of any joints.*
- *Fasten the centre buckle/strap first, followed by the one below and then the top one, to prevent the boot slipping down the leg.*
- *When removing, release the top strap first and work down.*

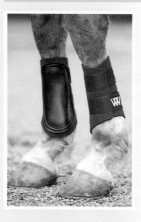

◀ **Brushing boot:** Protects the leg all round, from just below the knee to above the fetlock, with extra padding to guard the inside of the leg. Also sometimes seen with additional protection in the tendon area (front boots) and at the front of the leg in hind boots, for use when jumping solid fences.

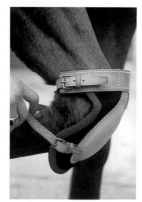

◀ **Knee boot:** If a horse stumbles, the area he lands on first is his knees. Often called 'knee caps', or 'skeleton' knee boots, these have a padded front to protect against falls when the horse is being ridden or travelled. They are fastened firmly above the knee but the lower strap must stay loose to allow the joint to flex freely.

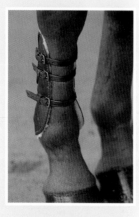

◀ **Tendon boot:** Fits around the cannon bone, with padding concentrated at the back to protect the tendons from being cut into by the toes of the hind feet when jumping or galloping. May have an open or closed front.

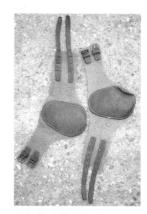

◀ **Fetlock boot:** A shorter boot which protects the inside of the fetlock joint from brushing injuries but offers no protection higher up the leg. Felt 'Yorkshire' boots or 'rubber-ring' or 'sausage' boots also give some protection to this area.

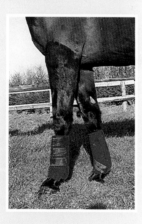

◀ **Combination boot:** The standard brushing and tendon boots have now been joined by a wide variety of 'combination' sports boots providing extended protection within one boot, reaching either higher up the leg to cover the inside of the knee or hock joint (known as 'speedy-cut' boots) or lower to protect the fetlock, pastern and even the heels.

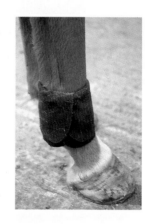 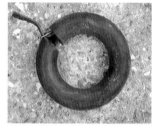

▲ **Sausage boot**

◀ **Yorkshire boot**

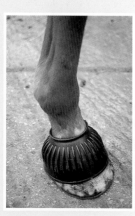

◀ **Over-reach boot:** Sometimes known as 'bell boots', these are fitted around the pasterns of the forelegs, protecting the back of the pastern and sensitive coronet and heels from being struck into by the hind feet, particularly during landing after a jump or in heavy going. Rubber varieties pull on over the foot.

Travelling boots: Combine the effects of all the above, offering padded protection from above the knee to below the coronet when travelling. Should cover the heel to guard against over-reaching (although can be used in conjunction with over-reach boots for this purpose). See page 192 .

Hock boot: Used for travelling to protect the hock joint from knocks. Fit is similar to knee boot (see above).

TYPES OF BANDAGE

All bandages, except tail bandages and some specifically designed stable bandages, need to be applied using a layer of padding underneath them such as gamgee, foam, or shock-absorbing pads. Fastening is usually via tapes or velcro.

Exercise bandages are made from a stretchy crepe-like material and are intended to support and protect the tendon area during work, without restricting joint flexion. Because of the degree of elasticity, care must be taken not to apply them too tightly. Poor bandaging can result in lasting damage to the leg.

Stable bandages are applied in a similar way to a veterinary or first aid bandage (see Chapter Two). This broad, thick bandage provides support, warmth and protection to tired legs in the stable or can be used when transporting. The whole of the lower leg is covered from below the knee or hock to the coronet.

Tail bandages are made from a similar elasticated material to an exercise bandage, and are used to smooth the top of the tail and protect against injury during travelling should the horse lean against the ramp or side of the lorry. It is important that tail bandages are not too tight, or left on for too long.

USING EXERCISE BANDAGES

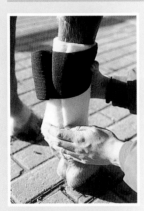

▲ *Unravelling about 4 inches (10cm) of bandage, hold it at an angle against the leg, below the knee.*

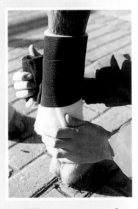

▲ *Wrap once around the leg to secure, and tuck in free end.*

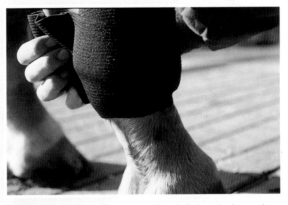

▲ *Continue wrapping around and down the leg, using a firm but even pressure. Cover about two-thirds of the previous wrap with each turn. Stop at the fetlock and work upwards again.*

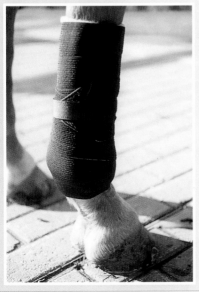

◄ *Aim to finish midway up the cannon. Fasten the bandage on the outside of the leg, never the front, back or inside. If tapes are used, make sure they lie flat before tying in a double bow, using the same pressure as the bandage, and tucking in the ends. Ties can be stitched for security or taped over.*

GENERAL BANDAGING POINTS

- Never kneel on the floor to put on bandages or boots – always crouch.
- Keep bandages clean. Roll up tightly and evenly after use.
- For applying stable bandages, see Chapter Two.
- Avoid leaving exercise bandages on too long, especially if they have got damp or wet. Remove by carefully passing from hand to hand as you unwind. Gently massage each leg to restore circulation.
- When an injury has been bandaged, the opposite leg should also be bandaged to help it take the extra strain.

CARE OF EQUIPMENT

Keeping equipment clean and in good condition is essential for both comfort and safety.

- Aim to clean and treat all leather at least once a week – ideally after each use. Always rinse the bit immediately after taking off the bridle.
- Have rugs cleaned regularly, re-proofing and making any necessary repairs before storing for the summer.
- Cotton girths and numnahs/saddle cloths, bandages, synthetic boots and headcollars can usually be cleaned in the washing machine, but avoid using perfumed or biological detergents.
- To clean synthetic saddles, brush off any mud and wash over with lukewarm water and washing-up liquid.
- Bridles can be given a quick clean hung on a hook, but should be taken apart completely on a regular basis.
- Take the chance when cleaning to check leather and stitching for wear and tear.

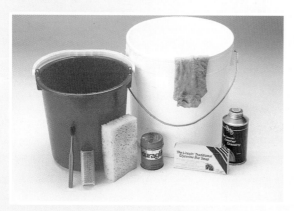

▲ *Items required for cleaning leather.*

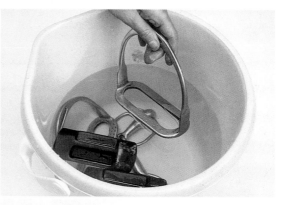

▲ *Undo all buckles and 'strip' the saddle. Place stirrup irons and bit in bucket of warm water and scrub clean.*

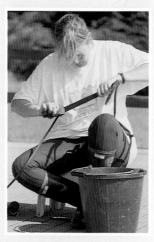

◄ *Use damp cloth or sponge to wipe the leather clean, taking care to ensure any 'jockeys' (lumps of grease) are removed. Avoid over-wetting.*

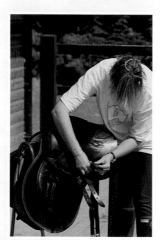

◄ *Dampen the saddle soap slightly and rub onto sponge or cloth. Work the soap into the leather, particularly the more absorbent, rougher side. Apply plenty to turns in the leather and areas which take pressure, e.g. girth straps. Neatsfoot oil or other leather preparations can be applied monthly to keep leather supple. It is particularly useful after the leather has got wet and has dried out. Avoid oil soaking stitching, however.*

Metal parts, with the exception of the bit, can be shined up with polish.

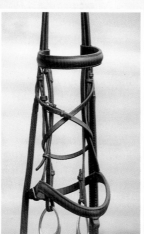

◄ *Finally, put everything back together again, using the correct holes, and put away, tidily. For long-term storage, leather is best kept in a cotton pillowcase, with straps undone and laid out flat.*

ADDED SECURITY

When riding across country, it is advisable to use PVC tape around boots and bandages to ensure that they do not slip or pull off in all the excitement. It is also possible to stitch the top layer of a bandage to the bottom layer with plaiting thread, working from top to bottom and taking great care not to prick the horse.

CLIPPING

Horses that are expected to work throughout the winter usually require some of the heavy winter coat clipping off, to keep them comfortable during exercise and make them easier to clean and dry off afterwards.

There are several set patterns of clip, allowing owners to choose the one which suits their horse's workload as well as his management regime. When deciding, remember that, depending on the extent of the clip, lost warmth must be compensated for by providing extra rugs, feed and stabling, so there is little point making work for yourself by clipping off more than you have to. It is not fair or advisable to give any kind of clip to a horse or pony which is expected to live outside full-time over the winter.

CHOOSING A CLIP

Choose a clip carefully, taking into account the horse's management regime as well as workload. A cold horse loses condition quickly. It is pointless to remove more natural protection than is necessary, only to have to replace it with rugs and additional feed. Once clipped, a horse should always be rugged. For a horse or pony which lives permanently out, do not consider any more than a neck and belly clip, together with the use of a deep rug.

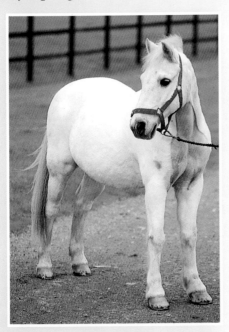

Neck & belly

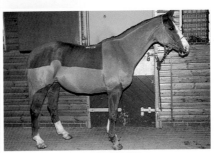

Trace

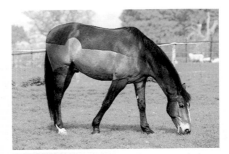

Blanket

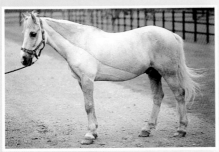

Chaser or Irish

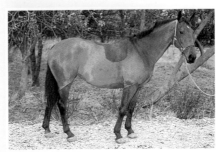

Hunter

Before clipping, run through the following checks:

- the blades are sharp
- the tension is correct
- the blades and clippers are well oiled
- all wiring is safe and correct and a circuit breaker is attached.

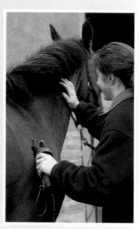

Clean the horse ▶ thoroughly and stand on a dry, non-slippery surface. A haynet will help occupy him.
Edges are best marked beforehand using some dampened saddle soap or chalk. Turn on the clippers and hold carefully against the horse until he relaxes.
Begin clipping, working against the direction of the hair. Start on a broad, flat area such as the sides or shoulder. Aim to take long strokes.

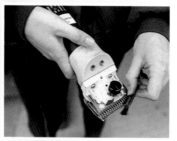

▲ *Switch the clippers off frequently for cleaning and to allow to cool. Brush clipped hairs off the horse's body and put a blanket over clipped areas to prevent chilling. Extra care is needed where the skin folds and in other sensitive areas such as under the belly. Ask a helper to hold up each foreleg and stretch it forwards to allow the elbow area to be clipped without nicking the skin. Many horses dislike the clippers around their head and ears. Sometimes blocking out the noise using cotton wool can help, or simply using quiet, battery clippers for this area. If restraint is necessary, refer to Chapter Two.*

WHEN TO CLIP

Unless there is a particular event which you need the horse to be smartly clipped for, wait until the winter coat is established and the horse is starting to get visibly hot during exercise before clipping – usually around late October. Depending on the horse's hair growth rate, the clip will need to be repeated every three to five weeks until early February. Clipping any later than this can interfere with summer coat growth.

You will need:
- A clean, dry horse
- A shelter area with power supply
- Plenty of daylight
- Clippers that have been regularly serviced and checked for safety
- Chalk, coloured pen or bar of saddle soap to mark out the clip
- Something steady to stand on if the horse is large
- Sharp clipper blades
- Clipper oil
- Small brush to remove hair clogged in the blades and filter
- Long extension cable
- Power-breaker socket plug
- Overalls, hat, face mask and rubber-soled boots for yourself
- Body brush, hay net, tail bandage and rugs for the horse
- An assistant
- Plenty of time.

Clipping is not a process that can be rushed. You will need to prepare the horse and your clipping area beforehand, stop several times throughout the clip to cool, clean and lubricate the clippers, and allow time to clean up the horse, clippers, yourself and the clipping area thoroughly afterwards.

FIRST-TIMERS

If you have never clipped before, watch others at work and see if it is possible for you to practise on a quiet horse which has already had the first clip and has clear lines for you to follow. Use long, firm, even strokes of the clippers, which should be the right size and weight for you to hold comfortably.

When it is your horse who is the novice, allow plenty of time to ensure that his initial experience is a good one. Horses which have become difficult to clip are all too common, so make sure that he is happy to be touched and groomed all over his body weeks before you attempt to put the clippers on him. Allow him to watch other horses being clipped and get accustomed to the sound of the clippers, and when his turn comes, turn on the clippers and hold them carefully against the horse until he relaxes before starting to clip. Take frequent breaks so that the blades do not get hot and he does not lose patience.

Numerous notices in tack shops, feed merchants and the equestrian press advertise the services of experienced people who will clip your horse for you if you do not own clippers or do not wish to do it yourself.

PULLING AND TRIMMING

Careful trimming and pulling of the mane and tail add the finishing touches to a neat, smart appearance and make the horse easier to keep clean. Do bear in mind, however, that all hair serves a purpose. Give careful thought to the amount of hair that it is fair to remove from a horse that lives solely or mainly outdoors, as his protection from the elements will be reduced.

Native types, who are designed by nature to survive in rough conditions, may have a great deal of coarse extra hair around their head and legs, while a fine-coated Thoroughbred may only need his mane tidied up a little to look very presentable. Breed societies and showing organisations have varying rules on what is considered 'correct' turn-out, so do some research if you plan to show. For example, registered native

---

TRIMMING

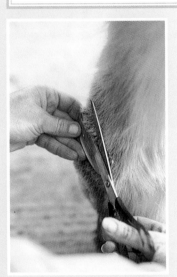

◀ *The backs of the legs and heel areas are trimmed of 'feather' using a mane comb and scissors rather than the clippers. To avoid a severe, 'layered' effect, lift small sections of hair with the comb, trimming off the stray hairs protruding through the comb teeth. Hairs around the fetlock and pastern do help to drain water from the legs, so it may not be advisable to remove these completely from a horse that lives out. Long hairs can be trimmed from the jaw line in a similar way.*

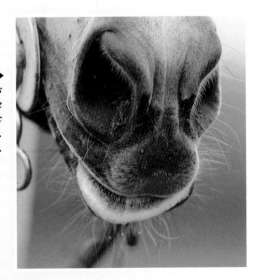

Show judges may prefer the 'streamlined' look of a ▶ trimmed muzzle, but the horse relies on these whiskers as an important aid to the sense of touch. Think carefully before removing whiskers for purely cosmetic reasons, as this is not in the best interests of any horse. Whiskers around the eyes should never be cut.

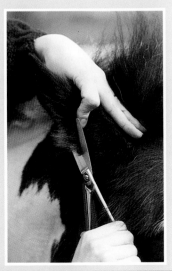

◀ *Do not trim hair away from inside the ears, where it gives essential protection from dust, flies and weather. Tufty hair can be trimmed back after gently pressing the edges of the ears together.*

Choose a warm day for pulling, or attempt it after exercise when the pores will be open.

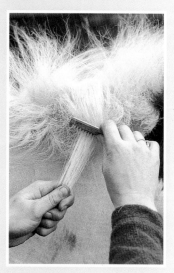

◀ *Thoroughly comb out the mane. Select a few long hairs from underneath and back-comb the remainder. Wrap the long hairs around the fingers or mane comb and pluck with a firm tug. To give a start, any very long excess mane length can be shortened by using scissors before pulling begins.*
Continue along the length of the crest, including the forelock, aiming for an even depth. Do not attempt to do too much in one session or to pull out too many hairs at one time.

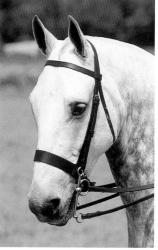

A 'hogged' or 'roached' mane has been removed completely, using clippers. It ▶ is often seen in cobs and polo ponies, or used for horses where a ragged mane spoils the appearance. Hogging needs to be re-done approximately every three weeks and will take several years to grow out completely.

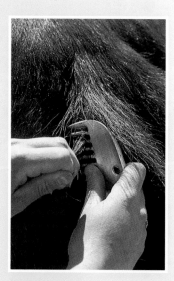

◀ *The top of the tail is pulled by taking a small number of long hairs from the underneath at each side, working down to around two-thirds of the way down the tailbone. The finished appearance is of a tail tapered at the dock but full at the base.*

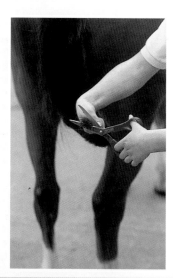

A pulled tail should be cut straight at the bottom, at around 4 inches ▶ (8-10cm) below hock level (known as 'banging'). Take care not to cut too high – the tail lifts naturally when the horse moves. Ask a helper to put an arm underneath to judge the required length. A tail left to grow naturally into a point is termed a 'switch' or 'swish tail'.

ponies are meant to be shown in their 'natural' state, cobs may need the entire mane clipping off (known as hogging) and pure-bred Arabs are exhibited with flowing mane and tail. Check before you set to work!

Areas suitable for trimming include the lower jaw (but not the whiskers around the muzzle, used by the horse as 'antennae'), down the tendons, fetlock and coronet, and any fluff poking outside the ear.

On the legs and along the jaw line, use a comb against the lie of the coat to lift small sections of hair away from the skin before cutting the hairs protruding between the teeth of the comb. Although this is more time-consuming than using clippers, it gives a far better, less severe effect. Some owners choose to clip out a 'bridle path' behind the ears to take the head piece of the bridle, but this is a matter of personal preference. If you do cut one in, do not make it too wide.

The mane and tail look much better if they are thinned out rather than cut with scissors, and this process is called pulling. Pulling can take the place of plaiting if done thoroughly, or it can make a very thick mane and tail easier to plait. Bear in mind that it is preferable to leave the mane and tail quite full if you wish to plait them for special occasions.

Most horses do not mind having their manes and tails pulled if a short section only is done each day, taking very few hairs at a time. For those sensitive individuals who do object violently, it is possible to buy specialised thinning combs which cut the hairs at root level rather than pulling them out and this gives a perfectly acceptable look.

SHOW PREPARATION

Correct turnout and tack varies according to the show class or discipline, so it is best to contact the relevant association or breed society for exact details before the actual day. Your horse will need to be healthy and physically prepared for whatever will be expected of him on the day of a show, so your fitness and stable management routine should take this into account weeks, if not months, before the event. Where hair needs trimming or pulling, do so in the week leading up to the show.

Regular grooming before the event should ensure that the horse's skin and coat are in good condition, but there are several extra measures that can be taken nearer the time, or on the day, to really make him stand out from the crowd.

BATHING

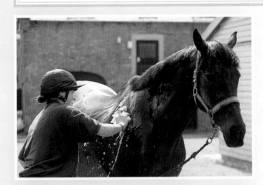

◀ *Tie the horse up on a well-drained surface. Brush clean the coat, mane and tail. Use warm water if possible – this is more pleasant for the horse and lifts grease more effectively. Dampen the coat all over and apply the shampoo according to the manufacturer's instructions. Use a specific horse or animal shampoo only and take care to prevent it going in the eyes. Rub the shampoo well in, using the hands or a rubber curry comb. The head is best wiped over with a sponge.*
Soap the tail by standing slightly to the side of the quarters and dunking it carefully in a bucket.

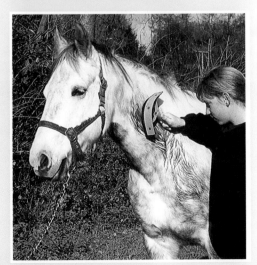

Rinse well ▶
with clean
water. If the
horse is
accustomed to
a hose pipe,
this can be
used in warm
conditions.

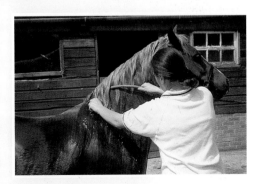

◀ *Remove excess water from the coat using a sweat scraper. Dry the lower legs and heels carefully with a towel. If the horse is quiet, help the tail to dry by standing to the side, holding the upper part and swishing around in a circle. Take care the horse does not chill as he dries off, by using a cooler or anti-sweat sheet or by walking around in-hand*

BATHING

Regular grooming is generally adequate to keep the coat clean and healthy. No matter how carefully and thoroughly a horse is groomed, however, it is almost impossible to remove all the dirt and grease, especially from the roots of the mane and tail hairs, without a good shampoo. Stabled horses in particular will appreciate an occasional bath, although bathing does depend to a large extent on the weather. In cold conditions make do by washing just the tail or any particularly dirty areas as quickly as possible. Avoid bathing animals who live outdoors as it will strip the coat of natural oils. Bathe only in mild weather and never when a horse has a full winter coat.

PLAITING

Depending on the class entered, breed of horse and level of competition, correct turnout may require you to plait. Plaiting is done for neatness and to show off the neck or the hindquarters of a horse with an unpulled tail. Plaits can also be used to train the mane to fall to the preferred side (usually the off-side).

- A few large, bigger plaits will suit a horse with a long, weak neck. A greater number of small, neat plaits enhance a thicker, shorter neck.
- Plaiting is best done on the day. Plaits which are left in overnight always have a 'slept-in' look! Never leave plaits in for excessively long periods.
- Plaits will be more symmetrical if the mane has been tidied and pulled slightly beforehand, but for a tail plait the hair at the dock must be long enough to get the plait started. Bear this in mind if you are pulling!
- Mane and tail hairs are slippery and difficult to plait after shampooing, so any washing should be done a couple of days in advance.

OIL, GLOSS AND QUARTER MARKS

Finishing touches for the ring include applying oil, gloss and quarter marks to help draw attention to particularly attractive features and to catch the judge's eye.

Coat gloss is usually sprayed on before a show class for added shine, but beware of using it on the saddle area before riding because it can make the horse's

PLAITING THE MANE

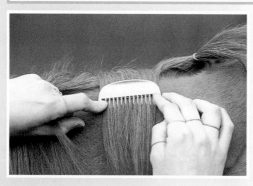

◀ *Ideally the mane should be pulled before plaiting, to create an even length without too much thickness. Comb thoroughly and then damp the mane slightly. Divide into equal sections using rubber bands.*

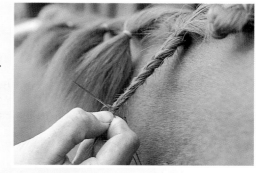

Starting at the top of the neck, take the first bunch of hair and separate ▶ *into three even strands. Begin to plait, lifting the bunch slightly away from the crest. Plait to the end of the hair, keeping a firm, even tension. If a needle and thread are to be used, loop the thread around the end of the plait to secure it. Now push the needle up through the plait from underneath, near to the crest, creating a loop. Fold as many times as necessary to create a neat shape, and finish by stitching through from the under-side.*

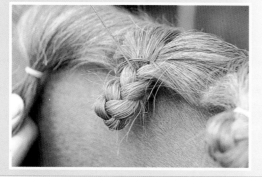

◀ *Rubber bands are a quick and convenient alternative to the traditional needle and thread. Use one band to secure the end of the plait, then double the plait up underneath, folding as necessary. Secure by looping one or more bands around the whole plait until it is tight.*

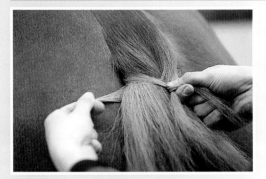

◀ *The tail must be full and unpulled, with at least three months' growth, to allow it to be neatly plaited. Take care when standing behind the horse, keeping slightly to one side. Dampen the hair. Either take three small bunches of long hair from the top, two from one side and one from the other; or take some from the middle of the dock added to one from each side.*

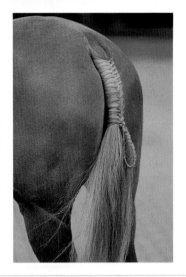

Begin to plait down the centre of the tail, taking a small number of hairs ▶ *from each side successively and incorporating them. Work downwards until three-quarters of the length of the dock has been reached. Finish plaiting the length of the hairs that are left. Secure the end with thread or a band and loop it back underneath itself. Sew firmly in position.*

For riding or competing in wet and muddy conditions, the tail can be put up. The plait is continued the full length of the dock and finished by incorporating the whole tail. Roll up neatly to the end of the dock and stitch firmly.

coat slippery. Baby oil or vaseline can be smeared lightly around the muzzle and outer edge of the eyes. Hoof oil is also generally applied.

Various patterns, known as quarter marks, can be brushed or stencilled onto the horse's hindquarters to draw attention to them.

TRAVELLING

TRAILER VERSUS HORSEBOX

There are basically two types of methods of transporting horses by road – horsebox (lorry) or trailer. The one chosen depends on a number of practical considerations such as budget, the number of horses needed to be transported at any one time, and how far and how often you intend to travel.

In general terms, a lorry provides a more comfortable, stable ride for the horse than a trailer and is easier for the driver to manoeuvre. A larger number of horses can potentially fit inside, and tack, storage and preparation space is less of a problem when going to shows and competitions. Owners who travel long distances or are frequently away over-night will find a lorry with a living area convenient and will save money on accommodation. With a lorry it is possible to check on horses in transit and make sure that all is in order. Lorries, however, can clearly cost a great deal to buy, run and maintain and require frequent use to keep the engine

in good working order.

A trailer is cheaper to buy, run and maintain than a lorry and takes up less space in the yard. It is a good choice if you only wish to transport one or two horses a relatively short distance from time to time. However, it does require a suitable vehicle to tow with and space for all your gear in the car. When only one horse is being transported in a trailer, he must always be loaded on the side nearest the centre of the road, not the kerb side, to avoid affecting the balance and handling of the trailer around corners.

TRAVEL CLOTHING

- Full leg protection from knee or hock to below the coronet band (use stable bandages with extra padding or specially designed travel boots). See page 182 for more details on fitting. It is a wise precaution to add over-reach boots to protect the vulnerable heel area.
- Rugs will depend on the weather conditions, but bear in mind that horses tend to get hot while travelling, so a lightweight rug or cooler is usually sufficient, even in winter.
- Tails can get badly rubbed while travelling, so always use a tail bandage and consider using a tail guard over it on longer trips.
- A leather head collar is better than nylon to prevent chafing, and the horse should always be

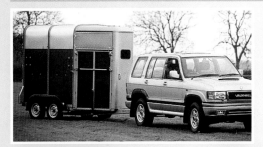

◀ *The mechanical condition and the floor of the horsebox or trailer must be checked regularly. The engine size and the weight of any towing vehicles should be well up to coping with the trailer when loaded and the towing hitch must be at the correct level. Check with the vehicle and trailer manufacturers for relevant weights, towing capacity and correct tyre pressure. Drive with the utmost care, particularly when towing, avoiding sudden braking or sharp turns.*

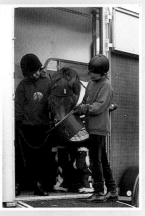

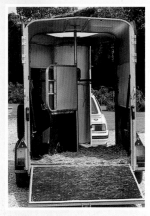

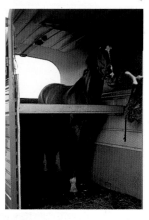

▲ *Even if regular transportation is not necessary, practise loading and travelling often. Introduce young or nervous horses to the experience gradually and sympathetically.*

▲ *The box or trailer should be light airy and inviting and appropriate for the size of the horse. A thin layer of clean, dust-free bedding or rubber matting aids grip. Partitioning must allow each horse plenty of space to adjust its weight and spread its legs a little. Avoid using partitions that reach right to the floor.*

▲ *Tie the horse securely but not too short - he needs some freedom to use his head and neck for balance. Provide a haynet for long journeys or the return home.*

Travelling is a hazardous business and a stressful time for horses, who have a knack of injuring themselves or treading on each other in transit unless they are well wrapped up. Protective gear increases comfort and avoids both major and minor scrapes, cuts or injuries. Even for the shortest of journeys, any horse in transit will require the following:

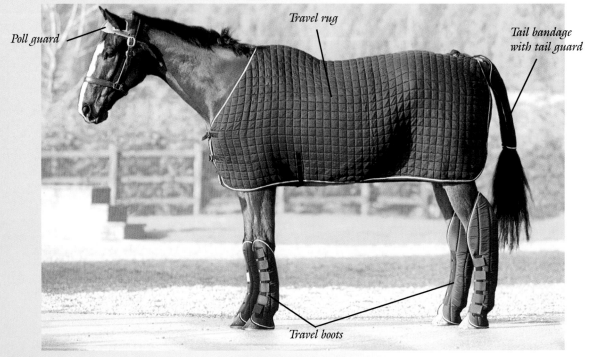

Poll guard

Travel rug

Tail bandage with tail guard

Travel boots

CLOTHING FOR TRAVEL

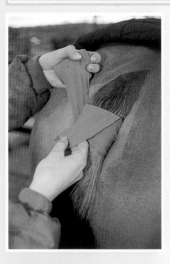

◀ *Dampen the top of the tail so the hairs lie flat. Lift the tail, if possible resting it over the shoulder. However, with nervous or unreliable horses, take great care and stand a little to the side.*

Unravel about 4 inches (8-10cm) of bandage and place at an angle to the top of the tail. Holding this in place, make one firm wrap, tucking the end in as you go.

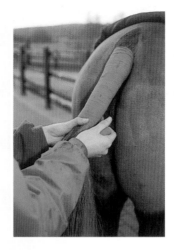

◀ *Wrap around at least once more to secure. Now continue down the tail, wrapping firmly and evenly and covering half of the previous turn each time.*

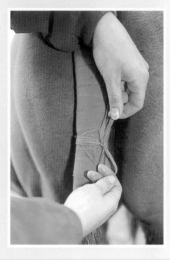

◀ *When the end of the tail-bone is reached,* ▶ *wrap upwards again, aiming to finish mid-way up. Tie tapes smoothly in a secure double bow and tuck in ends. A tail bandage can be removed by releasing the ties and pulling firmly from the top.*

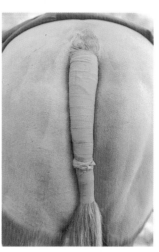

tied to the tie-ring with twine which will break in an emergency. He must be tied short enough to prevent him turning round or getting a leg over the rope, whilst still allowing enough freedom for him to use his head and neck to help with balance.

- A poll guard will protect the vulnerable area on top of the horse's head from knocks.

TRAVELLING & LOADING TIPS
It should always be acknowledged that entering a small, shady, enclosed space goes against every instinct a horse possesses. Considering that horses are naturally nervous and claustrophobic animals which evolved to rely on flight for their survival, it is remarkable that most are so tolerant of methods of transport where they are completely enclosed and constantly having to re-adjust their balance without warning.

The stress of the experience and the tolerance of equines are often under-estimated. Owners should strive to create travelling conditions that are both as safe and as stress-free as possible (see page 192).

It is well worth taking the time to teach a horse to load easily from an early age. Difficult loaders are all too common, and can be both frustrating and dangerous.

Practise familiarising a young horse with the vehicle at home. If he is properly halter-broken and leads easily then he should load, but be patient and allow plenty of time to achieve what you set out to do. Make sure there is bedding inside and down the ramp and that it is light and welcoming inside. Start by making small demands, such as loading him up with a friendly horse, running the engine and unloading again, before progressing to short trips.

Unloading can actually present more of a problem than loading to a youngster, especially if there is a steep lorry ramp to negotiate. These can appear quite intimidating from the top! Be ready for the horse to jump at least part of the way down on the first few occasions. With a trailer, ensure the horse is untied and that you are on the right side of the breast bar before you undo the breaching bar or straps behind him in case he goes into reverse and makes a quick dash for the exit.

193

There are a number of methods used to persuade reluctant loaders to go up the ramp, such as pressurising them from behind with lunge lines or a yard broom, but these are rarely humane or effective in the long term and can make matters worse, particularly for an already frightened animal. A more effective approach is to analyse why a particular horse is against the idea of travelling and go out of your way to make the whole experience as agreeable as possible. Time, patience, practice and very careful driving are usually the answer.

DRIVING WITH CARE
Horses in transit have no way of anticipating changes of speed or direction. The stress of trying to remain upright under these circumstances for an animal whose instincts make staying on its feet of paramount importance, can take a great deal out of it, even during a relatively short trip. It is, therefore, very important that you drive slowly and carefully, brake gently and swing wide around corners. Practise driving an empty lorry or trailer before trying with live cargo, as it this does take some getting used to.

Aim to arrive at your destination with plenty of time to spare to give the horse a chance to recover, and to ensure that you are not tempted to drive too fast because of time restrictions. On a very long journey ensure you have any passports and paperwork you will need so that the journey is delayed as little as possible.

CARE OF THE HORSE DURING SHORT JOURNEYS
Travelling is a stressful enough experience for the horse without unnecessary dietary changes, so always take a supply of his regular food and water. A hay net is a good idea, provided that the horse is drinking regularly; hay without water can cause gut blockages and colic. The horse should also have small short feeds at the usual times.

Dehydration is a significant danger when travelling, so check horses reguarly, offering water frequently and ensuring the vehicle is well ventilated. If the horse refuses to drink water on a long journey, see if he will take a sloppy mix of sugar beet, if beet is part of his usual diet.

On longer journeys unload at intervals, if there is a safe place to do so. Walk the horse around for half an hour, check he is a comfortable temperature and encourage him to have a pick of grass, drink, stale and do droppings. Muck out the lorry or trailer and add fresh hay and bedding before re-loading.

For further information on the travelling of performance horses, see Chapter Nine.

9 THE COMPETITION HORSE

FITTENING METHODS & SCHEDULES FOR THE COMPETITION HORSE

THE IMPORTANCE OF TRAINING ON THE FLAT

Flat training is of great importance for all competition horses. The description of one training system would be inappropriate here, but whichever discipline one is referring to – dressage, show jumping, cross-country, endurance or combined training events – balance, suppleness, manoeuverability and control lead to a better performance with reduced injuries, and to better jumping, as well as a better dressage test. Although the different disciplines are targeting at slightly different results, strength, fitness and condition are produced by flat work and are essential to all disciplines.

The importance of rhythm, suppleness, contact, strength and impulsion, together with collection, cannot be over-emphasised. The horse must be taught to yield to the leg and to the rein laterally, and to be able to shoulder-in, shoulder-out and haunches-in and haunches-out.

At all levels, a horse should be capable of working in a 10-metre circle off the centre line to produce flexibility, not only for a dressage test but also for the show jumping horse, to produce rideability and flexibility. Frequent transitions focus attention and help create a horse that is far lighter on the forehand.

The jumping horse needs to be able to increase or reduce its stride length and to stay balanced on its turns. Rein-back is important obviously in more advanced dressage tests; it is also important for

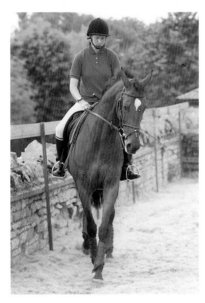

Whatever the competitive discipline, training on the flat is of vital importance both in terms of education and physical fitness.

horses of other disciplines. Correct work will produce suppleness and flexibility both laterally and lengthwise, allowing full use of the quarters, back and neck and developing the top-line.

Trainers and riders must always remember that flat work is often performed on all-weather arenas. The horse that is going to compete needs to be able to work on different surfaces, so do ground work on grass as well as on artificial surfaces. A horse must also be used to different types of going, including firmer surfaces, as, unfortunately, it will not always have an ideal track to jump off or compete on.

To avoid boredom, both mental and physical, fitness is hugely important during flat work for all disciplines. Fast work at three- to four-day intervals plays a central role in the correct preparation of a horse and one must assess pulse and respiration typically five to eight minutes after work. Do not

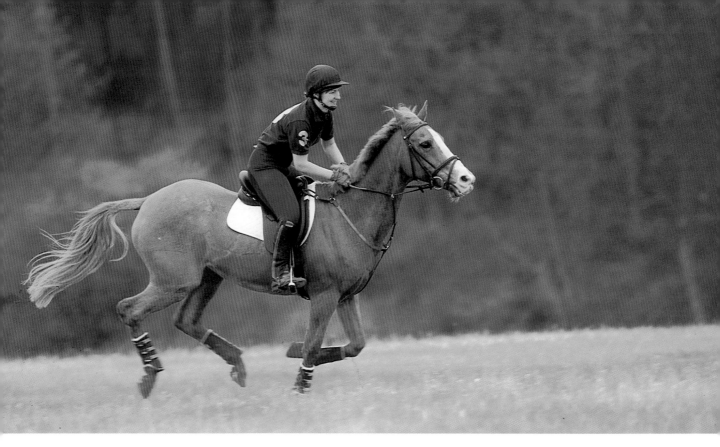

Interval training develops both anaerobic and aerobic muscular function.

forget that hills are useful training for those of us fortunate enough to live in areas with hills available.

INTERVAL TRAINING

Interval training is nowadays considered essential for competition horses to develop anaerobic as well as aerobic muscular function. The principle behind this method is that one works a horse near maximum speed, allows for partial recovery and then returns to fast work. This type of training is essential for three-day event horses and others expected to compete anaerobically.

It must be acknowledged that there are obviously risks involved in putting the body under stress. For the horses that are being used for endurance riding, anaerobic training may not be essential if one only wants to compete, but is important to those who wish to win.

Endurance horses require conditioning for physical and mental stress and the welfare and well-being of the horse must always be uppermost in mind. Metabolic, muscular, skeletal, and mental training have to go hand-in-hand, and nutrition also has an extremely important role to play. The time taken to train a mature horse for endurance riding is likely to be as long as six months, and much longer in a younger horse. Conditioning is a slow process. Group work may well be helpful for the lazy horse disinclined to push himself in training to the levels of effort required.

MONITORING

If, within five to ten minutes after exercise, the heart rate remains at 72 and above, the workload or speed of exercise is probably beyond the horse's metabolic tolerance. One would normally wait until the pulse rate is down to 64 before proceeding, and this should take no more than about 15 minutes. If it does take more than 15 minutes, the speed or amount of the workload should be reduced. This is the principle used in the training of an endurance horse.

The CRI (cardio-respiratory index) can be extremely useful in monitoring fitness. The pulse is taken and a 40-metre trot out and back performed, the pulse then being re-taken one minute after the first reading. A rise of more than four is an indicator that fitness is not satisfactory. This guideline is most useful if the pulse is initially between 64 and 80. As a method of monitoring this has been used regularly by endurance riders but is adaptable to other disciplines.

THE EVENT HORSE

Possibly the most complicated of our competition horses to get fit is the event horse. Originally a military discipline designed to prepare horse and rider to perform well in the battle field, eventing tests the ability of the horse at diverse exercises – dressage, speed and endurance, cross-country and show jumping. Each discipline requires specific, and sometimes contradictory, methods of training and fittening.

Unless competing only at a very basic level, the event horse must be able to exercise both anaerobically and aerobically. The horse's training must vary according to the level of competition expected. In addition, the complications of the varying physiological stresses have to be appreciated when planning an exercise regime. These obviously vary according to the target performance level – is it to be novice one-day events or advanced three-day events?

Horses competing at below three-day event status will be unlikely to have to reach sustained speeds of more than 500 metres per minute and so can largely perform aerobically rather than anaerobically. Thus a training schedule need not concentrate on anaerobic work to the same degree as a three-day horse, whose steeplechase will be well above the aenaerobic threshold, as will a demanding cross-country course. This is especially true of the course that is twisty or undulating or covers hilly terrain.

SHOW JUMPING TRAINING
When training for show jumping, it is essential to remember that the speed of approach to a fence will be greatly increased by the fence height, or in a jump-off situation. The energy expended by a show jumper can be extreme, even if it is only for a short period of time. In fact, this has been assessed as being the equivalent of galloping at 600 metres per minute.

In show jumping there is a marked cortisol rise. Although this is less than that seen in an endurance horse, the more experienced show jumper shows significant cortisol rises, and, once again, the importance of flat work cannot be over-emphasised. Many course designers use technical problems to sort out big fields rather than resorting to the size of the fence to solve the problem.

TRAINING OVER FENCES
Hand in glove with flat work, jumping is also an inherent ability to a large degree. It is therefore extremely difficult to train a horse which does not have the natural technique and aptitude to jump well.

Horses are trained to jump on the lunge, free-jumping down a lane of fences, and ridden. The use of ground lines is extremely important to foster confidence, as are poles at take-off and landing to improve the arc of the jump. Grid work is also used to produce precision and balance.

The process is not one that can be rushed. Time is required, as tissues are slow to adapt to the discipline. Consider three to six months as a minimum period for the adaptation of muscle tissue to jumping.

The type of jumping required from a horse varies from short course jumping to taking on a track such as that used in the Hickstead Derby, where aerobic respiration and anaerobic respiration are used. Where this element of endurance is introduced, show jumpers have, once again, adapted the principles of interval training to produce increased fitness.

POOR PERFORMANCE
Investigation of poor performance of the competition horse involves all the monitoring factors described previously, including blood samples for haematology and biochemistry, the use of endoscopes and treadmills to test respiratory function.

Discomfort, in the form of low-grade pain, soreness in the feet and joints when landing or hind-limb pain from the hocks when taking off, will clearly affect performance.

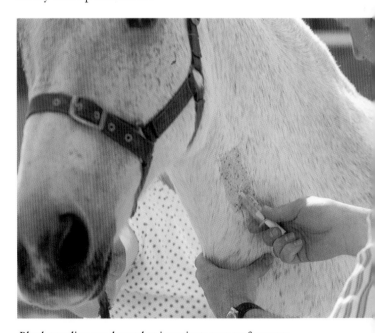

Blood sampling can be used to investigate poor performance.

When attempting to assess a drop in performance levels, it is often useful to administer a week's course of non-steroid anti-inflammatories and then to reassess the horse physically and clinically. This may be the only indicator that low-grade pain is playing a part in the reduced performance.

Studs may be required to help the horse keep a safe footing in varying ground and weather conditions. Studs, which can be of varying shapes and lengths, are screwed into a hole prepared by the farrier in the heel of the shoe. This job is made easier by the use of a special spanner or 'tap'.

- There are numerous lengths and sizes of stud, but as a general rule longer, pointed studs are used when the ground is hard and dry but possibly slippery, and larger, blunter, squared-off studs are designed for grip in wet, muddy conditions.
- Remove all studs immediately after exercise or competition to avoid the horse treading on itself (or its handler) and causing injury, and to minimise the unbalancing effect the studs inevitably have on the horse's leg and foot.
- Keep stud-holes free of dirt by plugging with greased cotton wool or screwing in flat 'dummy' studs.

PRACTICAL FACTORS OF PERFORMANCE

CARE DURING AND AFTER COMPETITION

Having spent a great deal of time and expense getting a competition horse fit, it makes sense to limit the risk of problems during competition by careful pre-planning and preparation.

SHOEING

- Shoe at least 7 to 10 days prior to competition to avoid problems created by nail binds or pricks or soreness from feet being cut back.
- Do not arrive with shoes that will require replacing during competition.
- Even with good preparation, shoes will come loose, so check daily.
- Take a spare set of shoes and studs, plus the correct size of nails, particularly when competing abroad.
- While mentioning studs, the author personally feels that long-term stresses and injuries can be created by using one stud only in the lateral branch of the shoe. Two studs should be used, one in the lateral and one in the medial branch of the shoe, for balance.
- Carry equipment to remove a shoe in an emergency and be able to use it (hammer, buffer, nail-remover and pincers). An Equiboot for temporary protection can be very useful and will double as a poultice boot.
- When considering preparation of feet for competition, remember that methionine and biotin supplements may improve hoof wall quality.
- Finally, always check the shoes and feet after work when performing the standard leg check.

VACCINATIONS

Vaccination provides important protection against virus infection risks such as equine flu and herpes and is especially important against tetanus (see Chapter Two). Immunisation against rabies is also routine in some countries.

There are also standard requirements for vaccination when competing under competition rules. It is important to check prior to competition that your horse's documentation is correct. If in doubt, ask.

FITNESS

The importance of fitness before competition and during competition cannot be over-emphasised and the fittening of a competition horse has been discussed in the first section of this chapter.

- **Monitor fitness** during competition and increase care when inspecting the horse for signs of injury or disease. Regular monitoring at the same time of day and at the same time of the exercise programme is important. Temperature, pulse, respiration and leg checks must be regularly performed both prior to and post-competition.

- **Blood sampling** for health status prior to and during competition provides useful information providing that regular pre-competition testing has been carried out to provide a base-line measurement.

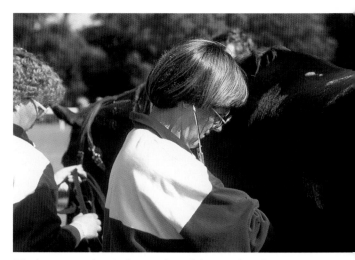

The heart rate of an endurance horse being monitored during one of several vet checks that are compulsory throughout the competition. All performance horses, in whatever discipline, should be assessed at regular intervals during the event.

- **Limb monitoring** before and after exercise is extremely important. An initial visual examination should first be done and then a manual palpation made, looking for swelling or temperature changes. Remember to perform these examinations before bandages are applied or cold water treatment has been performed.

- **Bandaging**   There is much debate about the use and value of stable bandaging. Obviously the monitoring of limbs is easier without.

Bear in mind that the absence of lameness does not mean that damage has not occurred. Failure to notice the early symptoms such as heat, pain and swelling can lead to disaster. Nowadays, monitoring the legs with ultrasonic scan and thermograph can assist in early diagnosis if trouble is spotted during limb monitoring.

NUTRITION
Monitor food intake before and during competition. Nutrition has been discussed in detail in Chapter Three; however, a few points are important to re-emphasise:

- If possible, take feed which the horse is used to from home. Change nothing in the run-up to or during competition.
- A laxative diet can be important during extended periods of travel.
- Never restrict water (apart from drinking very large quantities within an hour of fast competition).
- Make sure that the water is palatable by tasting it yourself. If you do not like drinking it, your horse will not, and this will lead to dehydration or colic.

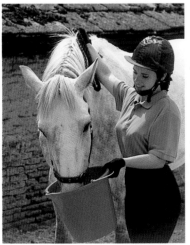

Horses under stress are at greater risk from colic. Make no abrupt changes to the diet before or during a competition. If possible, use feed from home that the horse is well used to.

Water filters can be useful, or in extreme circumstances, flavouring of water with apple juice, etc.

The idea that water is harmful close to competition is a fallacy. There is no harm in letting your horse drink small amounts of water (half a bucket) during competition (for example, during the 10-minute box in three-day eventing), between rounds (for example, in show jumping) and during long warm-up periods (such as in dressage). Drinking will also help to cool the horse down and reduce the effects of dehydration.

PROTECTION OF THE HORSE DURING COMPETITION

LEG PROTECTION
The use of bandages and boots for protection of the horse's legs is discussed in the previous chapter. In the opinion of this author, neither play any part in preventing strain or over-stretching. They may, if of good quality and properly applied, protect against physical injury during training and competition and therefore do serve a purpose in this way.

Where boots are used, it is important the correct type is selected for the competition or training in mind. For instance, some boots do have a tendency to funnel mud up between the boot and the skin and some types are more likely to rub than others. The correct material, design and size must be carefully chosen.

If bandaging is to be used, great care and skill is required so that the pressure exerted is sufficient to provide the protection required without slippage and without restricting circulation, which can cause extreme long-term damage to tissues.

SADDLERY
Well-fitting saddles and correct, properly-maintained bridles are obviously extremely important.

Always take spares; always check before and after competition and make sure that contact areas are kept extremely clean. Technology nowadays allows us to use new materials and some of these, for example gel pads, are particularly useful to provide extra protection for the back if necessary. Nothing can replace a saddle that is a perfect fit for the horse, however. An inadequate or poorly-fitting saddle will affect the performance of the horse, with or without a pad or numnah/saddle cloth. (For details, see sections below on back problems and on saddle fitting in Chapter Eight).

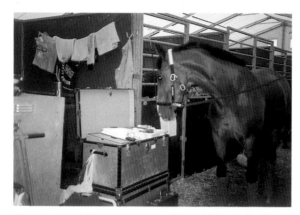

Temporary stabling at show grounds provides notoriously unhygenic, overcrowded and dusty environments over which owners have little control.

ENVIRONMENT

No matter how well you have conditioned your horse's respiratory system, if during travel or at an unfamiliar stable or show ground you expose him to an unsatisfactory and dusty environment, or use hay or feed that may be dusty, the horse's lungs will very quickly respond adversely, leading to a marked reduction in performance. Measures to avoid this include taking dust-free hay or haylage, damping all feeds, making sure the bedding is dust-free by use of shavings or paper, and ensuring there is adequate ventilation during transport and in the stable.

Finally, remember that however good the environment may be in your own box initially, dusty hay and straw in adjoining boxes will rapidly contaminate the air space and create a problem.

PRE- AND POST-COMPETITION WARMING UP
See Rhabdomyolis, below.

COMMON DISORDERS & INJURIES OF THE PERFORMANCE HORSE

RHABDOMYOLIS ('TYING UP')
(See also Chapters Two and Four)
Warming up, as well as warming down post-exercise, is particularly important for the three-day event, endurance or show jumping rider. One of the most common problems seen in these competition horses is rhabdomyolis, or 'tying up'. This is often seen in the three-day horse, post-steeplechase or on the roads and tracks. Clinical check-up in the ten-minute box for any stiffness in action is extremely important. The other time that it commonly appears

is at the end of the cross-country phase. In endurance horses, tying up is often seen quite early in competition, but may also occur in association with tiring and dehydration at any stage.

This condition is more common in fillies and mares than in their male counterparts and it is also more common in nervous horses.

Signs and causes: Clinical symptoms include mild to severe stiffness and alteration in gait, abnormal sweating and occasionally, mild colic symptoms. Raised muscle enzymes are found in blood samples. Causes are multiple and, as far as competition horses are concerned, viral compromise, electrolyte deficiency or imbalance or dietary imbalance, or excessive carbohydrates are amongst those listed. In recurrent cases, intrinsic abnormality and muscle function probably results from excess nitrogen storage and utilisation of the muscle and abnormal regulation of intracellular calcium in the muscle, causing the muscle fibres to contract and relax more quickly than in unaffected horses. Some researchers are investigating genetic links.

Treatment and prevention: Treatment should be immediate. The horse should be moved as little as possible and if necessary, transported by horse-box back to the stables. Fluid balance and renal function must be maintained, in acute cases by administration of intravenous fluids. The pain and distress must be relieved by the use of non-steroid anti-inflammatory drugs, perhaps with small doses of a sedative in an extremely distressed horse.

To avoid tying up, careful warm-up working-in and working-out of the horse before and after exercise, plus control of the diet, can be extremely helpful in preventing recurrence. Obviously, conditioning and fitness play an important part in this situation.

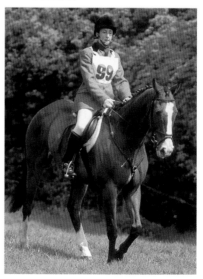

Careful working-in and working-down of the horse before and after exercise plays a crucial role in avoiding 'tying up', both at home and at competitions.

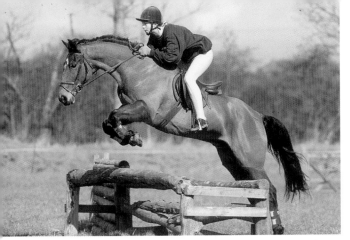

Freedom from discomfort is essential for the horse to make a good shape (bascule) over a fence.

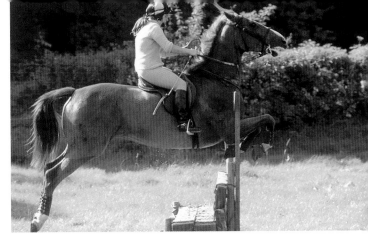

'Cat-jumping' is often an attempt by the horse to avoid or minimise pain from 'bad back syndrome'.

Remember that post-competition requirements will vary depending on the climate in which you are competing. Rugs/blankets must be available to prevent chilling in very cold climates, and the aggressive cooling described later must be available immediately after exercising in warm climates. The correct handling of the horse post-competition will have a considerable effect on its performance on the following days or weeks.

BAD BACK SYNDROME

Signs and causes: Cases of 'bad back syndrome' are usually reported to have a loss of performance, often involving a change in action both in their ground work and when jumping. This might include not making a good shape in the air, 'cat-jumping' or dropping a leg or legs. See also Chapter Eleven.

There are, in the author's opinion, several conditions responsible for this syndrome and any one or a combination of several may be responsible for the presenting symptoms. The problem can commonly be located in one of four areas, as follows.

PAIN IN THE WITHER AREA ON PALPATION
• often accompanied by mild fore-limb lameness which may only be seen on a circle or on flexion
• often the lameness is bilateral
• anterior phase of the stride is usually shortened jumping is affected, with horse being unhappy about landing.
Treatment: This often occurs as a secondary symptom to fore-limb lameness, and is due to the change in action created. If the primary cause is treated, the symptoms improve. Primary conditions might be due to infection (fistulas withers) or injury, such as fracture of the spinous processes. Saddles should be checked for correct fitting (see below and Chapter Eight).

PAIN IN SADDLE AREA
• pain on palpation of saddle area

• sometimes heat and obvious skin abrasion
• resistance when saddled
• occasional pain in area of girth.
Treatment:
• topical anti-inflammatory preparations
• systemic anti-inflammatory medication with antibiotics rest
• check saddle for fit and adequate padding (see Chapter Eight)
• use gel pad.

PAIN BEHIND THE SADDLE AREA
• muscle spasm
• pain on reflex of back
• unwilling to flex or 'make a good shape in the air'.
Treatment: Depends on cause. Radiography and bone scintigraphy will be required to diagnose the cause of the pain and spasm. The underlying cause may lie primarily in this region, e.g. 'kissing spines', or to trauma-induced local damage, or it may be secondary and a response to conditions of the sacro-iliac, or hind-leg lameness.

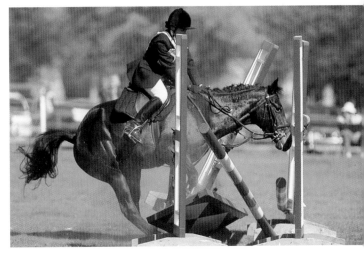

When persistent performance problems occur that cannot be attributed to rider error or inadequate training, the likelihood of some physical discomfort must be investigated.

Treat primary cause:
- rest
- anti-inflammatory drugs orally, systemically or by local injection
- muscle relaxants
- non-steroidal DMSO preparations
- heat therapy (infra-red)
- laser therapy
- ultrasound
- manipulation and massage (see Chapter Eleven).

PAIN IN THE SACRO-ILIAC REGION
- change in hind-leg action, which can vary from positive lameness to an inward swing of the hock
- flexion test may produce lameness
- pain on flexion
- palpable lack of uniformity of the sacro-iliac
- occasionally, crepitus (grating noise)
- muscle wasting on one side of quarters.

Treatment:
- manipulation and controlled exercise to build up the supporting muscles (not universally accepted by the veterinary profession!)
- rest
- local injection of sclereosing agents plus box rest.
- local injection of long-acting corticosteroids, possibly with controlled work regime.

PENETRATING WOUNDS

Penetrating wounds are amongst the most common injuries to which performance horses are susceptible. Wounds might involve either soft-tissue damage, joint penetration or tendon penetration, or a combination of these.

Fence-created injuries are common to all jumping disciplines, as are self-inflicted wounds, and both can be career-threatening. Prompt and accurate assessment of these wounds can make a huge difference to the athletic future of the horse.

OVER-REACH WOUNDS
- common sites are bulbs of heels, back of pastern/fetlock or tendon
- assessment must include search of wound for damage to tendons, ligaments, joints, or possible foreign bodies
- joint-flushing should be performed as soon as possible if penetration of the joint or synovial cavity has occurred. An inter-articular antibiotic should be used in these cases and referral to a specialist centre is advised
- whether to suture a wound below the fetlock, and

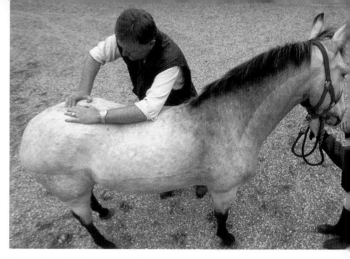

Palpation will frequently help to pinpoint the affected area of the back.

what form of support and dressing is required, depend upon accurate assessment.

CHEST AREA WOUNDS
These are created by striking the chest area with the extended jumping studs that are required particularly when surface conditions are slippery.
- careful repair is required as scarring in the girth area can be a major problem
- chest penetrations are often seen when horses run onto the wings of a jump
- good drainage is essential, as there is always significant tissue damage.

HIND-LIMB WOUNDS
Wounds to the hind leg tend to fall into the following categories:

- **Stifle injuries**
  Horses jumping fixed cross-country fences frequently drag hind limbs across fences resulting in stifle injuries. It can be difficult, in the absence of crepitus (scraping noise), to determine, in the acute phase, whether or not a fracture has occurred. Rapid development of severe peri-articular swelling, or distension of the femoro-tibial and/or femoro-patellar joint capsules may reflect a fracture. Lameness associated with bruising only is usually substantially better within 24-48 hours.
  Persistent lameness is highly suggestive of fracture and the joint should be X-rayed, including caudo-cranial and lateral-medial views, but also oblique views and a sky-line view of the patella. Even if fracture is suspected, support therapy is usually adequate until further investigation is performed. Stifle injuries can be created by metal cups on the wings. The same precautions must be taken as described above.
- **Brushing wounds**
- **Wounds and trauma to the front of the fetlock.**

DIAGNOSING BACK PROBLEMS

Problems with the neck and back are as common in horses as in people. The difference between our spinal structures and the mass of muscle and tissue overlying the horse's back bones, however, make it even more difficult to identify the exact source of the trouble in the horse.

Few X-ray machines are powerful enough to give anything but a moderate image of the vertebrae. And although the tips of the spinous processes can be felt emerging from the mid-line muscle, only a relatively superficial assessment can be made, particularly as the horse's back is naturally tensed to maintain its standing position. Ultrasound can assist in the investigation of ligament and soft tissue damage.

As the horse will try to compensate for any discomfort in his back, stress to joints in the back may show as problems in the limbs and feet. Horses do not suffer from slipped discs or trapped nerves, as there is no prospect of the disc (see diagram, Chapter Four) protruding from between the vertebrae and putting pressure on the nerve roots. Problems may involve muscles, ligaments, nerves, bones and/or joints. Bone disease falls into three main groups:

TRAUMATIC INJURY

Heavy falls may fracture one or more vertebrae. Usually the horse cannot get up and diagnosis may have to wait until the effects of concussion are overcome. Careful neurological examination can then establish if there is any paralysis of the hind limbs, which would indicate a likely fracture. Fractures may also occur in fragments of bone, which may recover temporarily but then deteriorate as bruising and internal bleeding affect the spinal cord. Few fractures heal completely, and secondary arthritis is always a risk. Most often the horse has to be put down.

Falls at speed can extensively fracture the pelvis. Recovery is not possible from such damage. Less severe stress fractures can also occur to the pelvic bones from strenuous exercise. As it is the wing of the ilum, well above the hip joint, that is usually involved, three to six months of box rest usually brings about a good recovery. Fractures of the bones of the sacrum, perhaps from a heavy fall directly onto the rear end, can damage the spinal nerves and lead to long-lasting paralysis of the tail and anus (see Chapter Six).

The other common pelvic injury is sacro-iliac rupture, where the fibrous junction between the pelvis and spine is torn on one side following a fall or the horse 'doing the splits'. Clear asymmetry can be seen between the one side of the pelvis and the other, viewed from behind. The horse may be acutely lame or only stiff. Ultrasound scanning and X-rays will confirm the diagnosis and extent of any twisting. Manipulation can bring improvement and box rest, to allow the joint to stabilise and become fixed, can result in a return to soundness.

INTRA-VERTEBRAL DISEASE

This is relatively uncommon and hard to diagnose accurately. Changes take place within the actual bones, e.g. abscess, infection or tumour, causing paralysis, stiffness and gait abnormalities.

INTER-VERTEBRAL DISEASE

Two types of disease commonly occur between the vertebrae.

In 'kissing spines' (spinous process impingement), the dorsal spines of the vertebrae rub together as the back flexes, causing inflammation and new bone growth that narrows the gap between vertebrae leading to reduced performance, reluctance to jump, erratic behaviour and stiffness. As these lie close to the surface X-rays can help with diagnosis, but must be considered cautiously as bone remodelling can take place between the vertebrae of normal horses. Most cases involve the thoracic vertebrae lying just beneath the saddle, where back flexibility is at its maximum. Injecting local anaesthetic into the space between the bones should produce a dramatic improvement. Treatment involves long rest, with physiotherapy and controlled exercise on pain-killers or surgical re-shaping of the vertebral spines. Interspinous injection of carticasteroids can be successful

Arthritis may develop between the joints of any of the vertebrae, but most commonly between the last lumbar vertebra and the sacrum, a highly mobile joint with three distinct articulation sites. Lumbo-sacral disease produces long-term stiffness and poor use of the hind limbs, resulting in dragged toes, reluctance to lift the hind feet and muscle wastage on the quarters. Pain-killers should reveal an improvement leading to diagnosis, but no treatment exists.

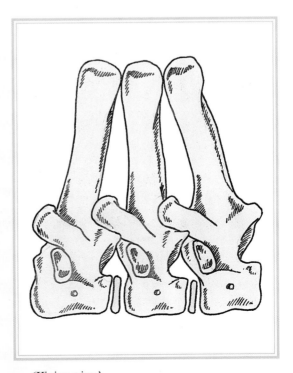

'Kissing spines'

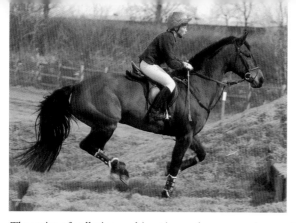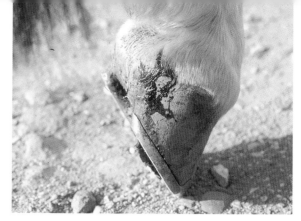

The action of galloping and jumping makes over-reach wounds common in performance horses. Even an innocuous-seeming wound must be treated seriously.

TENDON AND LIGAMENT DAMAGE

This may involve:

- flexor tendon strain/rupture (see Chapter Four)
- suspensory ligament desmitis (inflammation)
- check-ligament injury.

The importance of the initial anti-inflammatory treatment, combined with cold treatment (remember the frozen polystyrene cup for 20 minutes at a time!) and support cannot be over-emphasised. Beware of the mildly lame horse which has a slight lesion in the suspensory apparatus. Jumping with these lesions is disastrous.

FRACTURES

Fractures may involve:

- pedal bone
- navicular
- pastern
- fetlock
- cannon
- upper limb (rarely)
- skull.

Fractures of the pedal bone are relatively rare, the pastern of the fore-limb being the most common in the author's experience.

STRESS-INDUCED INJURIES

- 'Tying up' (rhabdomyolysis), see above.
- Colic, see Chapter Three.
- Bad back syndrome, see above.
- Navicular bursitis/sore heel syndrome, see below.

NAVICULAR BURSITIS (SORE HEEL SYNDROME)

The importance of good shoeing and foot balancing for all horses, but in particular for the competition horse, cannot be over-emphasised (see Chapter Four). Poor heel conformation is, unfortunately, all too common. The lameness that results usually has low-grade symptoms but can be sudden in onset if the bursa becomes acutely inflamed.

EXERCISE-INDUCED INJURIES

EXERCISE-INDUCED PULMONARY HAEMORRHAGE.

This is fairly common in the competition horse due to their environment which, even if good at home, is often poor on even our major show grounds (a cause for veterinary concern). Travel conditions also do not help. This is usually not a major problem, but certainly warrants detailed endoscopic examination to confirm diagnosis.

THORACIC VESSEL/ATRIAL RUPTURE

- Can cause rapid collapse and death and is often very dramatic

Also:

- Guttural pouch haemorrhage
- Exercise-induced asthma.

TRAVEL-INDUCED INJURIES

- Travel sickness
- Road traffic accident in box or trailer.

ENVIRONMENTALLY-INDUCED INJURIES

- Acute respiratory allergy (see Chapter Five).
- Acute urticaria (see Chapter Seven).
- Sunburn (see Chapter Seven).

OTHER

- Trauma (see Chapter Six)
- Eye injuries (see Chapter Six)
- Damage to the lip or tongue from the bit is a common competition horse injury and requires careful repair and time to heal.

THE HORSE UNDER STRESS

HEAT STRESS

Even in temperate climates such as Britain, summer temperatures can reach levels that may well affect a horse's performance. As, under certain circumstances, these can be life-threatening, no apologies are made for including the section below on Aggressive Cooling, which can be usefully applied to competition horses of all disciplines.

Dr David Marlin, leader of the Atlanta Project at the Animal Health Trust in Newmarket, has produced the following notes to assist riders.

WHY DOES THE HORSE GET HOT?
The horse's normal rectal temperature at rest is around 37-38 C (98.6-100.4 F). When muscles work, they produce heat. For every unit of energy used to make the muscles contract, around four times as much energy is lost as heat, because the process of conversion of energy to movement is not very efficient.

WHAT HAPPENS WHEN A HORSE OVER-HEATS?
Very high body temperatures (above 41 C) result in high sweat rates, large sweat losses (water and electrolytes), dehydration and consequently a reduction in performance, or more serious consequences such as heat exhaustion and even death. See Chapter Three.

HOW DOES A HORSE LOSE HEAT?
• **Convection**
The heat is produced in the muscles and then carried to the surface of the horse's skin by the blood. If the surrounding air is cooler than the horse, as the horse moves through the air or as air passes over the horse, heat will be lost by convection. The greater the differences between the horse's skin temperature and the surrounding air, or the stronger the air movement (natural breeze or fans), the greater the rate at which heat will be lost.

• **Evaporation**
Heat is lost when sweat evaporates from the horse. Sweat that drips from the body, however, does little to keep the horse cool and is essentially wasted fluid loss. Sweating is highly effective when the horse is in a hot and dry environment. In a hot and humid environment the rate of evaporation from the skin is much slower; this is because the evaporation rate depends mainly on the difference between the moisture level of the skin and that of the environment.

• **Respiration**
In the horse, around 15 per cent of heat loss can occur through breathing. This is part of the reason why horses may have high respiratory rates during and after exercise in hot, or hot and humid, conditions.

WARMING UP OR OVER-HEATING?
A moderate increase in body temperature is not a disadvantage. Muscles work more efficiently when they are warm. Bear in mind that when it is hot, the horse will warm up faster.

WHY COOL HORSES WITH COLD WATER?
The horse's willingness to exercise hard, and our previous lack of understanding of how different environmental conditions affect the horse, has led to a number of competitions where horses have suffered heat stress, including at the Barcelona Olympic Games (1992) and the World Equestrian Games in The Hague (1994). Regimes for cooling horses with ice-cold water at competitions in hot climates have been criticised, even though the cooling is beneficial; and some people have suggested this type of cooling may cause other problems such as 'tying up'.

Which horses will benefit from cold water cooling? Any horse at any competition or show at any level can suffer from heat stress – from event horses, dressage horses, show jumpers, racehorses, polo ponies, endurance horses and driving horses to horses or ponies in gymkhanas.

Horses that are hot (above 40 C or 104 F) and competing in hot environments (above 26.5 C/ 80 F), if cooled quickly during or after competition, are less likely to suffer heat stress, will recover more quickly, will not become as dehydrated and are almost certain to perform better.

COLD WATER COOLING TECHNIQUE
The cold water cooling technique cools horses using two of the three ways they normally lose heat – convection and evaporation.

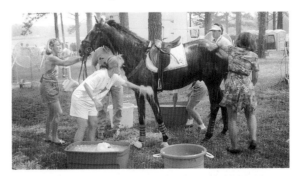

All that is needed are some large buckets to hold 40-50 litres of water and ice (and a supply of more water nearby), smaller buckets, giant sponges and three assistants - one to hold the horse and one person to cool each side. It is not necessary to remove the tack. Use a shady spot to carry out the cooling.

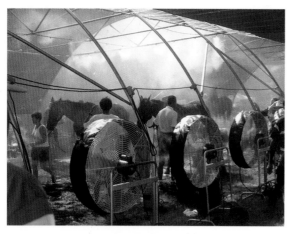

Start to cool the horse immediately it finishes exercising, whilst taking the horse's rectal temperature. Liberally apply cold water to all parts of the body including the quarters, as this is where most of the large muscles used for movement are located and so is an area that gets particularly hot. It is not necessary to scrape off excess water after each application; it is more important to continue to apply cold water. If you wish to scrape off the excess water, do so quickly at the end of each 30-second cooling period and while the horse is being walked between cooling periods.

Carry on cooling the horse for 20-30 seconds, walk the horse for 20-30 seconds and cool again. The walking and cooling sequence is important. The walking promotes skin blood flow and the movement of air aids evaporation. If possible, carry out the cooling and walking in the shade. Check the horse's rectal temperature at intervals. It should be possible to reduce rectal temperature by around one degree C in 10 minutes.

WHEN TO STOP COOLING
Stop cooling when:
• the horse's rectal temperature is less than 38-39C
• the horse's skin feels cool to touch (over the quarters) after a walking period
• if the respiratory rate is less than 30 breaths per minute
• if the horse begins to shiver.

HEAT STRESS AND THE RIDER
Mistakes and falls occur because of hot, tired horses – but the same applies equally to the rider. To cool the rider, remove their hat, sit them in the shade, wash their face with cold water (which makes them feel better, although is not very effective at reducing body temperature) and encourage them to drink an isotonic drink such as Lucozade Sport. An isotonic drink is at the same concentration as body fluids. The rider should also wear light-coloured, loose-fitting cotton clothing and ensure their hat is lightweight and a comfortable fit.

WHAT NOT TO DO
• Ice in the rectum does very little to lower body temperature. It makes it hard to assess body temperature and can hide a high temperature. Masking a high temperature from vets at events is unwise, as it will prevent a horse receiving appropriate cooling and other necessary treatments, which may result in the development of heat exhaustion and death. The chances of injury will also increase if the horse is allowed to continue when over-heated and dehydrated.
• Do not hold small bags of ice over the head, neck, under the tail, on the quarters, etc. Instead, concentrate on cooling as much of the body surface as possible. Holding bags of ice is likely to reduce cooling by stopping skin blood flow to the area under the pack.
• Do not place wet towels on the neck or quarters. Although at first the towel may be wet and cold, it soon warms and hinders the loss of heat, acting as an insulator.
• Excessive application of grease prior to cross-country limits sweating. The grease acts as an insulator, prevents sweating and limits sweat evaporation.
• Do not let horses stand still for prolonged periods. If cold water cooling is adopted, carry it out completely and not tentatively. The cold water on the skin will reduce the horse's sweating rate. This has the advantage that because the horse sweats less, it becomes less dehydrated.
• There is no harm in allowing horses to drink small amounts (half a bucket) during competition. Water should also be left in the stable until 15-30 minutes before exercise. Water is emptied very rapidly from the stomach. Do not give the horse ice-cold water to drink. Recent research has also shown that it is important to feed hard feed and some hay together, at least four hours prior to exercise.
• There is no evidence to suggest that cold water cooling causes other problems such as 'tying up'.

It is important that we learn to apply new ideas and findings from various studies so that we can maintain or improve the welfare of competition and pleasure horses at all levels.

TRANSPORT STRESS

Road, sea, and air transport all present their own problems. In the UK, as opposed to the USA, road transport is over much shorter distances and generally in a more temperate climate. Many top competition horses will be travelling to a different venue each week during the competition season. Long-distance travel by air, sea or road requires careful planning and preparation and allowing for the necessary recovery time on arrival before peak performance is expected. Certain principles apply, no matter how short or long the trip is likely to be. Clearly the length of the journey and the environment in which the horse is travelling will be the most important factors in the degree of stress created. What we must do is understand the stresses created and attempt to minimise these to help our competition horses achieve their best performances on arrival.

CURRENT METHODS OF TRANSPORT

ROAD TRANSPORT

Road transport of horses is first recorded in the eighteenth century. At that time, horses travelled in a form of horse-box pulled by other horses, the idea of which was to carry a racehorse to a meeting some distance from its home faster than he could be led or ridden, which was the usual custom. The horse would thus arrive in a better, fitter condition.

In principle, this is exactly what we are trying to achieve today, although our methods have changed considerably! Nowadays, horses are transported in heavy-goods lorries especially converted for horse transport, or in trailers carrying one, two or three animals, usually facing in a forward position, towed behind a suitable vehicle.

There is much debate as to the position in which horses travel best, i.e. the position which they find least stressful: backwards, forwards or sideways, with strong arguments in favour of rear-facing travel (although, due to the altered weight distribution, this

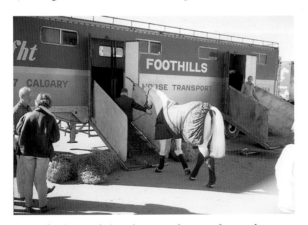

Large lorries are designed to carry between four and ten horses.

is not possible in trailers which are designed for forward-facing travel). Whatever the preference of an individual horse, it is likely that the travelling position is an important stressor. All horses need to spread their legs during travel and some will only travel happily in a much larger space than others. In all cases, avoid over-tight partitioning, particularly if it reaches down to floor level.

Larger lorries are designed to carry between four and ten horses with accommodation for grooms and storage space for feed and equipment. These lorries normally allow grooms to attend the horses in transit and to feed and water. New regulations within Europe carefully control the transport of horses, limiting travel times. On longer journeys the construction of the transport used is also regulated, with particular emphasis on ventilation.

AIR TRANSPORT

Over the past 20 years that the author has been travelling horses by air, there have been enormous improvements in the facilities and type of aircraft used. The modern stretch DC8 and jumbo jet have much-enhanced ventilation systems and are able to travel horses in a far greater degree of comfort. The jumbo jet in particular is an excellent platform for horses to travel on, the stalls used resembling those in a standard horse trailer.

SEA TRANSPORT

Sea transport nowadays is largely limited to roll-on, roll-off ferries carrying specially-designed horseboxes, and long-distance travel across the Atlantic by ship is a rarity. The stability of the ship is a major consideration. Exercise for horses on long sea journeys is a big problem, and happily this method of transport is not often used for performance horses.

REDUCING STRESS FACTORS INVOLVED IN TRAVEL

What are the stressors involved in travel and what can we do to reduce their effect?

The major stressors are: confinement (often for long periods of time); noise; air circulation and quality; movement sensation; changes in relative temperature and humidity; and exhaust fumes. Lorry design has now improved to the degree where vehicles can be very stable and incorporate forced ventilation systems and air conditioning. Air travel, as described above, has also vastly improved.

What can be done about the stressors described above?

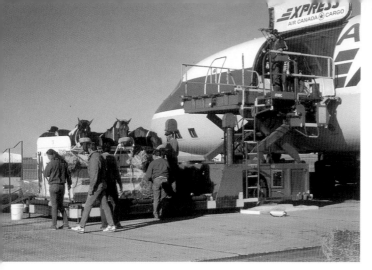

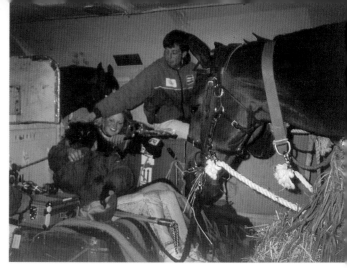

British team horses loaded on to stalls ready for the flight to the Atlanta Olympics, 1996.

Conditions inside the plane are very cramped, for both horses, grooms and vets. Good ventilation is essential.

CONFINEMENT

It is difficult to do much about confinement, which is obviously necessary due to the nature of travel. As described above, positioning, the arrangement of partitions to allow ample room for the horse to adjust his balance by spreading his legs, and avoiding tying up too short so the horse has some freedom of the head and neck, are all simple but important stress-reduction methods.

NOISE

Noise insulation of modern lorries has helped this, and noise has also been significantly reduced in modern aircraft.

MOVEMENT

This obviously depends partly upon the suspension of the vehicle, which should be adequate for the weight of horses carried and be well-maintained. The utmost care must be taken when driving, particularly in braking and turning bends and corners, to minimise the degree of adjustment to their balance that the occupants must make.

Clearly in sea and air travel, outside forces may well produce unpleasant movements that stress or frighten horses.

AIR QUALITY

In the author's opinion, air quality is one of the most important travel stress factors directly under our control. Drainage of urine and the use of products which absorb ammonia help reduce the contamination of the air breathed by the horses. Air-flow rates can be controlled by natural and artificial ventilation during travel. Regular air change is extremely important to prevent the build-up of noxious products and bacteria being breathed in. The use of haylage (e.g. Horsehage) and non-spore-containing hay can significantly reduce environmental problems. Dust-free bedding is essential.

Obviously the design of vehicle to some degree will limit exhaust fumes inhaled, although in heavy traffic this can be difficult unless the vehicle has air-conditioning.

CARE OF HORSES BEFORE AND DURING LONG DISTANCE TRAVEL

Short-distance transportation does not require any special dietary provisions. However, prior to long-distance travelling by air transport, a light laxative diet (e.g. bran mashes and not too much fibrous feed such as hay), should be used immediately prior to transport.

Pre-medication with antibiotics or respiratory medications should only be used in cases where it is specifically indicated, as the side-effects of these medications can sometimes outweigh the benefits. Treating horses with liquid paraffin prior to long journeys must be done with care, as excessive fluid loss through the faeces is not a good idea and dehydration can be a major problem. During transit give ad lib hay and offer water as regularly as possible. People talk about watering stops every six to eight hours, but in the author's opinion, it is far better to offer water every half-hour during long-distance transport.

Obviously, overnight rests are important. Horses are better fed on the floor to facilitate muco-ciliary clearance. Monitoring water consumption is essential, as it may be necessary to give fluids by stomach-tube, or intravenously if horses are becoming dehydrated. Monitoring cabin temperature is also important, as is measuring the body temperature of the horses. Recording this before, during and after travel can be extremely useful.

On arrival, clinical evaluation is must be made. Watch in particular for horses that are reluctant to eat or drink.

TRAVEL SICKNESS

Signs and causes: Stress is the predisposing factor in this condition, particularly the stress of travelling long distances by road, and especially by air. Sickness may occur during or up to several days post-travel. The horse, initially, will usually become depressed and stop eating or drinking. Other clinical findings include:

• depression
• off food and water
• raised temperature (usually 103-105 F)
• mild colic-like pain
• reduced gut sounds
• pulse is usually raised (50-60 bpm or more)
• sweating is often noticed
• occasionally, increased respiratory rate.

'Shipping fever' is a common problem in North America, where stress to the immune system on long journeys can increase the chance of viral bacterial infections, causing pneumonia.

Treatment and prevention:
• non-steroidal anti-inflammatory drugs, particularly phenylbutazone products
• antibiotic
• fluids and liquid paraffin by stomach-tube
• laxative foods.

Prognosis is generally good, providing early treatment and complete rest is undertaken. Pleurisy can be a serious complication of this condition.

Prevention involves:
• reduced travel times with good rest breaks
• improved travel environment (spacious stalls, good air quality and cool temperature in transport, reduced ammonia, etc.)
• reduced bulk feeds
• feed laxative feeds before loading
• supply small regular feeds and ad lib fresh water
• pre-medicate before long air trips (antibiotics, probiotic, electrolytes, laxative, and in special cases, clenbuterol).

10 THE NEXT GENERATION

THE REPRODUCTIVE SYSTEM

THE FEMALE REPRODUCTIVE SYSTEM

With the exception of the pituitary and pineal glands and hypothalamus, which are parts of the brain, the female reproductive organs are contained in the hind part of the abdomen and pelvis. The ovaries, oviducts, uterus and cervix are suspended from the upper body wall by broad ligaments which also carry their blood, lymphatic and nerve supply. The uterus, vagina and vulva form a Y-shaped structure, with the ovaries at the ends of the arms of the Y and the vulva at its base.

The following structures are involved in reproduction in the mare:

The **pineal gland,** a small, oval, red-brown gland sited between the two halves of the brain, which produces melatonin, a chemical secreted during the hours of darkness. Melatonin inhibits gonadotrophin-releasing hormone (GnRH) secretion by the hypothalamus, which is responsible for the onset of the cyclic oestrus (season).

The **pituitary gland** is attached to the base of the brain and produces the follicle-stimulating hormone (FSH) and luteinising hormone (LH). These control the activity of the ovaries, together with other hormones that indirectly influence the reproductive system.

The **hypothalamus,** connected to the pituitary gland, which produces other releasing and inhibiting hormones, such as GnRH, which affect the breeding cycle.

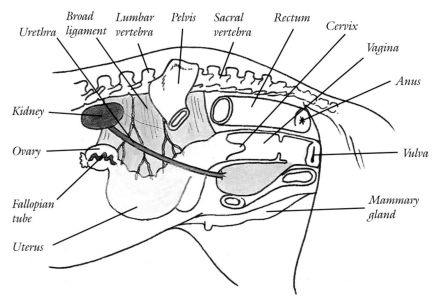

THE REPRODUCTIVE SYSTEM OF THE MARE

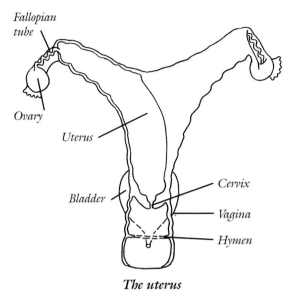

The uterus

The **ovaries** contain the female eggs (ova), many thousands of which are present in the two ovaries at birth. No more develop during the mare's lifetime. After puberty, ova are ovulated from the ovaries at intervals determined by the secretions of FSH and LH. The ovaries also act as glands which produce the hormones oestrogen, progesterone and inhibin.

Situated beneath the fourth and fifth lumbar vertebrae, the ovaries are typically bean-shaped. They vary in size depending on age, season of the year and individual variation from around 2-4cm long and 2-3 cm wide in winter to 5 by 10cm in older mares in summer. Although small, hard and inactive in winter, during the breeding season, due to follicle development, the ovaries grow in size and the follicles feel soft when ready to ovulate.

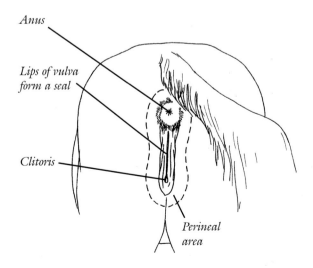

The external genitalia of the mare

The ovaries contain several hundred thousand small, primordial **follicles,** some of which are destined to develop into mature follicles containing ova. Several follicles develop just before and during oestrus, but one usually gradually enlarges whilst the others either 'wait' for development later, or regress. Development continues until this follicle reaches 3-5cm in diameter, filled with the enlarging ova and fluid containing oestrogen and inhibin hormones.

Ovulation occurs when the ripening follicle reaches an average of 4cm and its walls become thin. The mature follicle bursts, discharging its ovum through the ovary's ovulation fossa along one side, towards the open end of the **oviduct,** or Fallopian tube. The follicle now collapses and its lining thickens, growing into a clot to form the **corpus luteum.** Within 24 hours, this begins to secrete progesterone.

The oviducts, two narrow, tortuous 20-30cm tubes extending from the uterine horns to the ovaries, transport and store ova and sperm and are the location for fertilisation and early development of the embryo. Each tube is funnel-shaped where it meets the ovary (at the ovulation fossa) and have valves at the uterine end that selectively allow sperm to pass one way, and following fertilisation, the early embryo to pass into the uterus.

The **uterus** is a muscular tube that forms a continuation of the oviducts at its front, and opens at its rear into the cervix and vagina. It must provide an environment for transport of sperm to the oviducts, reception of the fertilised egg and maintenance of the developing and enlarging foetus throughout pregnancy. After foaling it must recover rapidly, repairing itself and reducing in size ready for the mare to start her first oestrus cycle at seven to nine days.

The uterus consists of two 25cm-long horns joined to an 18-20cm by 10cm body. Three coats make up the wall: an outer, protective layer; a muscular layer (myometrium) and inner mucous membrane (endometrium). The folded endometrium has a single-cell, layered lining containing coiled tubular glands and ducts that secrete hormones and nutrients in response to the stage of the oestrus cycle. A sterile environment, the uterus must be able to remove contamination from the outside that is introduced during mating, or infection can result.

The **cervix** forms a valve between the uterus and vagina. It must be capable of remarkable relaxation during mating and foaling, but tight closure during pregnancy. About 7cm long and 4cm in diameter, its wall contains a thick layer of circular muscle covered by a folded mucous membrane.

The **vagina** extends through the pelvis from the

cervix to the vulva and is around 20cm long and 12cm in diameter. Together with the cervix and vulva it forms another important seal between the internal and external environments. The **vulva** opens externally just below the anus and consists of two lips covered by thin, pigmented skin. Just inside at its lower aspect in a pouch of skin, is the **clitoris,** an area susceptible to infection if pathogenic bacteria grow in the cheese-like material (smegma) which tends to build up there.

THE MALE REPRODUCTIVE SYSTEM

The stallion's **penis** is located between his hind legs and, as in humans, it is a haemodynamic. That is, erection and relaxation is produced by blood flowing into and out of its erectile tissue, controlled by the action of valves that are in turn controlled by nerves. An average length of 44 by 5cm, the penis is enclosed at rest in the folded, pouch-like prepuce (sheath) but doubles in length and thickness on erection, producing the mechanism with which the stallion introduces sperm into the mare's uterus at mating.

The **prepuce** forms a protective pouch for the penis. Quite voluminous, it often produces a sucking noise during movement at the trot. Glands here secrete an oily substance that, together with skin debris and normal bacteria, form a red-brown substance called smegma which periodically dries and falls off.

The two **testicles** descend into the **scrotum,** situated between the thighs, at or shortly after birth. Normally measuring 6-12 cm long, 4-7cm high and 5cm wide, they increase in size with maturity up to the age of five. Testicles continually produce **sperm** and the male sex hormone testosterone. The **epididymes** lie above the testicles, and are complex

tubules in which sperm are matured after production, stored and transported from the testicles.

Extending from the epididymes, the **vasa deferentia** are narrow (0.6cm) tubes which transport the matured sperm upwards into the body to prepare for ejaculation and continue to the accessory glands cords. The spermatic cords containing the vasa deferens extend up through the body wall through the external and internal inguinal rings.

To produce sperm, the testicles must be at lower than body temperature and so are housed outside the body in the scrotum. The cremaster muscles in the spermatic cord contract to pull the testicles closer to the body wall when the stallion is excited and preparing to run, or when the external temperature is cold.

Located inside the pelvis, the accessory glands comprise the ampullae, bulbo-urethral glands, prostate glands and seminal vesicles, which secrete important nourishing fluids into the semen.

THE DECISION TO BREED

Careful consideration must be given to the decision to breed from a mare.

From a financial point of view alone, the costs of producing a foal are high and, outside of the world of racing, rarely recouped by the breeder. Even before a mare has conceived, stud and veterinary fees, travel and keep costs are already mounting up. Care of the mare during her pregnancy, veterinary attendance around the time of the foaling (together with any subsequent veterinary needs of the foal), when added to the costs of rearing the youngster for a further three years before ridden training can begin, mean

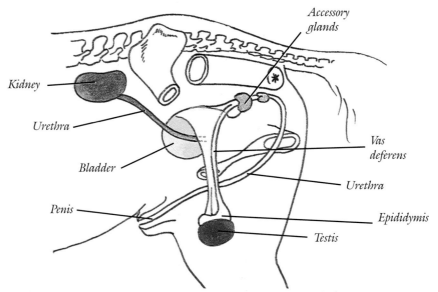

Kidney

Urethra

Bladder

Penis

Accessory glands

Vas deferens

Urethra

Epididymis

Testis

that it is invariably more economical to buy a nice young horse than to try to breed one.

It is a sad reality that the temptation to breed cheaply, often from unsuitable stock, has led to the over-production of poor-quality foals, creating many welfare problems and suppressing prices even for youngsters carefully produced for competition. Too many stallions are kept entire and used for breeding despite having no particular ability or desirable features. Similarly, many owners let sentimentality cloud an objective assessment of their favourite old mare and put her in foal without a great deal of thought for the future of the foal being created. Mares are frequently sent to stud not in a positive attempt to pass on desirable genes, but because they have no other 'useful' purpose. Stallions may be selected because they are inexpensive or local, whether or not they are a suitable match for a particular mare or will create a quality, marketable foal.

Nevertheless, breeding provides a unique challenge and thrill, and when success is achieved, the risk and effort become well worthwhile. Whilst there is no recipe certain to produce the perfect foal, careful thought given to the various aspects of breeding can significantly reduce the risk of problems arising.

PARENT SELECTION

The best can only be bred from the best. As a rule of thumb, it makes sense to only breed from a mare (or stallion) where all criteria point to the production of a good foal. There are three essential ingredients, which must be possessed by both parents. The relative proportion of each will depend largely on the intended career of the foal, but both mare and stallion should have the following qualities.

• **Correct conformation and movement**
A conformationally correct horse will be sound and useful, able to withstand work and perform athletically in any discipline.

• **Good temperament**
Few horses succeed, or indeed lead fulfilling lives in any sphere, if they inherit a difficult temperament. A willing horse is satisfying to own and more likely to fulfil its potential than the awkward animal who might require uncommon patience, skill and dedication to deal with and get the best from. Bear in mind the temperament of both parents when deciding to breed, but the mare's role as her foal's teacher and role model is particularly important. A mistrustful, unreliable mare will pass this attitude on to her offspring.

• **Ability**
Whilst matching two talented performers is no guarantee of producing the next champion (as Thoroughbred breeders well know), it nevertheless makes sense to breed from proven performers rather than from horses with no recognised ability in a chosen discipline. Animals with performance records have demonstrated their suitability and are likely to pass on those successful traits. Those who have shown no talent are unlikely to produce talented offspring. Whilst competition mares whose careers have been cut short through injury often become successful brood mares, it is a mistake to breed from a mare retired due to an unsoundness caused by some inherent weakness or fault. Many lameness problems have a hereditary predisposition.

AGE

Mares are considered to be at a suitable age to breed from between the ages of three and 12. Although many experienced mares who are in good health continue to produce foals well into their teens, conception is often increasingly difficult after this age, particularly for maiden (first-time) mares.

Not all mares, even of ideal age, breed easily or every year and this is not necessarily any fault of the stud or stallion. Careful choice of a well-managed stud and use of a vet with regular experience of stud work is advisable to maximise the chances of conception.

MATCH-MAKING

Given the wide range of stallions available, particularly in the UK with its numerous native breeds, a mare owner has ample chance to off-set minor weaknesses or poorer characteristics in her mare by the careful choice of a stallion particularly strong in these areas. In particular, consider conformation. Match, for example, a long-backed mare with a short-backed stallion, to counter the mare's deficiency rather than exaggerate it further.

Breeders must also bear in mind the type of foal they are aiming to produce and select a stallion most likely, when its genes are combined with those of the mare, to create a foal of that type. Details should be gathered from a range of stallions before making a final decision, and the mare owner should aim to visit as many stallions as possible in person, to assess both the stud itself and the stallion's 'presence' and personality.

ARTIFICIAL INSEMINATION (AI)

The increasing availability of artificial insemination

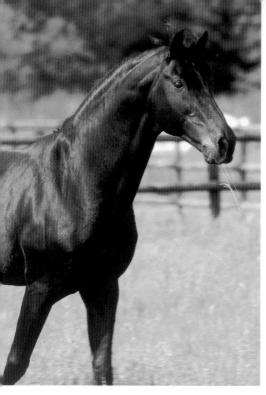

Mare owners must consider their choice of stallion carefully, bearing in mind not only his qualities, but their mare's strengths and weaknesses and the type of foal they wish to produce.

POSITIVE INDICATORS FOR BREEDING	NEGATIVE INDICATORS
For both parents:	
Correct conformation	Poor conformation
Pleasant temperament/intelligence temperament	Unstable
Straight movement & soundness	Permanent unsoundness known to be hereditary
Suitable age	Too old or young
Proven performance & trainability record	Lack of ability to perform
Good pedigree/blood lines	Pedigree unknown
Good example of the breed	Poor example of the breed
Good reproductive record (not known in maiden mares) and successful progeny	Record of infertility or progeny lacking success
For brood mares:	
Good physique for breeding (for brood mares – wide front, deep girth)	Poor physique for breeding
Good general health	Poor or inconsistent health, particularly connected to the reproductive system

now gives serious breeders an even wider choice of stallion, and in particular, of stallions still performing regularly in top-class competition. AI is not a simple or inexpensive option however, as it requires far more intensive veterinary input than natural covering. It carries both advantages and dis-advantages.

If proper precautions are taken, collecting semen under sterile conditions from tested and certified stallions only, the spread of disease and risk of infection can be less than that associated with natural covering. If not, both bacterial and viral venereal diseases can be very successfully spread by AI. Injury risks are lessened, making the technique particularly appropriate for over-enthusiastic or aggressive stallions, nervous mares or mares recovering from injury.

Conception rates for AI are not as good as for *well-managed* natural covering. The timing of insemination in relation to ovulation must be extremely precise, so mares may need a veterinary examination daily or every 2-4 times a day during oestrus. However, insemination can be repeated several times during this fertile period. AI also allows mares who travel badly to conceive without leaving home.

From a stallion-owner's viewpoint, considerable effort can be saved, as the amount of sperm usually produced for one ejaculation can be diluted and used to inseminate several mares. This allows minimum disruption by stud duties of a performance career.

Throughout most of the horse-breeding world (currently excepting the Thoroughbred industry and some breed societies, although this is under consideration), AI is now becoming more commonly-used. Experienced clinics and studs with staff skilled in the technique should be used, as it is

vital that the timing of insemination is accurate or valuable semen, and veterinary time, can be wasted. A good clinic should have a conception rate of around 75% with frozen semen and 90% with chilled semen.

Once the vet has confirmed the mare is in oestrus, the stud is contacted and semen collected from the stallion using an amenable mare and artificial vagina. Unless it is to be used immediately on-site, the semen is diluted ('extended') and either chilled or frozen and dispatched, in a temperature-controlled container, to the mare or the clinic, where chilled semen must be used within 72 hours. Insemination of the mare goes ahead immediately, the vet depositing the semen in the uterus, via the cervix, using a sterile pipette. If there is sufficient semen (two doses are usually supplied), the procedure can be repeated later or the following day.

Although frozen semen can be kept indefinitely in liquid nitrogen at an AI clinic, not every stallion has semen suitable for freezing and problems with the viability of frozen semen are only recently being overcome. In addition to the quality of the individual stallion's semen, the way the semen is handled and the preparation of the mare are crucial factors influencing the success rate of AI. Despite these difficulties, AI has made it possible for professional performance horse breeders to consider using stallions based much further afield – even in another continent, provided import regulations are followed – at a fraction of the cost that would have previously been involved.

As AI becomes more widely accepted by breed societies, it is an option worth consideration for experienced breeders under suitable circumstances. It must always be borne in mind however, that the most satisfactory and economical way for foals to be produced by inexperienced owners is to turn the mare out with the stallion at a well-managed stud i.e. the natural way.

REPRODUCTIVE BEHAVIOUR

Horses are seasonal, day-long breeders. The equine mating season is from April to September, with peak activity from May to August. Gestation length is 11 months and thus the majority of foals are born in April, May, June and July when the weather is improving and grass is growing.

THE MARE'S OESTROUS CYCLE
The age at which a filly becomes fertile is influenced by several factors. Well-nourished fillies born in the spring may be ready to breed at 12 months, whereas late-born fillies may take a further six months to reach puberty. Malnutrition, worm burden or disease may all delay the onset of puberty, but once it is reached the mare will then normally have oestrous cycles throughout her life-time.

The mare's reproductive ability is controlled by the seasons. During the breeding season (late spring and summer) she has regular oestrous cycles, timed to synchronise foaling to the spring and early summer when the foal has the best chance of survival. A mare is therefore described as being seasonally polyoestrous.

The oestrous cycle forms the basis of sexual activity. It has two components: oestrus ('heat') in which the mare is receptive, and dioestrus (the luteal phase), when she is sexually quiescent. The winter period when there is no cycle occurring is termed anoestrus.

The start of oestrus activity is mainly influenced by daylight length, mediated via melatonin and the pineal gland. Artificial lighting can advance the onset of the first ovulation by at least two months. Ambient temperature, food availability and pheromones are other factors that may have effects. Oral progestogens, stimulation and prostaglandi therapy may also shorten the transitional phase between anoestrus and oestrous.

The pineal gland controls production by the hypothalamus of GnRH (gonadotrophin-releasing hormones), which in turn influence the pituitary gland to produce the hormones FSH and LH, inducing follicular acitivity in the ovaries. The follicles produce oestrogens which cause typical changes in the tubular genitalia and oestral behaviour. Following ovulation, the ruptured follicle becomes luteinised and produces progestogens, suppressing oestrus behaviour.

The oestrous cycle typically lasts a total of 21 days (5 days of oestrous, 16 of dioestrus). It will recur throughout the breeding season unless the mare becomes pregnant, often being at its most intense behaviourally during the middle months. There is considerable variation in cycle length and character. During the transitional phase between anoestrous and the start of the seasonal oestrous, a cycle may even last several weeks ('spring heats').

THE STALLION'S BREEDING SEASON
From puberty (around one to two years), seasonal changes also influence reproductive behaviour in the stallion as they do in the mare. Although less obvious for the stallion, significant changes in reaction time, number of mounts per ejaculation and some seminal characteristics have been observed throughout the breeding season.

Environmental stimuli, in particular daylight length, stimulate the hypothalamus to produce gonadotrophin-releasing hormone (GnRH) which in turn stimulates the pituitary gland to produce the gonadotrophic hormones FSH and LH identical to those in the mare.

These changes in hormones stimulate the function of the testicles, controlling semen quantity and quality and sexual behaviour. FSH stimulates sperm production and LH the production and secretion of testosterone. Testosterone stimulates sperm production, development of the reproductive organs, descent of the testicles in the foetus or newborn foal, the development of accessory glands and the onset of puberty. It also influences the brain to produce normal sexual interest (libido) and behaviour and secondary sexual characteristics (i.e. personality, muscular development, 'cresty' neck etc.).

The cycle of sperm production (spermatogenesis) in the testicle takes around 50 days. A stallion produces approximately 800 million sperm a day by around five years of age, when the testicles have reached their mature size.

It takes, on average, ten days for sperm to travel from the testicles to the ampullae and a normal stallion keeps around 6000 million sperm in reserve, ready for ejaculation.

COURTSHIP, MATING & FERTILITY

IN THE WILD

In grassland environments worldwide, wild and feral horses live in small bands comprised of the basic equine social unit – the family group. This consists of one stallion (who is responsible for forming the group and is socially dominant), an average of four to five related mares and their foals. Subordinate young and old stallions form peripheral 'bachelor' groups and may help to defend the group's territory. They may try to abduct a mare, take over an unescorted mare or group whose stallion has died or lost contract, or oust a family stallion through combat or establishing long-term close contact.

The horse is naturally, therefore, a harem rather than territorial breeder. The stallion forms and maintains his group using ritualistic responses to urine and faeces, which he regularly approaches, investigates, paws and sniffs.

Free-running horses engage in prolonged pre-mating interactions, both stallion and mare playing active roles in mate location and pre-copulatory behaviour. For days before mating, the mare lingers near or follows the stallion, either alone or with other in-oestrous mares. She lifts her tail, frequently urinating and presenting her hindquarters to the stallion.

The stallion in courtship is an animal of great presence and beauty – an awesome spectacle. On recognising a mare in oestrous he fixes his eyes on her, arches his neck and restlessly paws or stamps his feet, drawing himself up to full height. He raises and stretches up his head, curling his upper lip (the Flehmen response, see Chapter Six) and may 'roar',

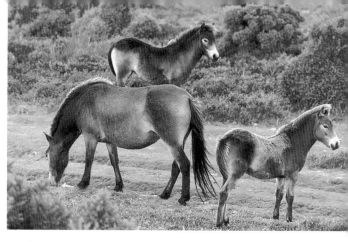

Feral ponies can live in small family groups and are free to follow a far more natural pattern of courtship and mating behaviour that their domesticated counterparts.

to which the mare responds with a nicker.

An approach is made to the mare's head or neck, nudging, 'talking' and sometimes biting her. The stallion progresses down to her flanks, buttocks and then nudges her vulva and clitoris. After a relatively short period of genital stimulation, with penis now fully erect, the stallion mounts. Mounting usually takes place from the left side, sometimes after the stallion has nudged the mare slightly off balance with his right shoulder, perhaps as a self-defence tactic against kicks! After entering, he will grip the mare with his front legs just behind the withers sometimes biting the mare's neck in an apparent attempt to gain stability.

Following a number of pelvic thrusts during which he 'dances' on his hind feet, the stallion ejaculates, pumping semen into the mare's uterus in a series of six to nine jets (accompanied by a rhythmic 'flagging' of his tail). He then rests for a short period on the mare's back before his erection subsides and he dismounts. Both stallion and mare frequently vocalise during mating.

IN DOMESTICATION

THE MARE

Domestication has resulted in major alterations in basic reproductive behaviour patterns. Mares are not continually in the presence of entire males and are only intermittently and variably 'teased', usually by entires of low value kept for this purpose. Man has taken over the role and responsibility of assessing the sexual status of mares and dictating when mating should occur.

There is a wide range of variation in the character and intensity of sexual behaviour between mares and so it is difficult for humans to interpret signs of readiness to accept the stallion, in particular because the mare-stallion relationship is based on smell in addition to sight. It is for this reason that 'teasing' is generally used as the most reliable method of assessing whether a mare is sexually receptive.

Signs of oestrous behaviour:
- mare appears docile
- often stands as if to urinate, for long periods
- lengthens and everts vulva, showing clitoris ('winking')
- raises tail and frequently passes bright yellow urine with distinct odour (containing pheromones that stimulate the stallion)

Signs of dioestrous behaviour:
- mare is hostile
- may kick, bite, flatten ears, swish tail and resent handling

Signs of anoestrous (transitional) behaviour:
- highly variable, but mare is usually indifferent

Individuals may show unusual or untypical patterns of behaviour, so it is important that owners and stud managers get to know these idiosyncrasies and are skilled at interpreting behavioural signs. Fortunately for human breeders, the size of a mare and arrangement of her anatomy makes internal veterinary examinations by hand and scanning by ultrasound via the rectum both practical options. These indicators, together with blood samples to measure hormone levels, can help stud managers mate mares at the right time for successful conception.

Pregnancy diagnosis is usually performed between 18-21 days following covering using an ultra-sound scanner and twins can be diagnosed with greater accuracy. Other traditional, but less reliable methods of diagnosis, include 'trying' the mare to see whether she is still receptive to the stallion, blood testing between 45 and 90 after service and blood testing

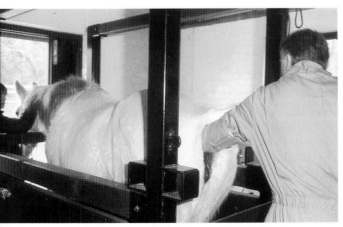

Examination stocks keep both mare, handler and veterinarian safe during examinations.

after 120 days. A manual examination only by the vet can detect a likely pregnancy at around 20 days, give a more reliable indication or detect twins by 35 days and diagnose with some accuracy by around 40 days. It is usual to check no early abortion has occurred at around 60 days.

Although temporary breeding failures are relatively common, few mares are truly sterile (i.e. incapable of breeding to a fertile stallion). A mare who is not pregnant at the end of the season is termed 'barren'. Barren mares should be thoroughly examined at this stage, before the winter, to investigate any potential abnormalities or infections which might require treatment or any changes in management that may be needed. Research does suggest there is a natural decline in the fertility potential of mares with increasing age.

Following the birth of a foal, the mare usually shows her first post-partum oestrous ('foal heat') at 7-10 days, usually preceded by a 1-3 day period of diarrhoea ('foal heat scours').

THE STALLION

In the wild state, a stallion will mate the same mare twice within a matter of minutes and repeat the mating many times during oestrous – up to ten times in 24 hours. He is able to 'tease' his mares himself and mate with them at will.

Modern systems of stud farm management (and to some extent, tradition) have made considerable changes to natural stallion behaviour in domestication. At commercial studs, mares and stallions are separated except for the act of mating and do not form a natural 'family' group. Teasing is usually performed by a separate entire horse. A quick, efficient mating routine, with little time allowed for courtship, is encouraged. The stallion becomes conditioned to the sight and sounds of the covering yard, where he may mate two or three times a day during the breeding season. He is only presented with mares shown to be in season by the teaser and veterinary examination, and which are restrained during mating to avoid physical injury.

A busy stallion may mate between 50 and 80 mares per season, covering each no more than twice per oestrous. Mating is limited in this way mainly to help maintain the stallion's libido, so it is important that mares are accurately assessed as being receptive before being presented to the stallion.

At most studs, the mare is restrained during mating to avoid injury. Felt boots are fitted to the hind feet. The tail is bandaged and held to one side. The genital areas are washed using clean, warm water. The

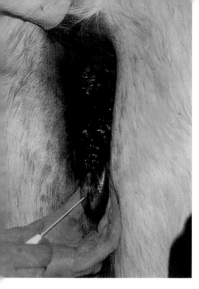

A swab will confirm the mare is free from sexually-transmitted infectious disease.

stallion is bridled and held on a long rein. The handler helps the stallion move into position for mounting and, if necessary, to enter the mare and maintain his position until the process is complete. After mating, the genitals of both horses are washed again with clean, warm water.

Although some stallions continue a performance career alongside stud duties, many retire from competition or racing to concentrate solely on stud duties and so must adjust to radical changes in management. This transition must be sensitively managed to prepare the stallion physically and psychologically and avoid confusion, particularly where a young horse has previously been discouraged from showing sexual behaviour in the presence of mares.

The establishment of a good personal relationship between the handler and stallion is essential for routine and successful performance at stud. The handler needs patience, understanding, intelligence and firmness.

Although probably no longer a competition athlete, the stallion must still be prepared for short periods of intense exertion. Stallions tend to be over-fed, leading to obesity and laminitis. The balance between food intake, work and exercise is important to maximise fertility and performance. Daily exercise, preferably turned out in a safe paddock, is essential, as is a large (6m x 6m minimum) and solid stable.

Regular attention to the feet and teeth are important, and stallions should be routinely vaccinated against tetanus, flu and equine viral arteritis (EVA). See Chapter Five.

FITNESS TO BREED

Once the decision has been made to send a mare to stud, she should be thoroughly examined by a veterinary surgeon to ensure her reproductive tract is normal, that she is free from venereal and other infectious diseases and that she is in good general health. Examination is particularly important for older maiden mares.

The examination consists of a check of the structure and condition of the ovaries, uterus and vulva. Faults in conformation of the perineum leading to (pneumovagina), to which older mares are particularly prone, can easily lead to contamination of the reproductive tract by faeces, leading to infertility. Careful surgical repair can correct this problem in most cases, by closing the upper part of the vulva together using sutures (known as Caslick's operation).

Swabs are taken to confirm that the mare is free from infectious sexually-transmitted diseases. These are insisted upon by most studs prior to covering in accordance with the Horse Race Betting Levy Board's Code of Practice. The sample from the swab is cultured in the laboratory and any bacteria present identified.

Results from the clitoral swab, which can be taken when the mare is not in season, are available in seven to ten days and will identify the presence of diseases such as Klebsiella, Pseudomonas and CEM (contagious equine metritis). The cervical swab and smear (uterine or endometrial swab) must be taken during oestrous, so many studs will accept a mare without an endometrial swab if the clitoral swab has proved negative. Preliminary results are usually evident within 24 hours and confirmed later. In addition, a blood test will reveal the presence of antibodies of EVA, a highly-contagious respiratory and venereal disease that causes spontaneous abortion in pregnant mares.

Infection by any of these organisms is extremely serious as it can be rapidly spread by a stallion to all mares which come into contact with his semen. If infection is shown to be present, a mare must be treated and cleared before mating. A mare with a uterine infection will not conceive (see Chapter Five).

FERTILISATION & THE DEVELOPMENT OF THE FOETUS

The gestation period of the mare is 11 months (on average, 340 days). Considerable variations are possible, with smaller breeds tending to have shorter pregnancies than larger ones. Ten days either way is not unusual and normal births can occur up to two weeks early or three to four weeks late.

Fertilisation takes place when the sperm fuses with the ova in the oviducts, each providing 32 chromosomes to create the full complement of 64. Ova die within 24 hours and are at their most fertile on entering the oviducts, so mares are best covered by the stallion before, rather than after, ovulation.

The fertilised egg, now termed the **zygote,** passes

into the uterine where it grows by dividing into an increasing number of cells and loosely attaches itself to the uterine lining. As differentiation of cells begins, it gradually changes from a single-celled fertilised egg to a clumped mass of cells, and eventually, by around day 40, becomes an embryo with equine features. From 60 days following conception the embryo is termed the **foetus**. After this time, development progresses mainly through growth and increase in size.

Membranes immediately begin to form around the developing embryo to enable the foetus to develop surrounded by fluids that cushion and protect it. The placenta, through which oxygen and nutrients are received and waste is removed, allows the foetal blood to come into close contact with that of the mother but not mix with it. The placenta connects the foetus, via the umbilical cord, to the lining of the uterus, and in the horse it covers the entire surface of the uterus. The umbilical cord contains two major arteries, a vein and a duct connected to the foal's bladder.

Although smooth early in pregnancy, by 70 days the placental surface is covered in minute finger-like projections known as microvilli, which enormously increase its surface area and the efficiency of exchange. By 150 days, a strong bond exists, consisting of a layer of six cells, three on the maternal side (epithelium, endometrium and blood vessel wall) and three on the foetal side (endoderm, mesoderm and ectoderm).

The placenta contains the allantoic fluid, consisting partly of waste material not yet removed. This fluid is separated from the foal by the amnion, another thin membrane that protects the foal during pregnancy and aids delivery during birth.

The amnion contains the amniotic fluid that bathes the foetus's airways and skin and is swallowed by the foetus to lubricate the stomach and intestine.

As embryo develops into growing foetus, the uterine walls stretch, but remain sealed from the external environment by the tightly-closed cervix. All internal organs are present by four weeks gestation, although, with the exception of the heart and some intestinal activity, most do not function until after birth.

Before birth takes place, the foal must become mature enough to function outside the uterus. All the body systems must be in place and in working order for chances of survival to be good. Premature, under-developed foals (usually classed as those born before 320 days) generally face serious problems.

THE IN-FOAL MARE
Most pregnant mares change in appearance after about six months' gestation, when their bellies begin to drop and they take on a swinging movement. The stronger uterine muscles of the maiden mare, however, mean these often show little signs of pregnancy. In contrast, older brood mares may take on an almost-permanent 'in-foal' appearance even when barren.

Healthy development of the foetus depends on the health of the mare, who should be kept in as good bodily condition as possible, neither lean nor carrying too much fat and with a shine to the coat. Avoiding

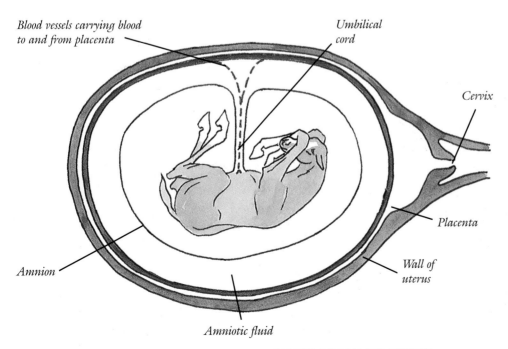

Blood vessels carrying blood to and from placenta

Umbilical cord

Cervix

Placenta

Amnion

Wall of uterus

Amniotic fluid

THE POSITION OF THE FOETUS PRIOR TO BIRTH

stress and trauma is crucial, as is correct nutrition at all stages.

Providing sufficient protein and amino acids is particularly important in the early part of pregnancy. Although good-quality grazing provides most nutritional requirements through the summer, a mineral supplement is advisable and poor doers, or those on poorer pasture, will need supplementary feeding. A proprietary brand of stud or brood mare mix or nuts will provide a correctly balanced concentrate ration. As winter approaches, quality hay, provided ad lib, will maintain the mare's condition. The provision of adequate shelter during winter is a necessity.

During the last third of the pregnancy the foal increases in weight three-fold and additional feed will be required to help provide for the needs of the rapidly growing foetus when the nutritional value of grass remains low. Protein is again important, both for foetal growth and lactogenesis (milk production), which begins at around two to four weeks before foaling. As foaling time approaches, the proportion of bulk feed is gradually reduced and a slightly laxative diet introduced to avoid constipation.

A regular worming programme, checking of teeth and keeping the feet trimmed are basics of horse care that should not be neglected for the in-foal mare. Natural exercise and movement should be encouraged throughout pregnancy. Mares can be kept in work for the first five to six months of gestation (some owners keep hardy types in work for even longer), though exertion levels should be gradually reduced.

THE BIRTH

The exact length of an individual's gestation is controlled by fotal gonadal steroid production. Maternal influence, however, ensures that the

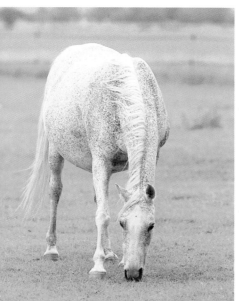

The healthy development of the foetus depends on the health of the mare. Care should be taken to provide the correct nutrition, avoid stress and maintain a regular worming and foot-care regime.

majority of foals are born at night, affording some degree of protection against predators. The mare is capable of 'fine-tuning' the exact time of parturition, if necessary delaying the process for several hours if interrupted (one reason why so many owners miss the event as soon as they leave to put the kettle on!).

Signs of imminent foaling include:
- Enlargement and swelling of the udder ('bagging up'). May occur up to two weeks beforehand, or occasionally, not until after the birth.
- Relaxation of the pelvic ligaments ('softening of the bones') may become obvious from around two weeks before foaling. Grooves may appear either side of the tail. Relaxation of the vulva and perineal muscles, swelling of vulval lips and increased vaginal secretions.
- Closer to the onset of labour, but again at a variable stage before the start, mares produce a waxy secretion at the tips of the teats ('waxing up').

FIRST STAGE LABOUR
This is signalled by anxious, restless behaviour, the frequent passage of small amounts of urine, drips of milk and signs suggesting low-grade abdominal pain. There is sweating, usually firstly around the brisket and behind the shoulder blades. Mares may repeatedly lie down and get up again and may sometimes roll. Contractions gradually become more frequent and intense, quickening from one every 5 or 10 minutes to around every 30 seconds.

The foal rotates so the forelegs, head and neck are extended and engaged in the birth canal, causing dilation of the cervix and relaxation of the vulva.

SECOND STAGE LABOUR
The end of the first stage, usually up to an hour from the first signs of pain, is signified by the rupture of the chorio-allantois ('first water bag'), as the foal's muzzle and forelimbs push through the weakest part of the placenta (the 'cervical star'). A gush of light-brown, yellowish liquid appears and lubricates the vagina. Though similar to urine, this is often released in large quantities and without the usual urinating stance.

Within 5 minutes, the whitish, glistening amnion ('foal bag') should appear at the vulval lips. The uterus contracts more strongly and the mare usually lies down at this stage, unless nervous or disturbed by humans, as she can then strain more effectively. Contraction of the abdominal muscles is clearly visible.

The mare may get up again and adjust position,

but repeated, anxious rising and lying down or continued unproductive straining indicate difficulties. Grunts are normal, however, and a series of strong abdominal contractions now gradually expel the foal. The foal is normally delivered with one foreleg slightly ahead of the other, and the head lying extended above or between the knees.

Once the foal's hips are clear, the mare may rest with the hind limbs still in the vagina for up to 40 minutes. The foal should now be lying on its side, with its legs in an arc. If the amnion has not broken, it should be carefully split and if necessary, the foal's head lifted clear of the fluid

The umbilical cord remains intact for now and a series of pulsations complete the transfer of placental blood into the foal's circulation. Normally within 8 minutes, a whitish constriction appears in the cord, 1-2cm from the umbilicus, and the cord naturally ruptures here as the foal begins to move. During the next few minutes, $1^1/_2$ litres of blood may be transferred from mare to foal.

From the breaking of the waters to the birth usually takes less than an hour, with mares that have foaled before often delivering in around 20 minutes. The cord should be broken within a further 30 minutes.

After recovering, the mare looks around, acknowledges the foal with the Flehmen response, and often nickers. She may then get to her feet and turn to smell and lick the foal. First-time mares can get quite agitated, as if surprised and alarmed by the foal, but maternal instinct usually prevails.

THIRD STAGE LABOUR
The placental membranes shrink and uterine contractions sweep towards the cervix to expel the placenta and any remaining fluid. This usually occurs within three hours of birth and should always be free within 10 hours. The after-birth should be checked to ensure it is complete, with nothing retained in the uterus that may cause infection.

INTERVENTION AND ASSISTANCE
Mares naturally foal outdoors, but for most domesticated horses control of management conditions and the commercial advantage of producing early season foals, means most mares foal in large, clean stables often designed and equipped for this purpose (foaling boxes). This allows close observation for valuable bloodstock, but there is no doubt that interference during birth can confuse natural behaviour patterns and if used injudiciously can be counter-productive and so should be kept to a minimum.

Most foalings go smoothly, but vigilance is needed to avoid potentially serious problems. Any significant delays in the timetable will require expert assistance. Careful recording of events will help if the veterinary surgeon has to be called in.

The most common problem during foaling is incorrect positioning of the foal. Intervention may also be necessary if the mare is becoming exhausted and the periods between straining are lengthening.

Before any force is exerted on the foal, its position must be determined to ensure passage down the birth canal is possible. As the canal is designed for the foal to be pushed out rather than pulled, excessive force should never be used, and exertion should only be made as the mare strains, never when she stops. Elbows, head and shoulders are all areas that commonly stick or cause problems.

After foaling, the foal must be observed carefully for any weaknesses or abnormal behaviour (see below). The immediate post-partum period is extremely important in the development of the mare-

Normal position

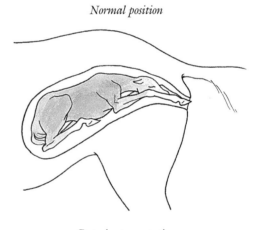

Posterior presentation

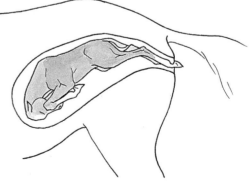

It is important to check that the foal is lying is the correct position. Abnormal positioning will require veterinary assistance.

221

foal bond, however, so mare and foal should be left to themselves as far as possible. If too much human interference occurs, mares have been known to reject or become aggressive towards their foals. Where, for reasons of illness, death or injury, it is necessary to artificially feed or supplement a foal during this period, foals may become attached to humans rather than the mare.

THE NEWBORN FOAL

Following a successful delivery, the newborn foal must adapt to its challenging new environment. At birth, the healthy foal with have:

- a bodyweight of approximately 40-50 kg
- a body temperature of 99-102 F (37.2-38.9C)
- a heart rate of 70-100 beats per minute
- a respiratory rate of 20-240 breaths per minute (70-100 during first hour).

The newborn first achieves respiration, with heaving movements of the thorax. Inflation of the lungs occurs, and sometimes fluid can be seen escaping from the nostrils. The foal shows shivering behaviour and often an apparently uncoordinated 'bobbing' of the head and neck. A regular breathing pattern should be established by 30-60 seconds.

The foal may respond to the mare's attentions by nickering. Licking and sucking behaviour soon starts, with a stretching and 'tunnelling' of the tongue in response to the mare's head, its own forelegs or objects close by.

Foals generally stand within one hour of birth. Repeated unproductive attempts may be made before standing position is achieved, in a rather un-coordinated way. The foal may fall down again several times before becoming fully coordinated and then actively seeking the mare. If the foal cannot stand within three hours of birth, veterinary advice is needed.

Licking and sucking becomes more aggressive, usually starting at the mare's forelegs and working backwards along her belly, eventually reaching the udder and teats. Occasionally foals may suckle as if ravenous and may cough or sneeze, ejecting milk from the mouth. This is normal, unless excessive.

Foals usually suckle within one to two hours of birth to obtain the nutrition, vitamins, fluids and antibodies vital for their health and well-being that is contained in the colostrum or 'first milk'. Unlike the young of many mammals, which transfer antibodies across the placenta before birth, the newborn foal is

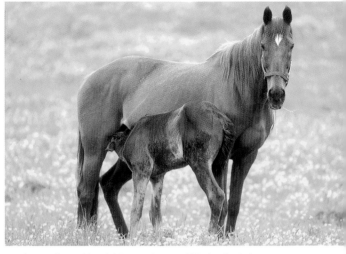

Foals usually suckle within two hours of birth, obtaining both nutrition, fluids and antibodies vital for their health contained in the colostrum, or 'first milk'.

dependent upon the colostrum as a source of passive immunity until it is able to build up its own immune system. The level of immuno-globulin proteins in the mare's milk falls dramatically after 12 hours, as does the foal's ability to absorb them.

At least 1 litre of colostrum is required within six hours of birth, while the foal's gut is still capable of absorbing these vital antibodies. If more than two hours elapse and the foal has not yet suckled, tactful direction can be tried and a vet consulted if there is no success. Normally suckling takes place 4-5 times per hour during the first week of life with each session lasting from a few seconds to several minutes.

The foal should pass meconium (faecal material produced in-utero) within its first 24 hours of life. Colts in particular often have difficulty passing meconium and an enema or small amount of liquid paraffin may need to be carefully inserted into the rectum if signs of straining are seen after 4 to 5 hours. Close observation should be continued during the early days for signs of further constipation, colic or diarrhoea (particularly when the faeces are dark).

Even when events have gone smoothly, a veterinary inspection of the mare and foal is advisable during the morning after birth, to check for early problems such as retained placenta and vaginal tears, and congenital defects or weakness in the foal.

THE FOLLOWING DAYS
If the weather is suitable and foal strong, the mare and foal can then be allowed outside for increasing periods. Only the most valuable or refined animals will need stabling over-night during a good summer.

Within the first two days the foal shows inquisitive behaviour, investigating its surroundings by smelling and licking. Coprophagia (chewing and swallowing the mare's faeces) is commonly seen by seven days of age and may be stimulated by the mare's pheromones. By eight to ten days most foals will be seen to nibble grass, though this is not eaten in much quantity for several weeks.

Good-quality pasture will provide most of the nutrition required for mare and foal over the summer months. The foal can gradually be introduced to a suitable concentrate feed, learning to eat by copying its mother and taking some of her ration. A correct, balanced diet is vital for the healthy growth and development of young stock. Worming at an appropriate dosage should commence at four weeks of age and continue regularly.

Together with suckling, periods of play and sleep take up the day of the young foal. While the foal is sleeping, the mare often stands with her head over it in a protective stance. As foals get older the periods of sleep become shorter and the distance with which they will play from their mother lengthens. Foals of a similar age will play together and indulge in mutual grooming, but when frightened immediately seek out their mother, often suckling for comfort.

Play develops co-ordination and balance, reinforces survival techniques and teaches the youngster social behaviour and discipline. Mutual grooming will reinforce friendships, but when frightened by humans or other horses, young foals show the 'menace reflex' (a characteristic 'mouth-snapping' behaviour), a behaviour that occasionally persists later in life (commonly in orphan foals).

FOSTERING FOALS

The fostering of foals is a difficult procedure requiring patience, understanding and experience. Mares can be induced, depending on their basic temperament, to accept alternative foals if their own foal is no longer present and if the smell, and to some extent the sight and sound of their own foal can be transferred or mimicked on the new foal.

Alternatively, or additionally, the mare's sense of smell may be confused by the use of powerful odours such as camphorated oils (e.g. Vick). In general

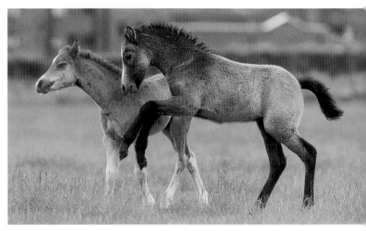

The youngster's day is taken up mainly with play, sleep and suckling. Play has an important role in developing coordination and balance, survival techniques and social skills.

terms, non-Thoroughbred mares make better foster mothers than do Thoroughbreds.

WEANING

If a mare becomes pregnant again, she will gradually wean her foal by showing progressively increasing aggressive behaviour from about seven, eight or nine months of gestation. If not pregnant, she may not actively wean her foal, and yearlings have been seen to suckle barren mares until puberty occurs at around nine to 12 months.

Traditional weaning of foals on stud farms is performed at around five to six months of age. In the past, it has been considered convenient for managers to divide mares and foals into batches, suddenly separating them in stables out of sight and hearing of each other, literally overnight. This traditional method is undoubtedly psychologically and physically traumatic. Injuries frequently occur, more commonly to foals, who may cut their legs or head in panic, frantically trying to escape to rejoin their mother.

Most studs now use a more enlightened and humane 'free-range' weaning system, whereby mares and foals of similar ages are kept in a paddock together to allow friendships to develop. Weaning is then performed in the morning, with one mare led away from the group at turn-out time. A foal quickly overcomes its distress in the company of friends and other mares. One or two days later another mare is withdrawn in a similar way, and this continues until all the mares have been separated.

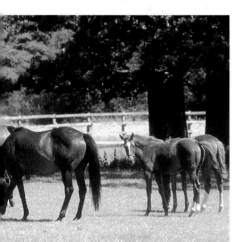

Good quality pasture generally provides adequate nutrition over summer months. Mares and foals turned out in small groups enjoy the benefits of company and lessons in socialisation.

CONDITIONS AND DISORDERS OF BREEDING AND THE REPRODUCTIVE SYSTEMS

CASTRATION

Most male horses are castrated or 'gelded' before they reach sexual maturity, which usually occurs between 16 and 20 months of age. Colts that remain 'entire' will often become a nuisance as they begin to show their natural male behaviour (aggression, fighting, mounting mares and other sexual behaviour) which may become dangerous without proper facilities and experienced handling. Young male horses that are not intended for a specific breeding purpose should therefore be castrated to avoid unwanted pregnancies and enable easier management.

STANDING CASTRATION

This is performed with the horse standing under intravenous sedation. Local anaesthetic is injected into the scrotal skin and testicles before the scrotum is incised and each testicle removed, using an emasculator to crush and cut each spermatic cord. This method is generally quicker and avoids the risks associated with general anaesthesia in the horse, but it is more difficult to keep the surgical site clean during the procedure. Certain post-operative complications, such as haemorrhage and eventration (see later), may be more likely using this technique.

CASTRATION UNDER GENERAL ANAESTHESIA

This can be performed under 'field' or 'hospital' conditions; it involves a full general anaesthetic, which enables thorough cleaning and preparation of the surgical site. More careful dissection of tissues and ligation of the spermatic cord are possible, which may help to control post-operative haemorrhage.

CRYPTORCHID HORSES

These horses can be a problem for the following reasons:
- The horse may be mistaken for a gelding but still is able to mate successfully with mares.
- Castration is more difficult, as the undescended testicle may be trapped in the groin or retained in the abdominal cavity.
- The horse may become a nuisance, showing stallion-like behaviour.
- The retained testicle may be more likely to become cancerous.

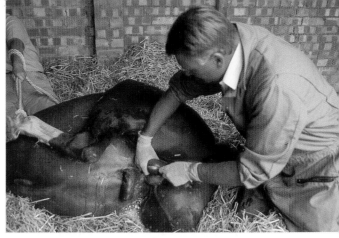

Castration is a common surgical procedure, which may be carried out under standing sedation or general anaesthesia. It is usually performed in the spring or autumn when there are fewer flies to contribute to post-operative wound infection. A preliminary veterinary examination will ensure that both testicles have descended correctly into the scrotum. If one or both testicles are undescended the horse is known as a 'cryptorchid', or a 'rig', and requires special treatment.

Blood hormone levels can be tested to prove whether a horse is a 'rig' or not. Castration of 'rigs' should be performed under general anaesthesia, ideally in a hospital environment to allow safe surgical exploration of the abdominal cavity if required.

COMMON COMPLICATIONS
- **Swelling:** The normal degree of swelling of the scrotum and prepuce may spread along the belly and cause some hind limb stiffness. Walking exercise will help to encourage this subcutaneous tissue fluid to disperse.
- **Infection:** Wound infections usually remain localised, causing excessive swelling, stiffness and sometimes a discharge. Antibiotics, non-steroidal anti-inflammatory drugs and good wound drainage is required. Delayed infection of the castration site may cause mushroom-like granulation tissue to protrude from the wound, known as 'champignon'. Chronic infection of the spermatic cord can cause fibrous thickening in the scrotal area and discharging sinus tracts, know as the scirrhous cord reaction. These more chronic conditions may not become apparent for weeks or months after castration; both require surgical removal of all the infected tissues for successful treatment.
- **Haemorrhage:** Occasional dripping of blood from the scrotal skin and subcutaneous blood vessels is common and usually stops spontaneously. Heavy continuous flow of blood can be serious and may require ligation of the bleeding vessels, although this can sometimes be very difficult.
- **Eventration:** This is where abdominal contents (guts, etc.) prolapse through the scrotal incision.

It is very serious. The veterinary surgeon should be called immediately if anything is seen to be dangling or dragging through the scrotal wound. A clean towel or cloth should be used to sling the viscera under the body of the horse in an attempt to minimise contamination. Surgical correction of the condition under general anaesthesia is required as soon as possible.

PROBLEMS AFFECTING FERTILITY

Fertility gradually decreases with age, but mares in good physical condition can breed into their twenties.

CHROMOSOMAL ABNORMALITIES
Some mares are genetically programmed to be sub-fertile or completely infertile, e.g. in Turner's syndrome. This can be diagnosed by specialised genetic testing. Affected mares may show erratic cycles or complete absence of cycles. The condition is not treatable.

OVARIAN ABNORMALITIES
Rectal palpation or ultrasound imaging of the mare's reproductive tract can help to diagnose some of these conditions.

Failure to cycle occurs whenever the ovaries are inactive. This happens:
- Out of the breeding season.
- In the transitional phase of breeding season
- Abnormality, during lactation – 'lactative anoestrus'
- In older mares, who may have less active ovaries.

Outside of these times, oral progesterone and light therapy may help to get a mare cycling.

PERSISTENT CORPUS LUTEUM (CL)
Here the mare shows long oestrous cycles. Treatment is via prostaglandin hormone injections.

CL FAILURE
The mare shows short oestrous cycles. This may be due to endometritis, which needs to be treated (see later).

OVARIAN HAEMATOMA
Haemorrhage after ovulation usually resolves naturally, but may rarely cause adhesions which can prevent eggs from passing into the uterus via the uterine tube after ovulation.

OVARIAN TUMOURS
The most common ovarian tumour is the granulosa cell tumour which usually affects one ovary only, in mares aged 5–7 years. Ultrasound scan of the ovary shows it to have a honeycomb appearance. The affected ovary may grow very large. Tumours can cause behavioural changes depending on the type of hormones created. If testosterone is secreted, the mare may act like a stallion and become aggressive. If oestrogen is secreted, the mare will act as though she is persistently in season. These tumours must be removed surgically.

OVARIAN CYSTS
These occur rarely in mares but may cause a failure to cycle or irregular cycles. Cysts may develop from follicles. Treatment is by an injection of the hormone HCG (human chorionic gonadotrophin) or GnRH (gonadotrophin-releasing hormone).

PROBLEMS ASSOCIATED WITH PREGNANCY

PREGNANCY FAILURE AND ABORTION
This is quite a common problem in the mare. Death of the embryo (less than 40 days old) or foetus before four months of pregnancy is usually followed by re-sorption; that is, the fluid is absorbed by the mare and expelled, usually unnoticed. The expulsion of the foetus before the 300th day of gestation is termed 'abortion'.

Loss of the foetus is a disappointing event, which should be investigated for a cause, as there may be implications for the mare's health and future fertility.

There is a wide range of infectious and non-infectious causes of pregnancy failure in the mare. Older mares are more commonly affected.
Signs
- Mare returns to 'oestrous' (i.e. shows signs of being in season). This may be the only sign if abortion occurs early in pregnancy.
- Foetus or foetal membranes made be found.
- Milk dripping from mare's udder.
Infectious causes
- Bacterial: endometritis (e.g coliforms or streptococci can both cause early pregnancy failure)
- Viral: (e.g. EHV1, or EVA, which is notifiable).
- Fungal: (Aspergillus – can cause late abortion).
Non-infectious causes
- *Twin conception.* Two ova are frequently fertilised, but only around 20% of twins conceived go to full-term. Those born often do not survive long,

or one foal is small and weak. Abortion of both foetuses usually occurs naturally at 6-9 months. Twin conception is therefore best avoided. A veterinary examination before service can determine whether two follicles are developing. Management is now directed towards early diagnosis by ultrasound scan and reduction to a single by manual crush.

- *Nutritional deficiencies,* e.g. starvation between days 20–30 of pregnancy, dramatic change of diet, or dehydration.
- *Disruption of oxygen supply to foetus,* e.g. from twisting of umbilical cord, blood pressure or heart problems in the mare.
- *Placental inefficiency.* Chronic endometrial degeneration may result in a decreased functional placenta, which may cause fatal malnutrition of the foetus.
- *Stress, trauma or over-exertion of mare.*
- *Hormonal imbalance,* e.g. inadequate progesterone production.
- *Foetal deformity.*
- *Side effects of certain drugs* (particularly during the first six weeks), or ingestion of toxic plants.

Treatment
Bacterial and fungal infections may be treated with the appropriate antibiotic. Infectious causes of abortion may be prevented in mares with poor perineal conformation, by good gynaecological management and, performing a Caslick's vulvoplasty. This operation involves putting sutures into the upper part of the mare's vulva in order to create an effective vulval seal, which prevents these mares from sucking contaminated air into their vagina, allowing ascending infection into the uterus.

RUPTURED PRE-PUBIC TENDON
Older mares (especially heavy draft breeds) in late pregnancy tend to be affected. The lower support to the abdominal muscles is lost and may prevent effective straining of the mare during the second stage of labour, so that an assisted foaling or a caesarean section may be required.

COLIC
Rupture of the caecum or colon and uterine torsion may be the cause of colic in the heavily pregnant mare.

UTERINE TORSION
Here the uterus twists along its long axis between 90 and 360 degrees. The condition usually occurs in late pregnancy. The mare shows signs of moderate to severe colic, and the foal may die due to the restricted blood supply to the placenta. This condition must be recognised and treated surgically as soon as possible.

ABNORMALITIES OF THE FEMALE REPRODUCTIVE SYSTEM

UTERINE TUBE

ADHESIONS
Rarely, an inflammation of the lining of the uterus spreads into the uterine tubes, where it can cause adhesions and prevent eggs from the ovary travelling into the uterus for fertilisation.

UTERINE HYPOPLASIA
The uterus is immature or underdeveloped, so that it is not able to carry a pregnancy.

UTERINE ATROPHY
Lack of endometrial glands becomes increasing likely with age, successive pregnancies and towards the end of the breeding season. Little can be done to treat this condition.

UTERINE CYSTS
These occur commonly in mares over 12 years of age and may be mistaken for an early pregnancy on ultrasound scans. If large and multiple, cysts may disrupt implantation of the embryo and the formation of the placenta.

Larger uterine cysts may be removed surgically.

UTERINE INFECTIONS (ENDOMETRITIS)
Acute infections can occur post-mating, after birth and in mares which have poor perineal and vulval conformation, causing contaminated air to be sucked into the vagina, cervix and uterus.

Mares with endometritis tend to have irregular, short oestrous cycles; they may have a vaginal discharge and tend to be sub-fertile. CEM (contagious equine metritis) is a highly-infectious venereal disease in horses. Caused by the bacteria *Taylorella equigenitalis,* it is spread at mating and causes profuse vaginal or penile discharge. Prevention of infection is by taking clitoral swabs of mares, and penile swabs of stallions, before breeding. Other bacteria known to cause endometritis include Klebsiella and Pseudomondoles.

Diagnosis
Endometrial swab for bacterial culture and sensitivity.

Treatment
Daily uterine infusions of antibiotic and saline solution for 3–5 days. Chronic uterine infections may develop from endometritis and cause a condition called pyometra, which can lead to permanent damage to the uterine lining and result in infertility. Wear and tear, rather than infection, can also be a cause.

With advancing age and repeated pregnancies, the number of endometrial glands decreases and the uterine wall becomes infiltrated with white blood cells, making the lining of the uterus unable to maintain a pregnancy.

SEPTIC METRITIS
This is a very serious condition in the mare and is often associated with retained foetal membranes. Toxins from the infection may be absorbed systemically, causing the mare to become seriously ill very quickly.
Signs
- Anorexia
- Weakness
- Depression
- Dehydration
- Increased heart rate and respiratory rate
- Laminitis.
Treatment
Must be aggressive, including intravenous fluids, antibiotics and non-steroidal anti-inflammatory drugs. The uterus should be thoroughly washed out with antibiotic and saline infusions.

CERVIX

ADHESIONS
A difficult birth may cause tearing and bruising of the cervix, which may then form adhesions.

INCOMPETENCE
If the cervix does not form a proper seal, it may allow infection to enter the uterus. These mares will be very susceptible to developing endometritis.

VAGINA
- Poor conformation may predispose to infection (vaginitits)
- Sexually transmitted diseases, e.g. Dourine (now eradicated from the UK), will cause vaginal discharge and can cause fever and death.
- Urine pooling in old brood mares may predispose to vaginal infections.
- Damage at foaling may form adhesions or scar tissue, which make subsequent matings difficult.

VULVA

SLOPING VULVA
Sloping vulval conformation forms an incompetent seal, predisposing the mare to vaginal contamination and infection. Caslick's operation can be performed, to improve the seal.

MELANOMAS
These are tumours effecting the pigment-producing cells (see Chapter 7, page *). Melanomas may affect the vulval skin and are most often found in grey mares.

HERPES VIRUS INFECTION
This can produce vulval skin lesions, which cause pain at covering. Treatment is with an antibiotic cream to avoid secondary bacterial infection and a rest from covering, to allow natural healing.

TEARING
Tearing and lacerations during birth may change vulval conformation.

PROBLEMS ASSOCIATED WITH FOALING

STANDING DELIVERY
A disturbed environment may result in the mare straining and even delivering the foal in a standing position.
Action
- Leave the mare undisturbed
- Dim the lights
- Keep environment as quiet as possible.
- Support the foal at delivery, to prevent it from falling. Try to keep the umbilical cord attached until the foal has started to breathe.

PROLONGED FIRST STAGE OF LABOUR
This can be caused by:
- An abnormally thick placenta, which fails to rupture.
- Human interference: a mare is able to postpone the second stage of labour by hours, or even days, when she feels threatened.

FAILURE OF ALLANTO-CHORION
The 'red bag' may be presented at the vulva lips. This should be ruptured by the assistant, either manually or using scissors.

ABNORMAL PRESENTATION OF FOAL
Leg flexion Flexion of one or both forelimbs under

the foal will increase the width of the foal's chest so that it cannot fit into the pelvic birth canal.

Elbow flexion One forelimb too far behind the other forelimb will cause flexion of that elbow, so that the point of the elbow can catch on the pelvic brim.

Head flexion The head and neck of the foal may be flexed to either side of the pelvis, or be flexed under the forelimbs, so that the head does not enter the pelvis.

Head down If the head is presented in the birth canal with the forelimbs lying above the head (i.e. the forelimbs resting above the ears), there is danger that the upwardly directed feet of the foal may tear the upper wall of the vagina.

Dog sitting All four feet in the birth canal with the head. The foal may be presented upright ('dog-sitting') or across the pelvis ('transverse'). Occasionally, only the spine is presented.

Breach This is quite rare in the mare. The hindquarters only are presented in the birth canal.

Hock flexion The flexed point of the hock is presented in the birth canal. The foal must be rapidly delivered.

'Wry neck' Neck muscles contract, to cause a fixed deviation of the neck.

Ankylosis This refers to the fusion of the knee and hock joints, so that the foal is unable to extend the limbs.

Correction of abnormal presentation The mare has very powerful contractions, so sedation, epidural anaesthesia or even general anaesthesia may be required to prevent straining and allow the foal to be pushed back into the mare and the malpresentation to be corrected. Soft ropes may be used as snares to help manipulate the limbs and head of the foal. Urgent vetinary attention is required at an early stage.

EMBRYOTOMY

This is where the body of a dead foal is surgically divided up as it lies within the mare and is removed piece by piece, to avoid further trauma to the mare.

TWINS

- Often detected in early pregnancy using ultrasound
- Most twin pregnancies abort by 7 months due to placental insufficiency
- If a twin pregnancy goes to term, both foals will be small
- The uterus may be over-stretched, so that it cannot contract normally
- One or both of the twins may be presented abnormally.

UTERINE TORSION

The uterus sometimes twists on itself during late pregnancy. This may cause colic and usually needs surgical correction or a caesarean operation.

UTERINE INERTIA

This is caused by an over-stretched uterine wall or a prolonged second stage of labour, e.g. due to mal-presentation of the foal. The uterine muscle is basically exhausted.

LARGE INTESTINAL RUPTURE

The caecum or colon may rupture during the first or second stage of birth causing reduced straining, shock and rapid death.

UTERINE RUPTURE

- This is rare and is usually fatal
- It may be a cause of uterine inertia
- It may only be discovered after the birth, when intestines may prolapse through the cervix and vagina
- Smaller tears may be treated surgically.

HAEMORRHAGE

Internal
- Major enlarged blood vessels supplying the uterus come under great strain during labour.
- Usually occurs within 24 hours of birth.
- More common in mares over 8 years of age.
- If bleeding is contained by the broad ligament suspending the uterus, the haemorrhage maybe controlled.
- Bleeding into the peritoneal cavity is usually rapidly fatal. The mare may show signs of colic, mucous membranes become pale, and heart and respiratory rate increase. The mare goes into a state of shock and collapses.

External
- Bleeding points for vaginal tears may be ligated (tied)
- Bleeding areas may be packed with sterile cotton wool swabs
- Antibiotic cover is advisable for vaginal haematomas (swellings).

PERINEAL LACERATIONS

The vaginal walls and vulval lips of the mare may be bruised and torn following the vigorous straining of the birth, especially if there has been an abnormal presentation of the foal. Tears may be sutured, or left to granulate.

RECTO-VAGINAL FISTULAS

During the second stage of labour, the foal's foot may be driven upward into the roof of the vagina and through into the floor of the rectum. If not corrected, the head may follow. Faeces are then able to pass into the vagina. Usually antibiotics are given at the time of the injury and the defect is then repaired surgically in two stages at a later date.

FRACTURE OF PELVIS OR FEMUR

This may occur as the mare gets up and down during foaling. A deep bed, non-slip floor and a quiet foaling environment will all help to avoid this.

UTERINE PROLAPSE

The large, soft, red, wrinkled organ is seen dangling behind the mare after normal or abnormal foaling.
- The organ is washed carefully in saline solution
- Epidural anaesthesia and sedation maybe required to decrease straining
- The uterus is manipulated carefully back into the mare
- Antibiotics are given
- Oxytocin helps the replaced uterus contract
- Vulval retention sutures are made.

RETAINED PLACENTA

If the placenta is not rapidly expelled (within 2–6 hours of birth), uterine infections and laminitis may result. Heavy draft horses are more susceptible. The placenta usually remains attached in the non-pregnant horse.
- Oxytocin, given intramuscularly or infused intravenously with sterile saline solution, is preferred to manual removal, which may scar the uterus or leave placenta tags behind
- Antibiotics
- Non- steroidal, anti-inflammatory drugs
- Careful monitoring for signs of laminitis
- Uterus may be washed out with antibiotic solution.

COMMON PROBLEMS WITH NEWBORN FOALS

PREMATURE FOALS

The normal term for a mare is 340 days (320–360 days). Early foals born after 300–320 days of pregnancy are said to be premature.

Signs
- Soft hooves
- Silky skin
- Bright red tongue and mouth
- Low birth-weight (may be associated with small placenta)
- 'Domed' forehead
- Tend to be weak and slow to suck
- Very premature foals may relapse after two days due to organ failure.

Causes
- Poorly formed placenta
- EHV1 infection of mare
- Developmental abnormality of foal
- Stress or illness of mare

Treatment
Careful nursing is essential. The foal must be kept warm, as it is less capable of regulating its own body temperature. Help the foal to stand and suckle the mare. Antibiotic cover is advisable, as premature foals are more susceptible to neonatal infections.

FOAL SEPTICAEMIA

Early recognition and treatment of infections of the newborn foal is vital to avoid serious complications or even death. Infection usually results from environmental bacteria, but can occur before or during birth from the mare's bloodstream or reproductive tract. Infections are usually generalised (septicaemic) and later become localised to specific areas (e.g. to the joints). Foals born with infections are weak and lethargic and can mimic foals with neonatal maladjustment syndrome (see below).

Signs
- Usually seen from 24 hours
- Foal becomes progressively weak and lethargic
- Gradual loss of suck reflex
- Foals with septicaemia tend not to suck frequently enough and quickly develop hypoglycaemia (low blood sugar). Distension of the mare's udder may be the first indicator that the foal is not well.
- Diarrhoea
- Pneumonia
- Neurological signs (e.g. coma, seizures)
- Swollen navel
- Swollen joints and lameness
- Body temperature may be raised normal or sub-normal.

Treatment
- Broad-spectrum intravenous antibiotics
- Intravenous fluids, if the foal is dehydrated
- Plasma transfusions, to provide antibodies
- Nursing: the foal should be kept warm (jumpers, hot-water bottles, infra-red lamps).

The foal may need to be helped to stand and feed from the mare. More severely-affected foals may need to be fed via a naso-oesophageal tube.

Prevention
- Good hygiene during and after foaling
- Ensure the foal has at least one litre of good-quality colostrum within six hours following birth. Foals which are suspected of not having sucked adequate colostrum should have their IgG (plasma antibody) levels tested.

NEO-NATAL MALADJUSTMENT SYNDROME (NMS)

This name is given to newborn foals which fail to adapt to their new environment. The exact cause is not known, but it is thought to be a dysfunction of the central nervous system, following oxygen starvation of the brain or brain haemorrhage during or shortly after birth.

Signs
- Foal may be normal at birth but develop signs usually within 12 hours of birth
- Most show a degree of respiratory distress and behavioural abnormalities, which may involve:
aimless wandering ('wanderer')
collapse ('dummy')
convulsions (convulsive syndrome)
a high-pitched grunting noise as foal attempts to gulp air ('barker')
sudden and complete loss of suck reflex.

Blindness usually precedes behavioural abnormalities.

Treatment
- Intravenous antibiotics
- Intravenous anti-inflammatory treatment (e.g. DMSO)
- Anti-convulsive therapy to control seizures e.g. diazepam
- Intravenous fluids to prevent dehydration.
- Tube feeding, as these foals are rarely able to suck the mare
- Huge nursing commitment is required, as these foals require constant support
- Nasal oxygen supplementation may be helpful in the early stages
- No improvement after 3–5 days of treatment suggests a poor prognosis
- Meconium may require removal.

Prevention
- Ensure good ventilation of foaling box
- Assist difficult foalings

- Avoid over-handling new-born foals, which may cause stress
- Resuscitate new-born foals if necessary.

MECONIUM RETENTION

Meconium is cell debris, digestive tract secretions and digested amniotic fluid. It is usually greenish-brown or black and may occur as hard pellets or as a thick paste. It is normally passed within 4–96 hours of birth and is followed by the yellow ('milk') dung. If not voided by 12–24 hours after birth, the retained meconium can cause discomfort and problems.

Signs
- More common in colts (narrower pelvis) or overdue foals
- Colic foal may roll on to its back
- Straining to defecate, the foal may also walk backwards with tail raised
- Appetite is not usually affected, but bouts of colic and pain may follow suckling.

Treatment
- Soapy water or liquid paraffin enema (performed gently to avoid rupture of delicate rectum)
- Analgesic (pain-killers)
- In more severe cases, liquid paraffin may need to be given by naso-gastric tube.

RUPTURED BLADDER

Signs
- Usually develops 3 – 4 days after birth
- Similar to retained meconium
- Blood in urine
- Gradual distension of abdomen may be noticed.

Causes
- Birth trauma
- Traction on bladder during rupture of the tough umbilical cord
- May be predisposed by congenitally thin bladder wall.

Treatment
- Surgical repair of the bladder tear is necessary. The tear is usually found on the upper surface of the bladder wall. Intravenous fluids and correction of electrolyte imbalance is vital before general anaesthesia is contemplated. Antibiotics to fight peritonitis.

GASTRIC ULCERATION

Signs
- Colic: the foal often lies on its back
- Tooth-grinding and excessive salivation
- Decreased appetite

- Pain after feeding
- More severe if the duodenum (small intestine) is also ulcerated
- The foal may die of peritonitis if the ulcer perforates.

Causes
- Stress
- Lactating mare on equipalzone treatment.

Treatment
- Gastric protectant (e.g. sucralfate)
- Drugs to decrease gastric acids secretion (e.g. cimetidine)
- Nursing: ensure foal does not become dehydrated
- Antibiotic cover maybe indicated.

Haemolytic anaemia

This condition is more common in Thoroughbred horses and more usual in mares that have had a previous foal. During the pregnancy the mare produces antibodies against the foal's red blood cells. After the birth, when the foal drinks the mare's colostrum, these antibodies are absorbed and start to destroy the foal's red blood cells, causing serious anaemia.

Signs
- Signs usually start 2–3 days after birth
- Loud, fast heart-rate
- Jaundice
- Pale mucous membranes
- Blood in urine
- Lethargy; foal yawns repeatedly
- Decreased appetite.

Treatment
- Blood transfusion
- Prevent foal suckling from mare for first 36 hours and strip all colostrum from mare's udder
- Nursing (fluids, warmth, etc.)
- Give foal donor colostrum
- Broad-spectrum antibiotic cover.

CONGENITAL DEFECTS

LIMBS

Contracted tendons   This varies in severity. The foal may just be a little bit upright, or knuckle over. Treatment may involve splinting or glue-on shoes with toe extensions. Severe cases may be treated with large doses of intravenous oxytetrocycline.

Sinking of fetlocks   This is caused by slack ligaments and muscles. It usually improves within the first few days of life. Box rest is advised whilst the foal 'comes

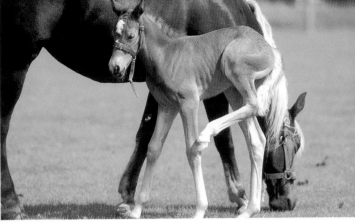

A very close eye must be kept on the foal for the first few days, particularly if it is premature or the birth-weight is low.

up' on its fetlocks. Support bandages may help. Foals with these problems may need help to stand and suckle.

HEAD

Entropion   Inward-turning of the eyelids, where the eyelids and eyelashes may rub against the inside surface of the eye and cause ulceration of the cornea. Manual correction may be all that is needed; it usually improves during the first two weeks of life as the foal grows but bad cases may need surgery (see Chapter Six).

Cleft palate   Milk is seen to bubble down the nose during suckling. This has a poor prognosis, and inhalation plus pneumonia is a common secondary problem.

Parrot mouth   An under-shot lower jaw may cause problems with adult teeth.
(see Chapter Three).

BODY

Umbilical hernia   This usually improves as the foal grows. Occasionally a loop of gut may strangulate in the hernia; this would need surgical correction. Treatment will depend on the size of the hernia.

Pervious urachus   Urine is seen to drip from the umbilicus, which will seem damp. It usually closes within two weeks, but may need surgery. Antibiotic cover is given and the umbilicus must be kept very clean. This condition may predispose to navel infections.

Heart wall defects   Loud murmurs, which persist beyond the first day of life and are associated with a weak foal or blue mucous membranes, may indicate a serious congenital heart defect. These foals will show a poor growth rate and may have breathing difficulties (see Chapter Five).

11 ALTERNATIVE APPROACHES

Despite the powerful armoury of modern chemical drugs, developed over the past half century and prescribed for use in horses for the treatment of disease, there is still strong support for, and provision of, so-called 'alternative medicine' methods. Much debate has taken place as to whether these methods should be called 'alternative', 'complementary', 'natural' or 'holistic'. Whatever the various merits and demerits of each term, what is clear, however, is that the appellation does not seriously matter. It is the methodology, science and philosophy behind the medicine which is important. The purpose of this chapter is to describe the main systems of natural/holistic medicine applied in a veterinary context, and to clarify the role each can play in the health of the horse, both on a curative and on a preventive basis.

The main feature common to the natural medicine treatments is that they work via the body's own mechanisms and should be applied according to holistic principles for best results. The objective is to stimulate, strengthen and direct the body's powerful natural healing processes, a much under-estimated and under-utilised resource. The body can then set about resolving the functional problems which have led to the symptoms and signs of disease expressed by the horse and observed by the carer.

HOLISM
The word 'holistic', which has been mentioned

Common to all 'complementary' therapies is their utilisation of the body's own powerful healing mechanisms. Health is the body's natural, balanced state.

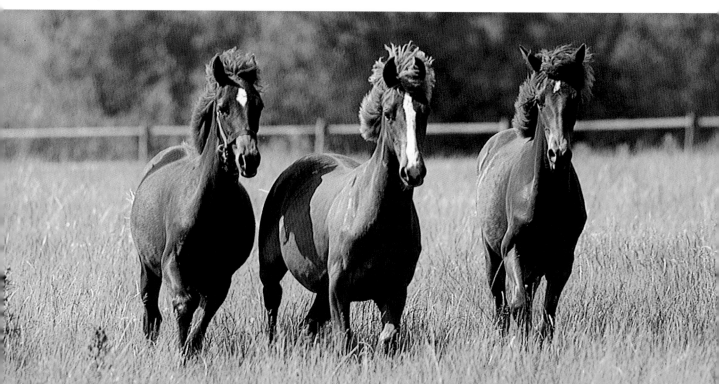

several times already, merits explanation. It is a term coined by Smuts (1870-1950) at the turn of the century, and implies an understanding of nature's tendency to create whole systems, functioning differently from the sum of the individual components of that system but depending upon each component.

Within any such system, not only does the whole depend upon the components, but each component depends upon the whole and upon each other component. No component can function separately and independently of any other. This applies to the universe, to the solar system, to our planet Earth, to each living thing upon the planet and to every compound, molecule or atom. From the macrocosm to the microcosm, no component is capable of independent function, free of the influence of the system or of other components. By the same token it is incapable of independent existence with no effects or influences being exerted by it upon the other components or upon the system.

We have, then, a concept of systems within systems within systems. Each is only a contributor to the function of the whole. The basic unit of such systems is, arguably, the atom and the basic force is energy. In living organisms it is better to think of the basic component as each individual living cell – but the driving force is still energy.

While the term 'holistic' had not been coined until the turn of the twentieth century, ancient systems of medicine nonetheless recognised the fundamental truth and the essential basic nature of the concept and its importance in health and disease. Applying those principles to the health of the horse, we have a concept of mind, body and spirit in harmony with each other and in harmony with their environment (the world). Within the horse, considered as a 'system', each component functions to the service of the whole and is, in turn, influenced by the whole. In this process, each component influences every other component and is, in turn, influenced by each other component. No part can function independently.

Whether considering the 'parts' to be mind, spirit or body, or as each internal organ, the same rule and fundamental law of nature applies. Any disharmony will create the need for compensation to maintain survival. This compensation process results in a shift of normal healthy function and the appearance of symptoms or signs of disease (dis-ease or disharmony). If the imbalance persists, then a chain of compensation develops in any component or among many components, whether in individual

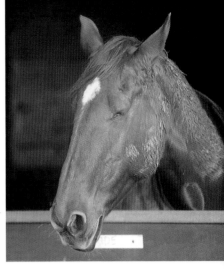

Any disharmony or imbalance in or between the parts of the system – the body, mind and spirit – will create the need for compensation. The result is a shift from the normal pattern of health and the appearance of signs and symptoms of pain and disease.

organs or in mind or in spirit or in all three.

Should this chain of compensation take place, the symptom picture can be far removed from the original compensation step and the trail of disease becomes harder to follow. What is certain, however, is that, in order to cure disease, we must pay attention to the concept of mind, body and spirit in the context of their environment (whether immediate environment or more widespread) and attempt to correct any imbalances or stresses in the system. Not only, therefore, are we to treat the horse itself as a whole (mind, body and spirit) but we must attend to feeding, lifestyle, management, working regimes, saddling, shoeing, harness, stabling, grazing, land management, routines and so on, in order to optimise these and to allow health to happen.

This is the great contribution to understanding that the natural medicine methods have made down the centuries: that if all factors are optimised then health will happen. In other words, there is a natural process of healing which is at work perpetually, day and night, in every body on this planet, tending towards health. If we free it from constraints and malevolent influences, it will win the day and the body will heal.

The medical sciences and philosophies that have grown up around this concept have developed skills and techniques for stimulating and enhancing the action of this health tendency, but they do not function properly without full attention to all the factors discussed above. For this reason, no one should set about treating the symptoms and signs of disease *per se* but should rather attend to all the factors that may impinge upon the ailing horse, to ensure that its healing capability is maximised.

No medicine (whether herbal, homoeopathic, acupuncture, aromatherapy, flower remedies or other) should be given without attention to the proper feeding of the horse for health, and the study of every factor impinging upon the horse which may be (and will be) contributing to its current state of health or disease.

Traditional Chinese Medicine, evolved over thousands of years, always had a very positive eye turned towards the diet, the lifestyle and the physical and emotional influences upon its patients. The concept is therefore not new. Herbal medicines have evolved with life forms since time immemorial and man has inherited an understanding and instinct for them. He has knowingly used them since the dawn of civilisation, recognising that the body functions within its environment, that the herbs alongside which the body has grown also function within the same environment, and that nothing can function independently.

This last point is especially poignant for horses, who have evolved to derive their entire nutritional input from herbage and plant material, water and soil. The idea of giving animal-derived material to a horse is not only repugnant from the point of view of ethics and morals but flies in the face of logic and reason. It denies both knowledge and understanding of holistic principles and the wisdom of observing the evolutionary development of a species. Equine supplements and veterinary medicines containing ingredients of animal origin (and there are many, surprisingly) should never be fed to horses on these grounds alone, let alone the questionable medical wisdom of doing so in the light of the recent BSE fiasco in cattle.

Having laid down the principles of holism and having described the underlying principles of natural medicine, it is now appropriate to describe the major systems of medicine which fall under this heading and which adhere to this philosophy.

The main headings are:

> Herbal medicine
> Homoeopathy
> Acupuncture and Traditional Medicine Chinese

Minor headings are:

> Aromatherapy (Essential Oils)
> Flower Remedies
> Radionics
> The supportive role of diet
> The supportive role of Chiropractic,
>   Osteopathy and Physiotherapy.

A small section explaining the relevance of these studies to natural medicine and the role they can play in the context of overall healing, is not only beneficial but is essential to a complete understanding.

HERBAL MEDICINE

As far as the sciences of geology and biology can tell us, plants developed as an earlier life-form than animals. According to our information, they were already well-developed, extremely varied and niche-adapted, prior to the emergence of animal life as we understand it now (in terms of large terrestrial and aquatic animals and, more relevantly to this text, land mammals).

Following this logic, the horse as we know him today, developed and evolved in the context of plant life. The horse has known no existence prior to plant life, and therefore it forms part of his environment and part of his life support system. It is simply not relevant to think of a horse separate from herbage and plant life. He is incapable of any existence without plants and the species of plants present in his environment during his development will have influenced the route of that development. His present form, structure and biology are therefore nothing other than a function of the plant life which surrounded him and supported him during his evolution.

When we consider the lifestyle of the modern domesticated horse, we can visualise, via this logical process of thought, that he is no longer kept in the environment in which he evolved and to which he adapted over the millennia of his time on Earth. He is denied the roaming to which he is attuned and he is denied access to the wide variety of herbage species that constitutes his natural fodder. Added to those 'penalties' of domestication are the factors imposed by modern agriculture and pasture management. The ground, on which the herbage he receives is grown, is no longer the same as nature devised. It is bombarded with fertilisers, pesticides and herbicides such that it is not of the same structure, nor does it support the same microflora and microfauna in its substance and it cannot support the same healthy plant life to which our horse should be entitled access.

Let us take the simple example of nitrogenous fertilisers to illustrate one of the ways in which modern husbandry can be detrimental to horse health. If chemical nitrogenous fertilisers are added to the soil, they will form ammonia ions ($NH4^+$). These preferentially bind to the clay micelles (the soil structure) and displace the positively-charged trace and major minerals such as copper (Cu^{++}), manganese (Mn^{++}), zinc (Zn^{++}), magnesium

The horse as we know him developed and evolved in the context of plant life. But many horses now live a life totally removed from the environment of equine evolution. Even those allowed free access to pasture are existing off ground that can no longer be described as being in its 'natural' state.

(Mg^{++}) and calcium (Ca^{++}), which are therefore left 'free' in the soil. When rain falls, those minerals are washed away in the ditches and drainage channels.

This effect is easily observable and quantifiable on each and every 'modern' pasture. It is not hypothesis but an established fact. After several years of this process, the soil structure becomes disastrously altered and its composition impoverished. The plants which grow in it become less nutritious and a vicious spiral of potential ill-health is created in the system. The horse cannot be independent of this process, for he eats his hay from such systems, grazes grass in such pastures and eats cereals grown in this way. In short, he depends for his basic nourishment, sustenance and renewal upon an impoverished resource.

Adding to that process the second example of how nitrogenous fertilisers, for instance, can be damaging to the system, let us look at the plant biology that occurs in grasses subjected to additional, soluble, nitrogenous material. Sugar content of the grass is altered and increased (a clear laminitis risk to our native ponies, to cite one disadvantage of this). Proteins and, more

importantly, toxic non-protein nitrogenous compounds, are increased in the grass, leading to metabolic imbalances and to risks of disease. Potassium levels are drastically increased, leading to risk of electrolyte imbalances and suppression of magnesium metabolism (and therefore alteration of nerve, heart and muscle function in grazing animals). The only 'advantages' that seem to follow from fertilising grazing land in this way are an increase in grass and a 'better' grass colour. There no increase in feeding value for horses – in fact the contrary applies.

The importance of herbal medicine, therefore, becomes more apparent in this context. It can serve a function not just as a means of helping the body to heal troublesome symptoms (although it is very powerful in that respect), but also as a positive background health and nutritional influence. Because we are thinking holistically, it is very difficult to separate the concepts of nutrition and medicine. When is a herb a medicine and when is it a food? That is a rhetorical question with no worthwhile answer, nor should we waste our resources on asking such a question. We should be considering a proper balance of indigenous herbs as a basic nutritional requirement in support of health. If we are needing 'treatments' for disease, we should turn to individual herbs or individually-tailored mixtures of herbs, containing the necessary mix of active principles to help a system back to health.

This picture sounds very friendly and perhaps a little precious and 'bland'. The power of herbal medicine must not be under-estimated as a result of this comfortable vision of benevolent plants in a utopian environment. The extraordinary power of herbal medicine has long been recognised by the modern pharmaceutical industry as a fruitful source of raw material for powerful modern drugs. The pharmaceutical industry makes its considerable profit from patented chemical drugs. A surprisingly large proportion of these started out as plant chemicals extracted, purified and modified in the laboratory, in order to create unique compounds more or less related to the original. The stated purpose of this work is to remove the impurities, instabilities and uncertainties inherent in nature and to create a more 'perfect' and active chemical. The result is a modified chemical which can be patented, unlike the original natural compound. The actual outcome of this process is to alter the 'safe' natural compound to one of less proven safety. The compound is removed from its natural context of other synergistic compounds contained in the plant, which ingredients could be argued to protect the patient by balancing and modulating the effects of the supposed 'active principle'.

Suffice it to say that herbal medicine has existed since the dawn of human civilisation and comprises the indigenous medicine of any society, primitive or modern. The instinctive collective wisdom of human society is oriented towards the use of herbs for medicine and this instinct is even stronger in horses, for whom herbage is everything and who have evolved entirely in the context of herbage. Their existence has therefore depended upon certain balances of herbage as a *sine qua non*, an indispensable ingredient of health and life.

ACTIVE PRINCIPLES

In order better to understand the medical use of herbs, it is useful to attempt a classification of 'active principles'. The constituents of herbs can be classified as:

acids	flavones
alcohols	flavonoids
alkaloids	glycosides
anthraquinones	phenols
bitters	saponins
carbohydrates	tannins
coumarins	volatile oils (it is these powerful substances which form the basis of aromatherapy).

Their medicinal action can be classified according to their main effects in the body. (These classifications are different from those used in Traditional Chinese Medicine – see later – since the way of considering the action of the body is so different in that practice):

alterative	diuretic
anodyne	ecbolic
anthelmintic	emetic
anticatarrhal	emollient
anti-emetic	expectorant
anti-inflammatory	febrifuge
antilithic	galactogogue
antibacterial	hepatic
antifungal	hypnotic
antispasmodic	nervine
aperient/laxative	rubefacient
aromatic	sedative
astringent	sialogogue
bitter	soporific
cardiac	stimulant
carminative	styptic
cathartic/purgative	tonic
chologogue and	vesicant
anticholagogue	vulnerary
demulcent	diaphoretic

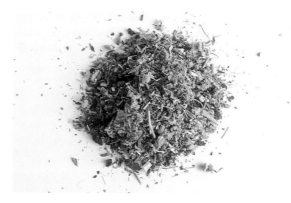

Herbal supplements must be treated as medicines. This applies both to the care with which they are produced and to their method of use. A pre-packaged supplement cannot be expected to have the precise effect of a formula prescribed by a vet specifically for a patient, after a thorough analysis of the individual's symptoms and needs.

In the major 'herbals' available to readers (books describing herbal medicines), reference is made to active ingredients of each herb, according to their chemical classification and their main medical effects. It is on this basis that herbs may be chosen for the treatment of disease. Combinations of herbs are designed according to the required balance of effects, compatibility with each other, and suitability for the individual patient in question.

It is of fundamental importance that herbs are correctly identified, before usage as medicines. They should be grown in a suitable healthy environment, without which husbandry they will not be healthy themselves nor can they be expected to have their proper therapeutic powers.

Proprietary preparations of herbal medicines are available, sourced and assembled with greater or lesser wisdom, care and traditional knowledge, depending upon the source. The products with a proper marketing authorisation have, by and large, been correctly tested and 'proven'. The companies who have undertaken the work necessary for granting of this authorisation have usually been in the business of herbal medicine for a great number of years, or generations in some cases, building up a proper tradition of knowledge and care. Many other products exist, marketed with varying vigour and showing varying regard for factual validity of implied medical claims and with varying care in the cultivation, identification, collection, mixing and preparation of the herbs for sale.

It is clear, if a product is pre-packaged for sale, that it cannot be tailored individually for a given patient and is therefore not being used holistically in the truest sense. For the best effects of herbal medicine, remedies should be formulated after a deep analysis of the patient's symptoms and individual needs. In the field of herbal marketing, the law protects neither the consumer nor the horse, so it is up to the consumer to protect himself or herself and thereby to obtain the best possible care for the horse in question.

SIDE EFFECTS AND DANGERS
When buying herbal products, it is important to observe manufacturers' instructions very strictly. If concurrent conventional drug medicine is being given, there is a danger of incompatibility or even of over-dosage of a particular ingredient, since many drug ingredients are related to herbal ingredients (see above). The administration of the more potentially toxic herbs, such as aristolochia, bryony, deadly nightshade, foxglove, hemlock, horsetail, lobelia, monkshood, mugwort and St John's wort should be avoided by the amateur prescriber, because dosage levels and application are of critical importance. Experience, skill and close monitoring of the patient are required for their safe usage.

DRUG RESIDUES
Since material doses of powerful medicines are being administered, it is highly likely that there is a potential for residues of chemicals to be found in blood samples of treated animals. For this reason, it is not always safe to use herbs in competition horses for a varying period prior to competition. Since the horse is also considered by European Union law to be a meat animal, residues in the tissues of dead horses are of potential significance and horses fed herbs prior to slaughter should not be sold for human consumption.

STORAGE
Herbs should be collected freshly each year and stocks should not be accumulated such that supplies over-run the year. Dried herbs should be stored in glass containers in a warm, dust-free atmosphere, protected from light and damp. They should not be tightly packed and should be properly dated. The damp feed rooms found as standard in many equestrian yards are not conducive to the proper survival of herbal medicines. The purchase of products without a clearly stated date of harvest, often in unsuitable containers, is to be discouraged.

MAJOR COMMON HERBS
There follows a brief and basic description of some of the common herbs (indigenous to the UK) which can be used in horse care, along with some of the major indications for use of those herbs. This list is far from comprehensive and should be taken as an indication of the scope and methodology of herbal medicine only, not as a manual of treatment. The disease conditions mentioned are only of a basic nature, those amenable for home treatment, but the exclusion of major, serious and complicated disease is not to be interpreted as an inability or inadequacy of herbal medicine, properly applied, to treat such diseases.

Camomile *Matricaria chamomilla* This herb, once common in hedgerows and pastures, has effective sedative and anodyne properties. Anxiety and over-excitement at shows or events are indications, along with 'anxiety colic' or facial pain (sinus or teeth). If the pelvis or spine becomes twisted, prior to a visit from a chiropractor it will help to relieve pain and to relax musculature, thus improving the effects of chiropractic manipulation. It is usually given internally.

Comfrey *Symphytum officinale* This is known as 'knitbone' in traditional circles, giving away its main use in the healing of injuries to bones. Do not under-estimate its ability as a general vulnerary, though, to aid healing of bruises and injuries of all types. It has recently been maligned as a potential liver carcinogen, owing to the presence of small quantities of a substance somewhat related to the poison found in ragwort. This is, in the author's opinion, an over-rated risk. Comfrey has been used effectively and safely for centuries, right up to the present time and the author has witnessed no side-effects consequent upon its correct usage. Beware of supplements intended for long-term use which contain it, however. Comfrey is used both internally, with the above caution, and as a poultice for wounds or leg injuries.

Dandelion *Taraxacum officinale* This deceptively simple and common plant is, in fact, a powerful medicine. It is diuretic, alterative, bitter and mildly laxative. It is deep-rooting and therefore brings up valuable minerals from the deep layers of the soil which are inaccessible to grass roots. Dandelion's reputation as a weed has seen its decline in many pastures, but the author believes its establishment in horse pasture should be encouraged. Used in cases of liver, kidney, skin or heart problems, it has powerful beneficial effects apart from its basic nutrient value. It is also rich in potassium, a valuable supplementary benefit in its application as a diuretic. The root is a more powerful diuretic than the leaf, and can be obtained as a powder. The diuretic and alterative properties make it one of the valuable herbs to be given in cases of laminitis.

Flax *Linum usitatissimum* Flax is the blue-flowered plant which gives us linseed and linseed oil. Linseeds (boiled for more than two hours in order to destroy the toxic prussic acid they contain) are a valuable nutritional supplement for protein and oils. For this reason they make one of the best conditioners available. Linseed oil may also be fed direct, but not too much or it may be purgative. Linseed oil is high in the essential fatty acids which are valuable as detoxicants and anti-oxidants. The oil even has a reputation for hastening excretion of heavy metal pollutants from the body, a potentially important

indication in today's toxic-waste-rich society. Many seed dressings contain mercury or other heavy metals, and pasture sown after cereals may be thus polluted, quite apart from the added risks of pasture on landfill sites or in industrial fall-out areas. Uses of the seeds are nutritional, laxative, conditioning, anti-inflammatory and emollient. They can also make a good poultice.

Garlic *Allium sativum* Garlic's increased use as a culinary herb in the UK over the last two decades has perhaps masked its tremendous medicinal value. It is expectorant, anti-inflammatory, anti-histamine, anti-bacterial, anthelmintic, anti-allergic, disinfectant, alterative and aromatic. The aromatic compounds are excreted via the skin and act as a valuable insect repellent. Its high sulphur content makes it useful for good hoof nutrition. The blood-cleansing properties make it a good supplement in laminitis and sweet itch, but its other many properties make it almost a panacea. Such is its value that the author recommends garlic for daily use, either as fresh cloves or, if this is impractical, as a pure powder. However, beware proprietary supplements that contain large quantities of inactive 'carrier' – an all-too-common occurrence.

Kelp *Fucus vesiculosus* This is a seaweed and brings with it the nutritional properties of the sea from which it is harvested. For this reason it is high in valuable minerals but also prone to marine pollution, so care should be taken in sourcing it (especially avoid North Sea or Irish Sea sources). Kelp is highly nutritious, making it a valuable dietary supplement. It is emollient and usable as a poultice. It is rich specifically in potassium and iodine. Calcified seaweed makes a very good land top-dressing in place of chemical fertilisers, providing humus and mineral nutrients in a valuable 'slow-release' balance. It is of particular use in goitrous conditions or in areas of the country known to be short in iodine (for example, Derbyshire).

Marigold *Calendula officinalis* This is another plant so decorative and common in the garden as to make it seem an unlikely medicine. Nothing could be further from the truth. It is anti-bacterial, antifungal, anti-inflammatory, vulnerary (to be given internally and externally) and, given internally, is a powerful digestive. As calendula lotion (used in homoeopathy and herbal medicines) it is an invaluable wound treatment, disinfecting and stimulating healing in a seemingly miraculous way.

Mint *Mentha spicata* Also: **Peppermint** *Mentha piperita*, **Horse mint** *Mentha sylvestris*, **Spearmint** *Mentha viridis* This common garden herb is very acceptable to horses and a much-enjoyed addition to their feed. It is often added to commercial feeds to make them highly acceptable, to mask less desirable flavours, to give the purchaser something nice to smell and to enable the manufacturer to put "with added herbs" on the bag as a strong commercial selling point! It is an appetiser, digestive, carminative and stimulant and is therefore a valuable colic treatment or supplement for horses with colic tendency. Peppermint is particularly antifungal compared with the more ordinary mints and is also a more powerful carminative and digestive. It is more highly flavoured and is the reason that horses are so fond of mint sweets (not to be recommended).

Nettle or stinging nettle, *Urtica dioica* This plant has such a reputation as a weed that its valuable nutritional and medicinal benefits are often overlooked. Iron, calcium and potassium are contained especially richly in nettles. As a rich source of Vitamin C, nettle is also of positive immune benefit and this also aids the absorption of its iron content. It is a powerful tonic and galactogogue. It is valuable as a daily nutritional supplement in lactating mares, laminitic ponies, arthritic horses and in cases of anaemia or poor condition.

DOSAGE OF HERBS
The dosage of herbs is not a simple dose-for-weight matter but depends more upon the medicinal purpose, the patient and the other herbs given in conjunction. Consult your veterinary surgeon for help with this. The reader should beware commercial herbal suppliers whose main interest is to sell a product and who are not legally enabled to prescribe or advise for horses.

Only a qualified veterinary surgeon is allowed to treat animals or advise on their treatment. A horse owner is only legally protected if a veterinary surgeon is consulted. It is also wise to be cautious about commercial products, vigorously marketed with quasi-legal medical claims or hints displayed on the label or in the brand name. These have not been specifically concocted for the particular horse in question and therefore may not be of much value and may even be unsafe. It is unwise to buy any product whose contents are not clearly listed on the package and any which are not clearly dated. Since it is clearly of importance to horse health not to source herbs from polluted areas (diesel, car fumes,

chemical sprays, industrial fall-out) then it follows that any supplier of herbs should be carefully vetted for quality. To pick one's own herbs from carefully chosen sites is an obvious safety measure but it is important to observe the laws relevant to wild plants and those relating to private property.

Western herbs   (examples)

Alteratives	e.g. burdock	(Arctium)
Antispasmodics	e.g. black cohosh	(Cimicifuga) (N. Amer.)
Aperients	e.g. flax seed	(Linum)
Astringents	e.g. golden rod	(Solidago)
Anthelmintics	e.g. garlic	(Allium)
Bitters	e.g. tansy	(Tanacetum)
Carminatives	e.g. sage	(Salvia)
Demulcents	e.g. comfrey	(Symphytum)
Diaphoretics	e.g. elder	(Sambucus)
Diuretics	e.g. dandelion	(Taraxacum)
Expectorants	e.g. vervain	(Verbena)
Febrifuges	e.g. angelica	(Angelica)
Hepatics	e.g. motherwort	(Leonurus)
Nervines	e.g. hops	(Humulus)
Rubefacients	e.g. nettle	(Urtica)
Sedatives	e.g. skullcap	(Scutellaria)
Stimulants	e.g. horseradish	(Cochlearia)
Tonics	e.g. elecampane	(Inula)
Vulneraries	e.g. marigold	(Calendula)

HOMOEOPATHY

Whereas herbal medicine is as old as human civilisation and animals naturally and instinctively 'practised' it before that, homoeopathy is only officially just over 200 years old at the time of writing. The principle was formally discovered in 1796 by a brilliant German physician and scientist, Samuel Hahnemann, who vigorously developed and improved the science over the rest of his life (he died in 1843). His discovery hinged on his experiments with cinchona bark, the raw material that gives us quinine, a useful drug in malaria. He found that, in small repeated doses, the bark could produce, in a healthy person, symptoms indistinguishable from malaria, a disease for which it is a very effective treatment.

This work was the basis of the 'law of similars' and gave rise to the name homoeopathy – 'similar to the disease'. As a result of his very scientific and meticulous development work, Hahnemann gave us not only a great many medicines, established and tested on the same principle of 'like cures like' as his original cinchona, but also the 'principle of dilution'.

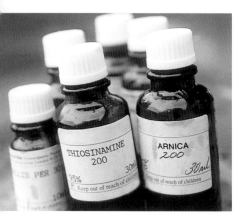

Homoeopathic remedies have proved effective in a variety of conditions, including chronic disease. Their influence is upon the imbalance that gives rise to physical symptoms, rather than directly upon the symptoms themselves.

He found that by serial dilution and succussion of the medicines, they became even safer and more powerful. This is one of the most perplexing of all medical paradoxes, but depends upon the harnessed energy properties of the medicine for its therapeutic activity rather than molecular or chemical interaction with a patient's body. It is not the purpose of this chapter to argue and reason through the logic and science that supports the practice of homoeopathy, but more to describe its use and its benefits.

The energetic and dynamic influences exerted by a homoeopathic medicine seem to help the body actively to re-balance its internal equilibrium. The holistic implications are strongly realised at this point. Balance implies mind, body and spirit in harmony with the environment. The medicines do not exert any direct influence on the symptoms but upon the imbalance that gives rise to the symptoms. They act upon mind and body as inseparable and integrated components. It goes without saying that the body must be able to respond to this stimulus and for this reason, for horses, a healthy diet, optimal saddling, shoeing, management and so on are essential. It is vital to remove those factors which may impede healing and which may, in many cases, have contributed to, or given rise to, the disease in the first place.

Homoeopathy is a valuable therapy for a great variety of diseases. It is as capable as modern drugs of handling even such emergency conditions as colic. It is uniquely able to help the body cope with and heal the effects of injuries of all sorts (especially see Arnica, Hypericum, Ruta, Symphytum later in this chapter) for horse (and rider!). It is able rapidly to resolve acute febrile and infective illnesses, often more promptly than the use of antibiotics but without the risk of side-effects. For these reasons it has become a valuable first aid therapy in horse yards.

It is in the treatment of chronic disease, however, that homoeopathy has really earned its reputation. Chronic disease is one in which the body and the disease exist in a sort of uneasy truce, often of long standing. Arthritis, skin problems, chronic diarrhoea, sweet itch, laminitis, allergic lung disease (COPD), navicular disease, spavins, tendon injuries, splints, chronic respiratory infection and many other conditions, many of which strike terror into the heart of the loving horse owner, are often successfully helped by properly applied homoeopathy in conjunction with the necessary management changes essential to the holistic method. It is important to remember that the body is constantly remodelling, involving resorption of tissues and replacement of them anew, on a steady, constantly rolling basis. This allows for healthy renewal where before there was disease, so long as the stimulus (homoeopathic medicine) is correct and the diet and management are favourable.

The name of the disease is not usually the factor which decides the outcome. More often it is the correct application of the method, treating the patient as a whole, combined with proper, supervised, long-term care.

HANDLING AND STORAGE OF MEDICINES

It is important to store and handle homoeopathic medicines correctly. Homoeopathic medicines are, by virtue of their dilution and finesse, very fragile. They therefore need to be handled and stored carefully, if they are to be of value over a number of years. There are several very simple rules to follow when handling and storing these medicines.

- Store in a glass bottle (preferably brown)
- Store in a dark cupboard
- Store in a normal temperature range
- Do not refrigerate, freeze or overheat
- Protect from sunlight at all times
- Store away from strong smelling substances such as perfumes, other toiletries, smelling salts, camphor, liniments, paints, polishes etc.
- Keep the lid on the bottle at all times when not in use
- Do not open more than one bottle at a time
- Avoid handling the medicines
- Do not return accidentally-handled medicines to the bottle.

SIDE-EFFECTS AND DANGERS

There are no side-effects attached to the use of homoeopathic medicines. They are completely safe, both from this point of view and because they do not create tissue or blood residues. There are, however, some potential undesirable effects. 'Worse before better' is one of those. As the body heals internally, the symptoms can appear worse at first. This phenomenon, usually only temporary, is termed 'aggravation'. Giving homoeopathic medicines can also cause old, unresolved symptoms to reappear, which can be both worrying and disappointing. It is usually, however, only an expression of the healing process at work and should, again, be a temporary problem, the body emerging completely healed at the end of the process.

COMPATIBILITY WITH OTHER MEDICINES
Homoeopathy, used properly, is a pure and powerful stimulus to the body. Ideally, it should not be mixed with other therapies. Modern medicines especially to be avoided are steroids, non-steroidal anti-inflammatory drugs, anti-histamines and strongsmelling substances (such as camphor). Vaccines can seriously affect the workings of the immune system and can adversely affect the healing mechanisms of homoeopathy. Acupuncture and homoeopathy, if used together, must be integrated very carefully and deliberately or they may clash and result in poor effects or damage. Many herbs should be used cautiously, or not at all, alongside homoeopathy. Aromatherapy should only be used with caution and under professional guidance, if it is to be used alongside homoeopathy.

AVAILABILITY
Homoeopathic medicines are available over-the-counter in many health stores and pharmacies, but usually only a limited range and only in the 6c potency. The 30c potency is often more desirable, for deeper effects, and is usually only available from specialist pharmacies or veterinarians. Such outlets would also hold a much wider range of medicines.

Only veterinary surgeons are allowed by law to treat horses with homoeopathy or advise on diagnosis or prescription. Many illegal or quasi-legal sources of homoeopathic medicines are only too ready to supply and to 'prescribe'. The horse carer is advised very strongly to avoid this risky practice. Medicines marketed in this way are not tailored to the patient in a holistic manner but are recommended or sold on a 'named disease' basis. This is an unwise, unsafe and often ineffective route to follow.

Vets are joining properly accredited courses in ever-increasing numbers. This trend is fuelled by consumer demand, by enlightenment, and by disillusionment with the inability of modern conventional drugs to solve chronic disease problems. Vets using homoeophy are therefore becoming more widely available.

SOME COMMON HOMOEOPATHIC MEDICINES
This section is not intended to be comprehensive, more to show the scope of a few common emergency remedies for use in the stable. It is good to develop complete confidence in the safety of the remedies and in one's own ability to use them, safe in the knowledge that they can only have a positive influence on the condition in question. Even if they are not fully effective in any single case, they will be of some help and benefit. Use of homoeopathic remedies as soon as possible at the onset of virus disease, injury or other emergency, is of great importance. They can never argue with any medicines a veterinarian may want to give, should a veterinary call-out become necessary and, in some cases, their use may render a veterinary visit unnecessary.

Aconitum napellus Fear, anxiety, terror, excitement, fevers of sudden onset, conjunctivitis of sudden onset, acute inflammatory reactions, all suggest this remedy. Conditions resulting from cold, dry winds.

Arnica montana A remedy everyone should have in the household and stable. It is the first remedy for any case of *injury, shock* or *surgery*. Use it to prevent or help problems from over-exertion. It can be used years after an injury, to lessen persistent after-effects. It is a powerful remedy to combat sepsis of wounds and can also be used in lotions and ointments. The sooner it is used after injury, the better its effect. It is not recommended for topical treatment of wounds. It may be used with other injury remedies, where applicable.

Arsenicum album Think of this in cases of anxiety or restlessness. Discharges are usually acrid and burning. Violent diarrhoea is characteristic of Arsenicum, especially after ingestion of spoilt food. There is often a thirst for frequent small drinks. Skin is dry and scaly with scurf. Allergic asthmatic conditions often respond well. Symptoms are worse for cold and wet weather and better for warmth. Symptoms are usually worse around midnight.
Belladonna This is a violent and sudden remedy.

Think of it in cases of fever, abscessation, inflammation, convulsions, violent temper. Symptoms are worse for noise or touch and better for warmth and quiet darkness.

Calendula officinalis Used mainly as a topical lotion or cream, it is a great healing remedy, speeding healing of abrasions, reducing suppuration and aiding first-stage healing of wounds.

Colocynthis This is a wonderful colic remedy. In typical cases, the back is arched and limbs pulled up. There is usually much agitation and evidence of pain coming in spasms. The horse grinds its teeth and is sensitive to noise. All deep, severe pains may be helped, wherever they are in the body (e.g. hip).

Euphrasia officinalis Euphrasia is an eye remedy especially for those showing symptoms of conjunctivitis, photophobia and watery discharge from eyes and nose. Symptoms are worse for warmth and bright light and better for dim light. It is used internally or in the form of eye drops. The plant's country name is 'eye-bright'.

Hamamelis virginica Venous congestion or pooling and extravasation of venous blood, haematoma and haemorrhage of dark blood fit the picture of this remedy.

Hepar sulphuris A very important remedy in suppurative conditions. It is useful as either a preventive or curative treatment in septic injury. Hypopion (pus in the anterior chamber of the eye) also responds. All purulent or septic conditions should suggest the need for this remedy, including infected wounds, whether surgical or traumatic.

Hypericum perforatum The homoeopathic 'painkiller'. Use this in cases of injury to extremities where nerve endings abound, particularly toe or tail injuries. Post-operative pain, spinal injury, lacerated wounds and puncture wounds all may show relief from this remedy. It has reputed anti-tetanus properties.

Ledum palustre Like *Hypericum*, Ledum has reputed anti-tetanus properties and is the first-choice remedy for puncture wounds. It helps them to heal effectively, from the depths outwards. It also has uses in arthritic pain of the small joints which are worse for heat or warmth. Nail injuries in the foot call for this remedy, after adequate paring of the sole.

Nux vomica Digestive disturbances following unsuitable food, constipation (sometimes diarrhoea) after over-eating, irritable temperament, sensitivity to noise, stuffed-up nose are all in the realm of Nux vomica. Symptoms are worse for noise and better for rest or in damp weather. The morning usually sees the worst symptoms.

Phosphorus This is a very 'sudden' remedy which is easy to remember when one thinks of the flare of a match, with phosphorus on the tip. The animal is sensitive to loud and sudden noise (e.g. thunder, gunfire, fireworks). Some respiratory problems respond to Phosphorus, particularly pneumonia. Jaundice and readily bleeding wounds are helped. Disrupted nerves stand more chance of regenerating with the help of Phosphorus. Symptoms are better in the dark, in open air and for rest.

Rhus toxicodendron Rhus is a remedy which is mainly of use in the skin and musculo-skeletal system. The skin shows small red papules and sometimes vesicles. The rheumatic/arthritic symptoms are its greatest sphere of success, where it is the first-choice remedy for symptoms that are worse for cold, wet conditions and for first movement after stabling. Conditions are better for continued movement and for warmth. Excessive exercise again produces a worsening. Where there is damage to muscles, think of Rhus tox.

Ruta graveolens Ruta is the sprain and dislocation remedy. Where any tendon, ligament, joint or bone is injured, turn to Ruta. It also helps rheumatic symptoms which are similar to Rhus and can be used in conjunction with that remedy.

Symphytum officinale Comfrey, or knitbone, has an unsurpassed reputation in the speeding and regulation of bone healing. Use it also in injuries to the eye area (orbit).

PREVENTION
In addition to its very powerful ability to treat acute, infectious, traumatic or chronic disease in the horse, homoeopathy is also able to act in a preventive capacity. For this purpose we usually use Nosodes, which are homoeopathic remedies made from disease material. They are in the same extreme dilutions as the usual homoeopathic medicines, so are completely safe. They can be considered in the same light as vaccines but without the dangers and without the proof of efficacy (the author will not

perform animal experiments, which would be necessary fully to prove the efficacy of these medicines).

Nosodes exist to aid with prevention of influenza, herpes, shigella, staphylococcal disease, strangles, bastard strangles, ringworm and many other infectious diseases. It is important to consult a veterinarian about the use and availability of these medicines and thereby obtain the necessary advice on their proper use.

SUMMARY

To summarise, homoeopathy is a safe, gentle, powerful and effective therapy which operates via the dynamic energy processes of the body. It is able to produce benefits or cures in a great many troublesome and rare conditions, many of which are considered incurable or as having a hopeless prognosis in conventional modern veterinary medicine. It is a valuable modality to consider, either as a first-line treatment or as a follow-up to conventional input in chronic, difficult cases. Its use has prevented the need for antibiotics in the author's equine practice and has enabled the return to work of a great many 'hopeless' cases – a very rewarding result for the necessary hard work to be expected in the learning of homoeopathy.

ACUPUNCTURE (AND TRADITIONAL CHINESE MEDICINE)

Acupuncture is not a stand-alone therapy. It is commonly used in the modern western world as if it were, however, and this has led to rather poorer results than can be expected from using acupuncture in the holistic context of Traditional Chinese Medicine.

The ancient Chinese used acupuncture as part of a very holistic approach to health and disease, supporting it with proper dietary, lifestyle and herbal medicinal advice. All these strategies were used together to re-establish a proper balance in the body

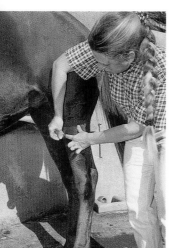

The objective of acupuncture is to re-establish a correct flow of energy within the body by releasing blockages within the energy channels, or 'meridians'.

and to maintain that balance (Chinese Medicine was always very strong on the maintenance of health, rather than just the treatment of disease).

THE THEORY

Chinese Medicine and philosophy does not separate medicine from nutrition, nor does it define boundaries between medicine, nutrition, philosophy, religion and a study of the world and cosmos. Man and animals take their place as an integral part of the whole and the holistic understanding is comprehensive. It is, however, couched in very different terms from those of western education and understanding – thus it can seem strange to the 'western' mind.

A 'life energy', Qi (which is pronounced 'chee'), is postulated which is continuous with universal or cosmic energy. It is composed of a balance between Yang and Yin, terms which can, broadly speaking, be translated as 'positive' and 'negative'. They are the eternal opposites. Without one, the other cannot exist. Light cannot exist without dark, and vice versa, but one does not cause the other; they merely flow into each other in a constant and rhythmic cycle. Evil cannot exist without a concept for good. Male cannot exist without female. High and low are not independent concepts, each depends upon the other and so on. Now we can see how simple and how comprehensive is the idea.

Qi or 'Normal Qi', the body energy, is made up from original Qi (derived from mother and father) and a combination of air Qi and grain Qi. Here then is revealed the concept of the genetics from each parent and maintenance of life by food and air (which mix gives energy), one totally compatible with modern western science but hammered out thousands of years ago.

Thus Qi in the body, for health to be possible, must be in a good yin-yang balance and must flow through the body in a regular 24-hour rhythm, following certain channels or routes (often called meridians). These are mapped out in the diagrams overleaf, showing meridian positions as proposed by the author. There is still disagreement about exact routes, so these are only drawn in their approximate positions.

As can be seen, the meridians relate to different organs, most of which are recognisable in western medical terminology. Their function is related to those organs but not exclusively so. If energy does not flow evenly through the meridians, then blockages exist and the concept develops of excesses and deficiencies on either side of the blockage.

APPROXIMATE POSITION OF THE PRINCIPAL MERIDIANS (ACCORDING TO AUTHOR)

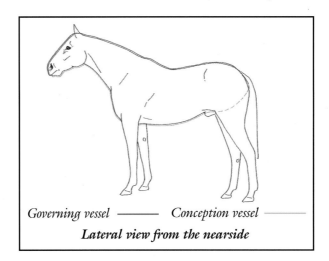

Governing vessel ——— Conception vessel ———

Lateral view from the nearside

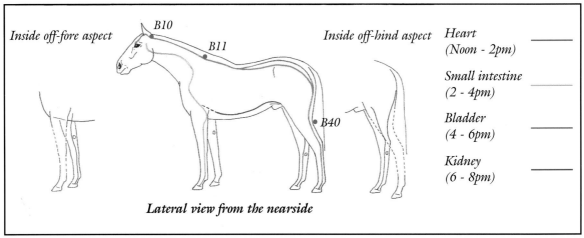

Inside off-fore aspect

Inside off-hind aspect

B10

B11

B40

Heart
(Noon - 2pm) ———

Small intestine
(2 - 4pm) ———

Bladder
(4 - 6pm) ———

Kidney
(6 - 8pm) ———

Lateral view from the nearside

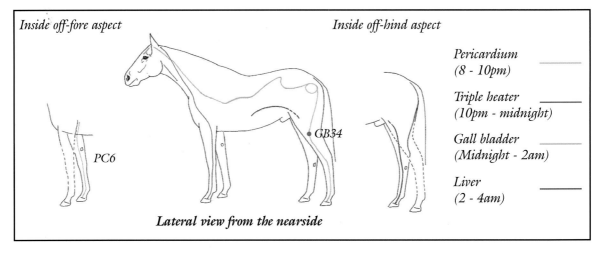

Inside off-fore aspect

Inside off-hind aspect

PC6

GB34

Pericardium
(8 - 10pm) ———

Triple heater
(10pm - midnight) ———

Gall bladder
(Midnight - 2am) ———

Liver
(2 - 4am) ———

Lateral view from the nearside

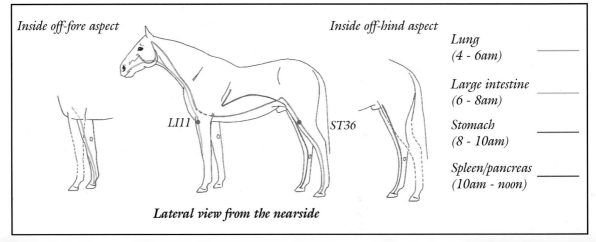

Inside off-fore aspect

Inside off-hind aspect

LI11

ST36

Lung
(4 - 6am) ———

Large intestine
(6 - 8am) ———

Stomach
(8 - 10am) ———

Spleen/pancreas
(10am - noon) ———

Lateral view from the nearside

Disease is postulated simply as an imbalance between yin and yang and as an interruption or alteration of the normal energy flow pattern. The objective in therapy is to try to re-establish a correct yin-yang balance and a correct rhythmic flow of energy.

The techniques used to correct the imbalance are foods, which energise yin or yang as needed, herbs which do likewise and which have relationships with the meridians and organs, and stimulus of the meridians at certain points (called acupuncture points), depending upon the site and nature of the imbalance. Lifestyle and other external influences will be examined in full and modified as necessary for health.

From this it can be seen that therapy of an individual patient is not according to the supposed name of a disease or condition but more according to the individual patient's needs, in an entirely holistic manner. Beware the 'quick fix'!

There follows a short list of some major acupuncture points with some of their indications. Some basic examples of Chinese herbs are listed, showing Chinese name, genus, family and Chinese indication.

Point	Chinese name (debatable)	Major effects
B 11	**ta chu**	bone/arthritis treatment
LI 11	**chu chi**	fore-limb, immune problems
GB 34	**feng long**	vertigo, paralysis, spinal problems
B 40	**yang ling**	hip, lumbar, hind-limb problems
B10	**tien chu**	head, neck and throat pain
ST 36	**tsu san li**	digestive, abdominal distension, tonic point
P 6	**nei kuan**	chest and stomach problems, hysteria.

Some conditions which lend themselves well to holistically-applied acupuncture therapy are back disorders, lameness, nerve damage, laminitis, colic, skin disorders, allergy, respiratory disease and behavioural problems.

COMPATIBILITY WITH OTHER THERAPIES
Acupuncture is compatible with homoeopathy and with Western herbs, so long as proper care is taken

Chinese herbs

gui zhi	(Cinnamomum – lauraceae)	Release externally
da huang	(Rheum – polygonaceae)	Purge down
zhu ye	(Phyllostachys – graminae)	Clearing heat
huo xiang	(Agastache – labiatae)	Transform moisture
che qian zi	(Plantago – plantaginaceae)	Facilitate urine
du huo	(Angelica – umbelliferae)	Expel wind damp
chuan wu tou	(Aconitum – ranunculaceae)	Warm interior, dispel cold
long nao xiang	(Dryobalanops – dipterocarpaceae)	Open spirit gate
mu li	(Ostrea – ostreidae)	Calm the spirit
xie	(Buthus – buthidae)	Calm the liver
chen pi	(Citrus – rutaceae)	Manage /discipline Qi
dan shen	(Salvia – labiatae)	Manage/discipline blood
shan zha	(CratAEgus – rosaceae)	Digest and guide
ban xia	(Pinellia – araceae)	Melt mucus
ren shen	(Panax – araliaceae)	Repair & tonify emptiness
rou cong rong	(Cistanche – orobanchaceae)	Yang tonic
he shou wu	(Polygonum – polygonaceae)	Blood tonic
sha shen	(Adenophora – campanulaceae)	Yin tonic
shan zu yu	(Cornus – cornaceae)	Withdraw and hold back
bing lang	(Areca – palmae)	Drive out worms

to integrate the therapies correctly. Individual homoeopathic medicines and Western herbs have properties and effects which can be related to yin and yang, to meridian theory, to the 'pernicious influences' of traditional Chinese theory and to the 'five elements' theory. Use them incompatibly and clearly there will be antagonism and failure to achieve the desired effect. There may even be negative effects, resulting in detriment to the patient. The author advises extreme caution therefore, when 'mixing' therapies.

LEGALITIES AND CAUTIONS
Apart from the cautions mentioned with regard to concomitant use of other therapies, it is important to stress that acupuncture is an act of veterinary medicine and, as such, in the UK comes under the Veterinary Surgeons Act 1966. No one without veterinary qualifications can be allowed to give acupuncture to a horse, under the terms of the Act. To do so renders the perpetrator liable to prosecution and, if a problem arises, the owner too could be liable for prosecution under the Protection of Animals Act 1911.

Acupuncture carried out without compatible internal medicine, dietary work and sympathetic saddling advice will fall far short of its potential. Trying to correct an energy imbalance by needles alone, when total imbalance is a result of many internal and external influences, is bound to result at best in temporary alleviation of symptoms. At worst it will be totally ineffective or even damaging.

AROMATHERAPY (ESSENTIAL OILS)

The use of essential oils in medicine dates at least from ancient Egyptian civilisations. The essential oils are often the most pharmacologically powerful and active ingredients of plants. For this reason it is important to view aromatherapy as a powerful, effective and potentially dangerous system of medicine. It is, again, not to be performed by non-vets, since it is an act of veterinary medicine to select and use the oils or combination of oils.

By and large it is best not to use aromatherapy and homoeopathy concurrently, since the very powerful stimulus of the essential oils can over-ride or confuse the body's response to the subtle and pure stimulus of homoeopathy.

Some useful examples of essential oils for use in horses:

Lavender	Analgesic, anti-convulsive, antiseptic, deodorant, nervine, sedative
Rosemary	Adrenal cortex stimulant, antiseptic, astringent, carminative, digestive, diuretic, stimulant, vulnerary
Tea tree	Antiseptic, immune stimulant, disinfectant, vulnerary
Sandal wood	Anti-depressive, antiseptic, astringent, carminative, diuretic, tonic
Bergamot	Antiseptic, deodorant
Eucalyptus	Analgesic, antiseptic, expectorant, febrifuge, rubefacient
Geranium	Anti-depressant, diuretic, haemostatic, sedative, tonic
Clary sage	Antiseptic, astringent, diuretic, sedative
Melissa	antispasmodic, carminative, cordial, digestive, febrifuge, nervine, tonic.

FLOWER REMEDIES

Remedies made from flower essences, distilled in sunlight (or by other means), are common throughout the world. Arguably the best known are the Bach Flower Remedies. These are used according to the pattern laid down by Edward Bach, an English physician of the twentieth century.

Flower remedies are used to help the body via the spirit and mind, more than vice versa. For this reason, they are prescribed mainly on the basis of mental symptoms noted by the veterinarian. Again

these medicines can only legally be prescribed by vets in the UK, but can be used by a horse owner for his or her own horse.

Some examples of Bach Flowers for horses:

Agrimony	Hides mental stress behind cheerful appearance
Aspen	General fearfulness
Elm	Feels weight of responsibility and owner's expectations
Gentian	Easily discouraged and generally melancholic
Gorse	Convinced that condition is hopeless
Heather	Over-concerned about own problems
Impatiens	Hasty, rash, impatient, nervous
Larch	Self-confidence is very low, constantly needs encouragement
Mimulus	Fearful of certain objects or situations
Olive	Exhausted and drained, mentally and physically
Rock Rose	Panic situations leading to abject terror
Scleranthus	Unable to concentrate on task in hand, variable moods
Star of Bethlehem	Helps in shock situations, both mental and physical
Vervain	Extremes of tension, mental & physical
Vine	Dominant animal, intransigent behaviour
Walnut	Prone to undue influence from situations and atmospheres
Willow	Deep-seated resentment of physical or mental misfortune or abuse
Rescue Remedy	General shock and fright remedy.

RADIONICS

The art and science of diagnosing and healing via the etheric energy patterns which pervade the entire atmosphere in which life exists, is termed radionics or radiaesthesia. Other terms of relevance, applied to this method, are 'black box' and 'dowsing'.

The study of radionics is a very esoteric area and this short chapter can neither relate the theory nor explain the mode of action nor justify its validity. Suffice to say that this method is used by a great number of horse carers, employing the services of radionics practitioners, with some extraordinary results (in conventional terms).

The method is to 'analyse' a 'witness', whether that be a sample of hair, blood, photograph or other material from the patient, and to highlight where energy patterns are dysfunctional. 'Treatments' can be sent by a reversal of the technique.

Needless to say, this is working entirely on the

plane of etheric energy, and conventional science finds it very hard to accept the method as valid. The reader is left to draw conclusions without comment from the author, since there is not space for a fuller discussion. Suffice it to say that the author has employed the technique in many patients, often working with bona fide practitioners.

There is some debate as to whether the practice by a non-vet is legal in the UK, but where the author has a problem is in the illegal sale and supply of medicines by a non-veterinary practitioner on the basis of radionics diagnosis. This practice produces profit for the practitioner and removes the impartiality and independence which is otherwise so important in the proper practice of the method.

THE IMPORTANCE OF DIET

The food your horse eats is the basis for daily energy and for constant renewal of the body. It is clear that, if the food is of poor quality, or not compatible with the horse's needs, the daily energy or the repair function or both will suffer.

General principles are easy. The opening words of this chapter, and of the herbal section, refer to the need to seek food which is compatible with the horse's evolved needs. For this reason any products

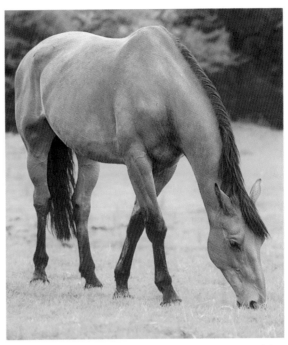

The horse is essentially a digester of low-quality fibre. Rich, fertilised grass and cereal grains are not optimum feeds.

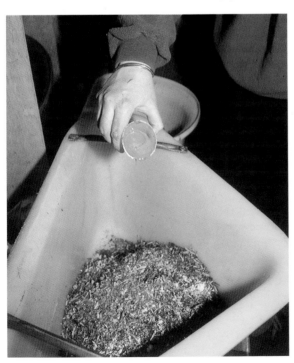

For health, horses require food compatible with their evolved needs. Supplements, in particular, must be chosen with care. Those containing products of animal or artificial source should be avoided.

of animal source should be rejected. We can include under this heading such feeds and supplements as cod-liver oil, gelatin (in many hoof formulae and usually derived from pigs), cartilage products (for the treatment of arthritis), beef proteins (found in at least one famous supplement) and bone meal. We should avoid artificial colourants and flavourings, which are also common ingredients of popular supplements. Artificial antioxidants (such as Ethoxyquin and BHT) should be avoided, since it is not clearly known what these do to the essential bacteria and other organisms found in a horse's gut.

The most widely used and unsuitable ingredient of horse feeds and supplements is molasses or other sugar material. This is both unnecessary for the horse and potentially harmful, affecting the proportional populations of different micro-organisms in the bowel, causing changes in metabolism to which a horse is not adapted. Millions of years of evolution cannot be defied in a few decades in this way, without penalty.

Generally speaking, organic food is best, as it is as free of chemicals as we can obtain. In the case of carrots this is essential. The author advises against feeding any carrots which are not cultivated organically and certified accordingly.

Because the horse is, by evolved nature, a fibre digester, the more fibre in his feed the better. Rich, fertilised grass or cereal grains are not optimal feeds. Hay, straw, older or unfertilised grasses, herbal material (and minerals if necessary, without molasses) are the ideal food for the horse. If cereals are necessary, owing to the energy demands put upon the horse, then they should be kept to a minimum and, ideally, not have been microwaved (micronised). Pure alfalfa (not a molassed, branded product) is a very good protein and energy source. Linseed oil or boiled linseed is also a useful supplement, as is seaweed (or kelp).

Vitamins should ideally be derived from herbage, not artificially manufactured, and minerals likewise plant-derived, but can be fed in 'straight' form, as required (e.g. limestone flour, manganese sulphate, magnesium chloride or acetate, zinc sulphate, etc.), according to local or specific needs.

MANIPULATIVE THERAPIES

The three practices of manipulative treatment of most importance are chiropractic, osteopathy and physiotherapy. The first two of these are therapeutic systems in their own right but are also very good adjuncts to homoepathy, herbal medicine or more particularly, acupuncture. The third, physiotherapy, is a method of mobilising and exercising muscles and joints and is not a stand-alone therapy. In the author's opinion, physiotherapy should only be used when all other factors are corrected, e.g. spinal misalignments, diet, etc. A brief description or comparison of these manipulative therapies is useful.

Chiropractic adjusts spinal and other skeletal relationships, via techniques of high-velocity, low-amplitude application of a gentle force. It is thought to operate by a sudden release of the damaging muscle spasm which created the misalignments, thereby releasing pressure or inflammation around nerves to and from the spine. For this reason it is able to affect the workings of the entire body and is holistic when used correctly (that is, by qualified McTimoney animal chiropractors who undergo lengthy training).

Osteopathy, on the other hand, uses a technique of low-velocity, high-amplitude force (the long lever principle) to achieve similar objectives.

Physiotherapy works directly on the muscles and mostly, it seems, takes no account of spinal misalignment. Used alongside other therapies, it can aid and speed musculo-skeletal healing. Most

manipulators are generally non-veterinary, but can operate via a veterinarian (they are not legally allowed to act otherwise in the UK).

PHYSIOTHERAPY AND MASSAGE

Chartered physiotherapists are members of a profession allied to medicine. They train for four years studying anatomy, physiology and the science of cells to a level comparable with radiographers, occupational therapists, respiratory therapists and a host of other medical support groups recognised by both doctors and veterinarians as essential back-up for their work. Physiotherapists learn the effects on cells of electricity, magnetism and light, produced by a host of 'therapeutic machines'. They also study bio-mechanics and are trained to re-educate movement by the use of exercises, hydrotherapy, resistance, passive movements, passive stretching and active patient participation. Their human patient load is interactive with the entire range of both medical and surgical conditions.

In 1984, physiotherapy skills were offered to the veterinary profession in the UK by a small group of chartered physiotherapists who had themselves been working with veterinary approval for a number of years. At the same time, Paddy Downer in the USA published *Physiotherapy for Animals*.

Chartered physiotherapists in the UK are entitled to suffix their title with MCSP (Member of the Chartered Society of Physiotherapists), FCSP (Fellow of the Chartered Society of Physiotherapists), and, if qualified to work with animals, are allowed to call themselves Members of ACPAT (Association of Chartered Physiotherapists in Animal Therapy).

TWO PHASES OF PHYSIOTHERAPY	
MACHINE	**REHABILITATION**
Removes pain	Re-educates movement
Stimulates muscle repair	Active muscle strengthening

The general public, both animal lovers and animal owners, are generally unaware of two very important facts. First, as has already been emphasised earlier in this chapter, in the UK, European countries, most of the states in the USA and in Canada, it is illegal to treat an animal without first consulting the animal's veterinarian. This is not to achieve exclusive rights for the veterinary profession to work with

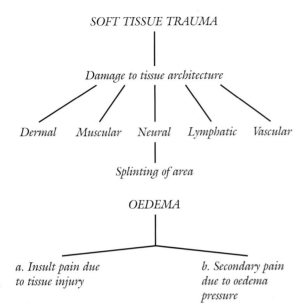

SOFT TISSUE TRAUMA

Damage to tissue architecture

Dermal   Muscular   Neural   Lymphatic   Vascular

Splinting of area

OEDEMA

a. Insult pain due to tissue injury

b. Secondary pain due to oedema pressure

animals, but to safeguard the animal patient. A human patient consults with whomsoever he or she chooses – they can reason and know if the 'therapy' has helped and may change their mind and go elsewhere. An animal is forced to accept the therapy – it has no choice.

The second point not generally considered is, just as chemical medicine administered as pills, powders or liquids acts upon cells and changes their behaviour, so do all therapy machines. These machines deliver 'electrical medicine' and over-ride naturally-produced body electricity. In 1981, Pilla proved and stated: "A variety of living cells are capable of functional response to weak electrical currents." This scientific discovery led to the development of many new therapeutic machines and, as the marvels of cellular behaviour continue to be exposed by on-going research, so the machines and the therapy they deliver will change in order to keep pace with new discoveries. A person over-dosing on chemical medication does not recover; they become sick from the chemical side-effects. Likewise, electricity, magnetism and light, incorrectly applied, can destroy tissue rather than assist in repair.

Physiotherapy is not a DIY technique and should never be attempted by the untrained, unless under strict supervision following a diagnosis made by a professional. Only then can the appropriate therapy be selected.

TISSUE DAMAGE TO THE MUSCULO-SKELETAL SYSTEM
Physiotherapy for the animal is concerned with the tissues of mobility: the skeleton, joints, ligaments, muscles, nerves. None of these tissues can function in the absence of adequate blood flow (circulation), adequate nutrients (digestion and respiration), adequate waste removal (bowel and bladder) and adequate protection (lymphatic system), not to speak of the liver, kidneys, spleen, brain, thermal control and so on. As outlined in the introduction to this chapter, the list is endless, covering all the systems which contribute to creating a living being. Tissue damage is, therefore, a multifactorial affair.

All life has its own in-built planned reactions, enabling tissue to repair. Therapy can enhance these repair programmes if the correct stimulus is given at the appropriate stage of recovery. Therapy will never accelerate recovery, merely enhance recovery.

Repair of all soft tissue has three distinct phases: inflammation, proliferation and re-modelling.

INFLAMMATION
Inflammation is the immediate response to damage. Leaking vessels are sealed off, chosen cells are directed to the area and excess fluid is produced, each action with its specific function. This occurs 30 to 50 hours after damage, the time dependent on the chemical signals from the damaged area. Amongst those cells which migrate to the area are 'mast' cells which orchestrate tissue recovery. If inflammation is curtailed, or ceases due to therapy interference, the eventual healing of the tissue will be of poor quality. When dealing with a new injury it is sensible to control the inflammatory stage but not to reverse, curtail, or eliminate this essential reaction.

PROLIFERATION
Once the mast cell has migrated to the area of damage and has assembled the necessary cellular 'repair gang', a temporary repair is effected. Tissue is laid down in a random manner to ensure the temporary maintenance of a 'steady state' and avoid continuing breakdown.

REMODELLING
As the name suggests, cells 're-make' most disorientated tissues in a near perfect match to the original. This process can take up to 18 months in the case of muscles and much longer if nerve tissue is badly damaged. Tendons and ligaments never re-gain their original architecture.

Appropriate therapy should commence when proliferation is established, the aim being to avoid massive scarring, retain joint range and maintain muscle credibility. As remodelling commences, aggressive therapy can be introduced, incorporating both machine therapy and controlled activity.

PAIN

Pain is secondary to any tissue damage. Just like inflammation it should be controlled but not eliminated. Control ensures that the animal is comfortable and not sweating, distressed or miserable. Pain has a reason in the scheme of recovery – it guards injury. The presence of pain ensures fragile tissues with diminished tensile strength are not over-stressed.

Physiotherapy, as the name suggests, is 'physical therapy'. Active participation on the part of the patient ensures a good end-result following trauma, whether this be from accident or disease. The machines used are merely an adjunct to the whole of physical therapy and, therefore, a treatment regime must consider two features: the machine phase and the active, or rehabilitation, phase.

MODALITIES

> **MACHINE**
> Massage, magnetic field, muscle stimulator
> Therapeutic ultrasound, cold laser
>
> **REHABILITATION**
> Pool, treadmill, walker, work in school

MASSAGE

An owner-friendly therapeutic modality, massage has two major therapeutic effects: it reduces pain but will not, as do some of the machines, totally remove the sensation, and so leaves the necessary guarding mechanism intact. The pain reduction with massage occurs due to release by the tissues of natural body-manufactured opiates, in response to the 'rubbing'. Anyone who knocks into a sharp object or bangs, for example, an elbow, will rub the sore area and get immediate relief as the body opiates have been released.

Every body tissue activity necessitates delivery and removal of nutrients, oxygen, cellular components and waste, to name but a few. This delivery and removal is achieved by the flow of arterial blood (the 'porter' liquid) and venous blood (the 'dust cart'). As a result of each heart-beat, arterial (porter) blood is, under pressure,

forced through the maze of arteries with exchange of goods and waste taking place in small, terminal vessels known as capillaries. Waste-laden blood moves from capillaries to veins and venous blood moves slowly back towards the central loading areas of the body. (For further details on the circulatory system, see Chapter Five).

There is little or no pressure in veins: the blood moves through the veins aided and in response to the compressive and relaxation forces of muscle contraction, with back-flow prevented by non-return valves. Following injury, due to pain guarding, there is a lack of local muscle activity with reduction of venous flow. Correctly applied massage in part replaces the compression and relaxation normally achieved by muscle activity, so that massage aids the venous flow. If a rhythm is established, the long, slow stroking also achieves general relaxation through commands from sensory nerve endings located in the skin itself.

Massage strokes

Effleurage

The hands can be used singly, as a pair, or contact with one hand is followed, as the stroke ends, by repetition of the stroke with the second hand. The direction of the strokes must always be towards the central body mass. To work away from the centre is counter-productive, as the masseur is pushing against the returning blood. The hands must be moulded to the underlying tissues and an even pressure exerted.

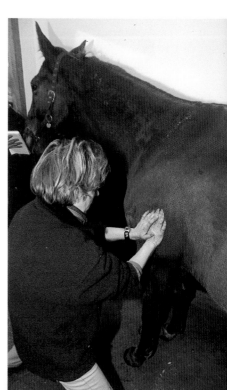

The hands can work singly or as a pair, always working in a direction towards the central body mass.

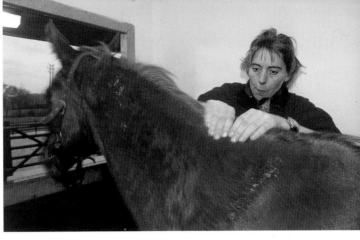

Localised techniques can focus on an area of chronic injury.

Petrissage

Petrissage strokes achieve a local compression and relaxation and are used following effleurage to ensure a greater depth of pressure over large muscle masses. One hand reinforces the second, or the backs of lightly-clenched fists are employed to push deep into the muscle mass, then to relax, allowing the mass to return to its normal contour.

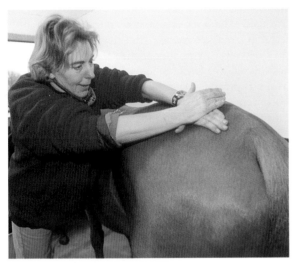

▲ *Petrissage strokes are used to produce a greater depth of pressure over large muscle masses.*

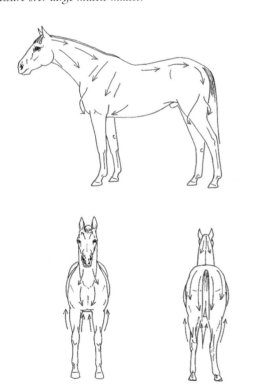

Direction of massage strokes

Frictions

Frictions are localised techniques, the aim of which is to reintroduce the inflammatory phase in an area of chronic injury, or attempt to mobilise scar tissue formed in an inappropriate area following trauma. The technique is effected by placing the underside of a finger tip over the area to be treated, reinforcing the pressure by using the tip of a second finger and working across the long axis of the underlying tissue. The skin must also move or a blister will form.

For those who have never massaged or had a lesson in massage, first go to have a massage yourself. Then, before 'punishing' your horse, massage a friend, who should comment on the depth of pressure you achieve, the contact pressure, whether one hand is more active than the other, and also the pressure applied by fingers and thumbs. It is also essential to know if the hands are moulded to the underlying area.

MAGNETIC FIELD THERAPY

Magnetic field therapy is another owner-friendly modality. Magnets are not new; their use is recorded down the ages in common with massage. The ancients, whose medicine involved a trial and error approach, discovered (no-one quite knows how) that certain types of rock appeared to help sick people. They ground lode stones (also used for navigation) and used the powder applied either in a paste or as an infusion.

Today science is beginning to give reasons for the possible benefits of MFT. Fractures (bone breaks) reluctant to heal can be persuaded to become active in the presence of magnetic fields applied at an appropriate gauss and frequency. Random parameters are not effective. Bone research led to an explosion of magnetic field devices. Treatment protocols, unsupported by scientific investigation, were published and all manner of injuries subjected to magnetic bombardment.

Every individual cell is dependent for efficient metabolism (function) on the maintenance of a balance of positive-to-negative electrons across its membrane. Disturbance in this balance changes the behaviour of the cell, leading to numerous associated problems. It appears that cells may be able to attract missing electrons to stabilise themselves, if a source of free electrons, as supplied by magnetic field devices, is available.

The type of magnetic devices purchased by owners should follow professional consultation. Strong fields can cause cell malfunction rather than restore function. Magnetic wraps producing static magnetic fields are now replacing electrically-created, alternating magnetic fields. Alternating magnetic fields cause cell vibration which in turn produces a local temperature rise. To offset this and return the local temperature to the normal 'steady state', circulatory flow in the 'treated' area shows a temporary increase.

Magnetic field therapy is also claimed to reduce pain. The mechanism by which this happens is thought to be associated with the proven fact that certain nerve fibres reduce conductivity when subjected to repetitive cycling vibrations. Physiotherapists have successfully used magnetic fields disguised by other names to achieve heating of deep-seated tissue for many years (the technique known as diathermy), but treatment always follows a diagnosis, enabling the therapists to be specific rather than random in their selection of frequency, gauss and treatment time.

PROFESSIONAL MACHINES

Tens Machines

There are a mass of differing TENS machines on offer, designed to reduce pain. TENS deliver small electronic signals which, provided the pads are correctly placed, will reduce the ability of nerves to record pain or, in accordance with the type of signals, command pain-killing mechanisms in the brain to release naturally-produced pain suppressants (in particular, a substance known as seratonin). In human medicine these machines are used to help persons suffering the pain caused by such conditions as chronic back lesions, many of whom have become resistant to the effects of chemical pain-killers. Some are designed for the pain caused by bone cancer in patients who have also become chemically resistant.

The effects of TENS machines on the horse have not been scientifically investigated, although claims made of miraculous recovery following their use are published. The questions, "Do you want the pain?" and "Is it safe to remove it without having a reason

for its presence?", should always be asked before random usage of any pain-killing modality. The role of pain was illustrated recently when an animal at international level of show jumping was noticed, by an untrained therapist, at competition. It was obvious to all that the animal in question did not flex the left hock as efficiently as the right. No diagnosis, no veterinary examination, yet the animal was winning at top level without therapy. The rider was offered therapy and a type of TENS machine was used. The hock was treated and the horse went to jump a practice round. After three perfect jumps the rider was ecstatic, but at the fourth fence, as the hock flexed to a level not allowed by the body when pain was present, the muscles running from dock to hock were put under a stretch they had not experienced for a considerable time. With an audible crack, they tore, and the horse landed on three legs, his career at an end.

Therapeutic Ultrasound

A sound wave above the human audible range but within that of canines and equines is applied to the soft tissues via contact with the head of the applicator known as a transducer. The passage of the sound wave through the tissues in the path of the beam achieves a cell vibration.

This effect is used for a variety of conditions: mobilisation of scar tissue, absorption of swelling, to reduce the viscosity following a haemarthrosis (bleed into a joint), to promote healing of indolent wounds, to fragment calcified deposits and to aid re-absorption of excess tissue exudate.

Unfortunately, therapeutic ultrasound is often inappropriately applied. One of the conditions that does not benefit from it is sore shins. The periosteum, (the outer covering of bone), fails to recognise the heat created at the bone interface as

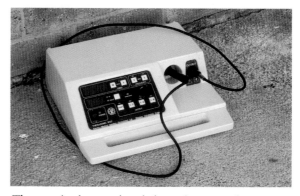

Therapeutic ultrasound works by passing a sound wave through injured tissue to produce vibration of the cells.

the ultrasound bounces back, doubling the local dosage. Heated bone becomes very fragile. It has been shown in the laboratory that therapeutic ultrasound delivered incorrectly will achieve bone breakdown. Also, if the bone is in the process of repair, ultrasound can reverse the repair situation, the new bone breaking down, with ensuing tissue chaos. Therapeutic ultrasound incorrectly used is tissue-destructive. It also reverses certain processes occurring during soft tissue re-build.

Low-level Lasers

Exposure to natural light is essential for life, and light in various forms has been used therapeutically down the ages. Ultraviolet, a part of the spectrum of light, is currently used to treat some skin conditions. Until recently, patients were burned by the use of a Cromayer lamp, a treatment used as an attempt to relieve chronic pain by re-introducing a secondary pain.

The low-level cold laser is the latest in the field of light therapy. Einstein theorised as to the possible therapeutic uses of certain beams of light, but it was the family Mesner in Budapest who developed the theory, leading to the range of low-level lasers currently available. The light source is achieved by the activation of molecules of certain elements. The helium neon laser produces a light wave band of 620nm and was the first device to become commercially available. This was closely followed by the galium arsenide laser, producing a waveband of 720-820nm. Multi-diode lasers were the next to be commercially produced for sale, devices that were said to have several laser beams incorporated in a square head, enabling a larger area to be irradiated.

It is known that certain tissue reactions require photons of light, for example the production of vitamin D. Quite what the process of the photons delivered by the helium neon and gallium arsenide lasers was in the scheme of tissue recovery is still unclear. Tissue is very selective, choosing essential components and rejecting others. The wavebands 620-820nm have been demonstrated to improve cell constructional ability, yet 820nm and above, have, in some instances, interfered with the process of cell reconstruction (this work has been published by Baxter in Belfast).

The most impressive ability of low-level lasers to date is the apparent ability of nerves to respond, re-establishing conductivity in damaged neurons following laser therapy. A further use, provided the energy levels are appropriate, is the application of

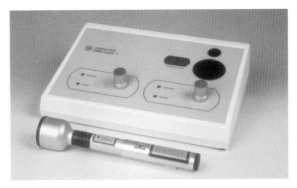

The cold, or low-level laser, is the latest development in the field of light therapy. Its increased use has revolutionised the treatment of damaged nerves and tissue.

low-level lasers for acupuncture point stimulation in place of the traditional needles.

Lasers are dangerous to use near the eye. Devices should never be pointed toward the naked eye, as temporary and even permanent blindness can be the consequence of exposure to the beam.

Fortunately, tissue and the body systems appear to be able to absorb, without adverse affect, gross over-dosage. While the effect on open wounds appears spectacular, with the wounds closing rapidly, the tissue laid down has poor-quality tensile strength and time must be allowed for the remodelling phase to occur. Closure of knee wounds in the horse is a classic example. A horse falls on the road, cutting the knees wide open. Treated with a low-level laser there is a rapid wound closure. All is well until the horse commences activity, when full knee flexion often splits the apparently 'healed' area.

Muscle Stimulators

Faraday demonstrated the ability to achieve a muscle contraction using an electric stimulus and this device was to become known as Faradic stimulation.

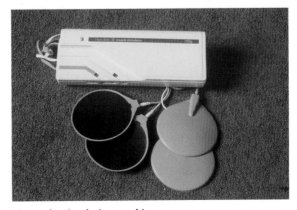

A muscle-stimulating machine.

Muscle deteriorates following direct trauma to its own architecture, but also as a result of damage to any bone, joint, ligament or tendon with which it is intimately associated. This loss, or atrophy, disturbs the normal balance between groups of muscles, in turn creating both mechanical stresses and uneconomic movement patterns.

In the last decade, a new type of muscle stimulator has been developed. As knowledge of the events involved to achieve muscle contractions have widened, so it has been possible to produce electrical signals to mirror those delivered during normal activity, by commanding its nerve centre, the motor end plate.

To use these devices to advantage, weak muscle must be identified, then stimulated. Care must be taken not to over-build muscle during recovery. If this should occur, mechanical stress will still be present due to a strong muscle working against a less well-developed opposite. The placing of the electrodes correctly requires both anatomical knowledge and considerable expertise.

REHABILITATION

In the case of the equine patient, rehabilitation concerns the re-education of movement patterns lost during trauma or pain. The horse has a brain designed to record movement patterns, which might be likened to the programming of a computer. The horse readily re-records those patterns, replacing the original economic patterns with those dictated by pain. These new patterns then become the accepted 'norm'. It requires knowledge of equine bio-mechanics, equine conformation and a trained eye to spot the incorrect movement patterns and to re-establish, by exercises and activity, the natural economic patterns. No machine will ever do this.

These re-education processes are best done with the horse in long reins, when the movement patterns can be observed by the person working the animal. Recourse to the movements used in the classical schools of Europe produce an excellent exercise programme for re-building muscle, re-establishing coordination and re-educating the horse. The outdoor arena becomes the equine gymnasium. The use of poles and cavaletti can also be introduced – poles on the ground placed at equi-distant intervals one from the other to ensure that equal stride-length will be achieved by the animal as it works down the grid.

The design of the rehabilitation programme required will vary with the type of injury that the animal has suffered, its state of recovery, its conformation, its ability to respond to the exercises required and to its eventual discipline. The programme needs to be tailored with all these facts in mind.

The recipe for successful physiotherapy necessitates:
• Being given, or making, a diagnosis in company with a veterinarian.

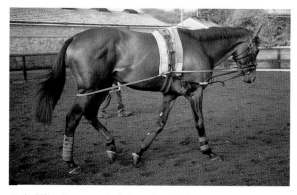

Rehabilitation exercise is best done in long-reins, so that the handler can carefully watch the horse's movement.

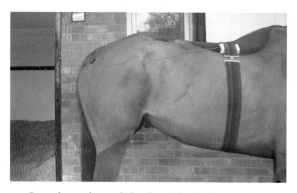

▲ *Once the weak muscle has been identified, a muscle stimulator can be used to help rebuild it.*

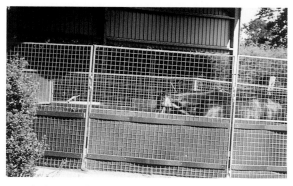

▲ *The horse walker is an invaluable aid to rehabilitation following injury.*

- Understanding the phases of tissue recovery.
- Choosing the appropriate machine at the appropriate time.
- Having an in-depth knowledge of the discipline to which the particular animal must return.
- Incorporating appropriate active rehabilitation with the appropriate machine therapy.

Owners attempting DIY therapy can usefully apply massage and weak magnetic field therapy. Advice should be sought from those trained before attempting to use machines, even those sold as safe and infallible, as they are in fact complicated and dangerous. Remember that whenever any machine therapy is used, electrical medicine is being delivered, taking over and commanding the body's own natural pattern for repair that is in-built in all species.

Rehabilitating of the injured

animal requires

team work

Owner/Rider

Trainer	*Veterinarian*
Groom	*(Veterinary nurse)*
Farrier	*Physiotherapist*
Harnessmaker	

CHIROPRACTIC

Manipulative techniques have been used for centuries in various medical systems far older than our own. Arabic woodcuts dating from well before Christ, show scenes of very specific pelvic manipulation, even if the apparatus used is rather gruesome. The Chinese used not only an elaborate herbal system and even more elaborate acupuncture system, but advanced and complex manipulative techniques.

So manipulation is not new – ever since man has had a skeletal system there has probably been someone prepared to tinker with it. And doubtless, if man has tinkered with his own skeleton, he has done the same with his animals.

Like many other traditional therapeutic systems, manipulation became submerged under the rapid advance of modern scientific medicine, its importance being overshadowed by startling advances in the scientific field that seemed to presage the end of disease as it was known at that time. The potential and uses of manipulation were swept aside in the rush towards the expected 'magic bullet'. When that panacea patently failed to materialise, interest in the more traditional forms of therapy began to be revived, and it is as a player in this restoration that chiropractic has performed an important role for both animals and their owners.

WHY IS MANIPULATION NECESSARY?

Physiological systems are, by their very nature, dynamic – that is, they are in a continuing state of change. The musculo-skeletal system is no different. Throughout life, be it two-legged or four-legged, the skeletal system changes constantly. In early development, these charges are large and comparatively rapid, so we see and hear of growth abnormalities in children, foals and puppies. But even after the skeletal mechanism has settled and the majority of bone development has been completed, there is a constant altering of the mechanics of the body in response to both internal and external influences.

Physiological systems are very sensitive to change – chemical, electrical and, the one which principally interests manipulators, mechanical. Calcium metabolism, for example, is very sensitive to mechanical stress, altering the amount of calcium excreted or retained within the body in a matter of hours to cope with changed circumstances.

Not only is bone in a constant state of change, but the skeletal system as a whole is also very plastic, deforming and re-forming in response to stresses both from within and from outside. Whilst it is usual to think of the skeleton as largely changeless, it is in fact constantly changing. This is both a disadvantage and a godsend, since it offers opportunities not only for pathological change but equal chances for therapeutic change.

We can see, therefore, that simply existing and moving about can cause negative changes to occur in the position of bones relative to their articular neighbours. In addition to this, body usage can be a particular problem, and asymmetric use tends to generate asymmetric muscle development, leading to uneven stress on the skeletal structure.

If we then add to this the inevitable incidents and accidents that happen from time to time in daily life, the possibilities for pathological change become even greater. Racing, or competing a horse in National Hunt races or three-day events, broadens possibilities into probabilities. Hitting the ground at upwards of 20 miles per hour is not a recommended practice for any structure and many vertebral dysfunctions are a direct result of falls, or partial falls, at speed. That much is obvious, but some of the foregoing has, I hope, illustrated that it is not absolutely necessary to have had a fall for dysfunction and its attendant muscular change and skeletal distortions to occur.

HOW DOES IT WORK?

There is much controversy about manipulation and its mode of action. It has been stated by well-respected veterinary researchers that it is unlikely to be possible to move a horse's vertebrae with manual manipulation, and that it is rather some form of muscular release caused by the action of manipulation that achieves the observed effect.

Chiropractors remain convinced, however, that vertebral movement – rotation, to be precise – is the key to many varieties of spinal dysfunction. The amount of vertebral rotation may only be of the order of a few degrees at the spinal axis, but this amount would be quite sufficient to have a marked effect on the complex inter-relationship of bone, muscle, ligament, blood vessels and nerve tissue of which the vertebrate axial skeletal complex is composed.

Failing further research on the live animal, a staggeringly intricate proposal which is currently exercising the minds of the veterinary scientific community, we can only forward our current hypothesis, which seems to fit observations to date. This is, that many disorders of the animal spine are brought about by minute rotational displacements of the vertebrae. These lead initially to protective and adaptive reactions in the muscle system, and ultimately to more severe forms of musculo-skeletal breakdown. Ignored, such reactions can lead to

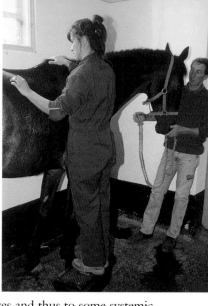

Manipulative therapy involves physically rotating a vertebra, in relation to its near neighbours, to restore correct function.

neurological interferences and thus to some systemic abnormalities.

It is obviously dangerous to extrapolate individual case histories to cover the whole animal population, but the increasing evidence from a growing number of McTimoney manipulators is that manipulation is a field in which we have only just begun to scratch the surface. With luck, and given the more active dialogue that we have been pursuing with the veterinary profession both in general practice and in research, we should be seeing some more positive pointers by the first years of the new millennium – better late than never.

Manipulative therapy involves physically moving the vertebrae, one in relation to its near neighbours, in order to restore correct function. This is done in a number of ways, depending on the training of the manipulator. Sometimes, with the slower type of manipulation which allows time for the animal to resist, the horse may require sedation to achieve good results. The high-speed, low-amplitude manipulations characterised by chiropractic techniques do not usually require any sedation unless there is great pain, or a very nervous animal. Although this section is specifically relating to chiropractic, there are many osteopaths in the equine field doing excellent work in a slightly different way.

HOW DO WE RECOGNISE WHEN MANIPULATION IS NECESSARY?

There are many indicators that manipulation is necessary – some dramatic and obvious, some subtle and often fleeting. Because of the body's ability to adapt, a certain amount of vertebral misalignment can be absorbed and accommodated by the skeletal system. This absorption and adaptation is a natural process by which the body copes with skeletal stress, continuing to function so that the animal does not become dinner for some alert predator.

In evolutionary terms, an animal whose mobility was impaired by a single musculo-skeletal change

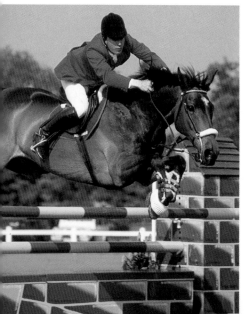

Merely existing and moving about can cause changes to occur in the position of bones relative to their neighbours. The extremes of physical activity we ask of our performance horses often broadens the possibility into a probability.

would not last long in the wild – their species would soon die out. Alternative modes of action and movement had to be available for those occasions when stress or accident brought about less than favourable conditions for body flight or fight movements. These alternatives allow the animal to cover up its shortcomings, so the early stages of musculo-skeletal stress can easily be missed.

When an animal presents with a severe, spinally-induced lameness or lumbar muscle spasm, a careful scrutiny of the case-history will often reveal early indicators, many months or sometimes years before the final, severe symptoms. It is important to identify these so that they are not ignored in the future, and early treatment can be applied to prevent long-term problems.

In ridden horses, the process of identifying problems quickly can be relatively easy, since the weight of the rider is added to the stress on the spine and so can highlight spinal problems early on. Depending on the sensitivity of the rider, the slightest change in the horse's gait or action can be detected, noted and rectified if necessary. It is important to stress that there are many causes of change in gait, and for this reason (and to stay within the law) chiropractors should work only with the full knowledge and approval of the animal's veterinarian.

Where a lameness is the result of causes other than the back, we believe it is vital to have the spine checked when the causative factor has cleared. In this way, any adaptive changes that have taken place due to the animal's altered movement (and there will be some), can be dealt with at that time rather than waiting for those changes to cause a further problem later on.

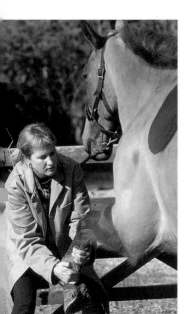

The chiropractor works with the whole skeleton, not only the spine.

PREVENTION RATHER THAN CURE

Another important aspect of the chiropractor's work is that of preventive treatment. Since most vertebral misalignments take place over a long period of time, vertebral misalignment is, in fact, a process rather than a single event. It follows that preventive treatment can be given at an early stage to avoid future problems.

As with all preventive treatment, it is difficult to prove its effect. Would the animal have become lame, or is all of this just an elaborate hoax to sustain the therapist's income? Only time will tell incontrovertibly – time, and research. All that can be said at the moment is that the principle of preventive treatment, when applied to our human patients, has been proved to our satisfaction and that it is definitely a worthwhile procedure to follow. The author believes that, in the future, it will prove itself in the animal field to the satisfaction of all.

EARLY INDICATORS TO IMPENDING BACK TROUBLE

- Sensitivity to touch, pressure or brushing on the low back muscles, particularly if that sensitivity is on one side of the spine only.
- Asymmetric muscle development, where one muscle has more bulk than its partner on the other side of the body.
- Difficulty going up or down hill. This action will highlight problems in the lower back.
- Change in gait, shoe wear patterns or muscle development.
- Change in behaviour patterns, particularly in jumping, or in performance habits, for no apparent reason.
- Unexpected and inexplicable changes in eating behaviour and/or temperament. Consequent change in food absorption and assimilation – the animal suddenly becomes a 'bad doer'. Pain can cause strange symptoms.
- Sudden change in movement, fitness and stamina. A three-mile horse will only stay two miles, for example. Or the fluent jumper suddenly becomes a lethal weapon. See Chapter Nine.

If ignored, these indicators may turn into a more severe lameness and will become much more difficult to deal with. Not all of the above signs are definitely caused by back pain, but if all else has been eliminated, consider the spinal column and its musculature.

In the future we hope that, far from being a 'last

resort' therapy, to be used when conventional means have failed, manipulation will be considered as a first stage, and to that end we hope to collaborate in research projects to identify the most likely conditions to respond to manipulation. It is gentle, non-invasive, comparatively straightforward and safe when used by properly trained people, and has a remarkable success rate, if empirical evidence is to be believed.

In brief, McTimoney chiropractors believe that spinal alignment and correct function is vital to overall health, but particularly to the health of the musculo-skeletal system, in all vertebrate animals. Repeated successes by almost 40 practitioners in the McTimoney group are beginning to make in-roads into the prejudice that has bedevilled animal manipulation in the past. More dialogue with members of the veterinary profession and all those concerned with animal health is proving most productive in allaying many of the fears of people to whom the word 'manipulation' conjures up all sorts of negative images.

IN SUMMARY

Natural therapies are becoming much more popular in our current times. Providing an effective 'alternative' to conventional drug therapy, they operate on holistic principles to achieve healing in the deepest sense. They do not suppress signs of disease, when used correctly, and can provide healing in cases often considered beyond hope in conventional thinking. Since the body is perpetually renewing itself, the scope for healing is enormous and there should be no reason to fear laminitis, COPD, navicular disease, sweet itch, recurrent ophthalmia or arthritis in as pessimistic a fashion as is often the case in traditional thinking.

The horse is a sensitive creature and is a very rapid and effective responder to the subtle stimuli of natural medicine. What is needed is wider education of veterinarians in the practices of natural therapies, a more open-minded approach to the integration of such methods into daily practice, and a re-writing of the text books in terms of prognosis of many of the currently most dreaded diseases of the horse. It is also important to recognise that not every disease in every horse can be cured, whatever means is employed, and that experience of practitioners will vary widely.

Medicine can only be practised on horses in the UK by qualified and registered veterinarians, except in the case of a carer treating his or her own horse. It is commonly believed that a non-vet can treat an animal if no fee is charged, but this is incorrect. Veterinarians are now very willing to call in colleagues who are more experienced in specialist areas of all types and they are also becoming much more willing to co-operate with manipulators or call them in to help.

Above all, the welfare of the horse should be paramount and nothing should be done to compromise that most important goal.

12 IDENTIFICATION & DESCRIPTION

CLASSIFICATION OF HORSES

BREEDS AND TYPES

Horses come in all shapes, sizes and colours, but although there are a huge number of different breeds, all fall within three separate categories depending on their origin: hot-bloods, warm-bloods and cold-bloods (see also Chapter One).

Hot-bloods are of oriental or eastern origin and are typified by the Arabian, Thoroughbred and Anglo-Arab. These are the handsome athletes of the horse world – as a general rule intelligent, speedy and sensitive with fiery temperaments. Hot-blood types are not usually suitable for novices, although there are always exceptions to every rule.

Cold-bloods are the workers, bred for size, strength and pulling power, such as the Shire or Percheron. These are usually slow but sure and when crossed with more hot-blooded types can produce a kind and docile riding horse.

The warm-blood is a mixture of hot- and cold-blood, ideally exhibiting the best of both worlds. These types should have a touch of the class, movement and athleticism of the hot-bloods yet some of the strength and reliable temperament of the cold-bloods. Examples of warm-bloods are the French Selle Francais or the American Quarter Horse.

There are also some 'breed within a breed' classifications : for example, there are three types of native Welsh pony divided into Sections A, B and C, while the Welsh Cob is known as a Section D. 'Types within a type' might include a light, medium or heavy-weight hunter.

Only animals that have met specific, laid-down criteria may be registered into the Stud Book of a

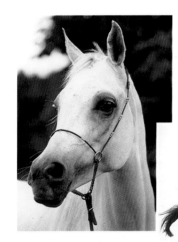

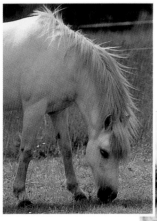

The Arabian (above) and Thoroughbred (right) represent the hot-bloods.

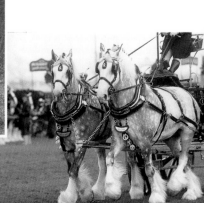

Pony (above) and draft breeds (right) are classed as cold-bloods.

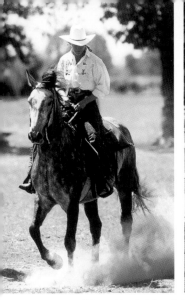
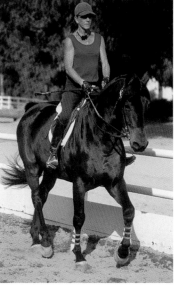

Warm-blooded breeds include all whose origins contain a mix of the other two types: the American Quarter Horse (left) and German Holsteiner are two examples.

particular breed and so be officially accepted as belonging to that breed. Unless those criteria are met, the animal must be described as being of that 'type' only. Certain types are accepted as belonging to an actual 'breed' with its own register in the United States but not in the UK, examples being the colours palomino and pinto.

CHOOSING A BREED OR TYPE TO BUY
The breed or type of animal you choose is partly a question of personal preference and partly a matter of your individual requirements. The type you want is not necessarily the type you need! Riders intending to show at a serious level, for example, must buy an animal that is a very good example of its breed or type, showing all the attributes and none of the weaknesses.

For those simply after a 'fun' horse, breeding is generally less important than the right size, age, temperament and ability. This type may not be a pure-bred horse at all. The 'mongrels' of the horse world can make fabulous partners if they suit your requirements!

Some advertisements for horses for sale will make it clear where the horse's talents lie; for example, 'Riding Club all-rounder', 'ideal first pony' or 'event prospect'. Consider also the following when trying to decide on a breed or type to suit your needs.

BUDGET
A well-bred, quality horse costs more, especially if it comes with the relevant papers and has breeding potential. Rare or 'fashionable' breeds will also attract a premium.

SIZE AND WEIGHT
The height of the horse does not necessarily reflect its weight-carrying ability. A short, stocky type with a good width of bone and muscular back, neck and quarters, such as a cob or native breed, can carry more weight than a tall, spindly Thoroughbred.

ABILITY AND LEVEL OF EXPERIENCE
Generally speaking, 'hot-blooded' types such as Thoroughbreds and Arabs do not have temperaments suitable for novice riders and owners. 'Cold-blooded' types, on the other hand, may not have the speed and athleticism required in a riding horse, so a cross-breed may be a suitable compromise. Also take into consideration any other people who may ride or handle the horse. It is not practical for you to be the only one who can do it, because there is sure to come a time when help is needed.

MANAGEMENT REGIME
Owing to their desert ancestry, hot-blooded horses, or warm-bloods with a high percentage of hot-blood in their breeding, are thin-skinned and fine-coated. This means they require extra feed and care and are likely to need stabling in winter. The robust and hardy native type which has adapted to survive in a colder, tougher climate should deal better with adverse weather conditions (see Chapter One).

FUTURE PLANS
The horse must be physically capable of the work the rider intends to ask of it. The percentage of hot-to cold-blood in his breeding has a strong influence on this. Arabians are sought-after by endurance riders, Thoroughbreds are designed for the race-track, while a dash of cold-blood will add strength and power but detract from speed and possibly stamina.

HORSES FOR COURSES
While it is not always possible to generalise, certain types and breeds have definite characteristics which act as a general guide to help potential owners find a suitable horse. A large show is a good place to compare lots of different breeds and types. Here horses can be divided according to breed, type, age or colour, and are shown ridden or in-hand, from show or working strains.

HUNTER
In the UK this is a type, not a breed, and for show purposes there are three different categories: light,

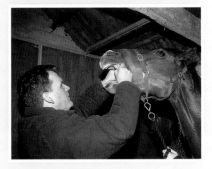

◀ Stage 1: Preliminary examination

The whole body is looked at from all angles and assessed for general condition, conformation and symmetry of the limbs, body and head. It is felt all over for signs of disease, previous injury or abnormality and any lumps or blemishes. The mouth and teeth are examined and approximate age estimated. The heart and lungs are listened to and the feet examined in detail, including with hoof testers.

Stage 2: Trotting up ▶

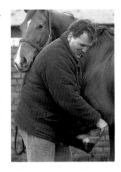
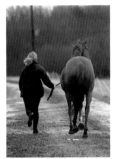

The vet observes the horse walking and trotting in a straight line on a hard, level surface and possibly also on a circle. It is made to walk backwards for a few steps and also turn in several tight circles in each direction: movements which help to detect certain nervous diseases and check the flexibility of the back. Flexion test are carried out on all four legs by holding up each leg with the joints firmly flexed for one minute and then immediately trotting the horse away. This can detect trouble brewing in a joint. If a flexion test proves positive, further investigations, e.g. X-rays, may be needed.

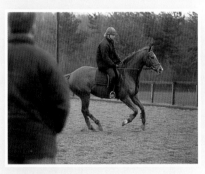
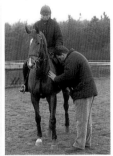
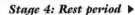

◀ Stage 3: Strenuous exercise

The horse is ridden or lunged actively for at least 10 minutes to enable the vet to listen to the heart and lungs under exertion and for any noises that might indicate respiratory obstruction in the larynx. It is also a chance to assess the horse's gait and movement at all paces.

Stage 4: Rest period ▶

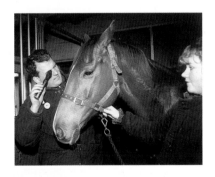

The horse is untacked and allowed to cool down and recover for 20-30 minutes, after which any stiffness or lameness brought on by exercise will show. The heart is monitored for its recovery rate and the eyes examined in detail in a darkened stable. Individual identification details, e.g. markings, whorls, brands etc., are usually put on the examination certificate at this point.

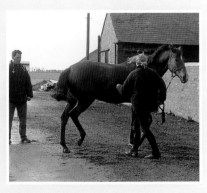

◀ Stage 5: Second trotting up

The horse is trotted up and turned in circles again to check for lameness. The legs are examined for any signs of heat or pain following exercise.

Point to consider:

- The vet works on behalf of the buyer, not the seller. He examines the horse for its suitability for the purpose the buyer intends to use it for, so this should be made clear from the outset.
- A buyer should use their own specialist equine vet or, in another part of the country, one recommended by him.
- Further investigations such as X-rays, ultrasound or endoscopy are not generally carried out at pre-purchase examinations, although they can be by prior request. Blood samples can be taken to store for future analysis in case the horse should show lameness shortly after purchase.
- The report lists any significant abnormalities and states the vet's advice as to whether these will affect the horse's suitability for the buyer. A 'perfect' horse is rarely found! The examination cannot detect symptoms not present on that day, such as intermittent lameness or seasonal conditions such as COPD or sweet itch. Obtaining an additional written warranty from the vendor is always advisable, covering soundness and freedom from vice, allergies and any potential problem areas to do with performance, e.g. behaviour in traffic, clipping, loading, shoeing, catching.
- Height measurement is not part of the examination. Where documentation does not exist, the age of the horse assessed by dentition is only an estimate.

medium or heavyweight. This classification refers to the amount of weight that a horse is capable of carrying and is judged by the thickness of the cannon bone below the knee. There are no stipulations about his exact size; the table below shows the approximate height, build and weight-carrying capacity of the different categories.

Whatever his category, a show hunter's paces, conformation and manners should indicate that he would be ideally suited to hunting. In 'working hunter' classes, horses must show ability both on the flat and over a course of rustic fences.

COB

The stocky, short-legged cob should be between 14.2hh and 15.1hh, with quality as well as weight-carrying ability. These are expected to be sensible, generous types that give a comfortable ride. In show terms, a cob should be a suitable ride for an elderly gentleman!

MOUNTAIN AND MOORLAND

Britain's nine native pony breeds are described collectively as 'Mountain and Moorland' breeds and their physical hardiness and good temperament make them a popular choice, particularly as children's ponies. To be entered into a show class for their breed, ponies must be registered in their relevant breed Stud Book. A pony or small horse generally described as a 'family all-rounder' suggests it is well-schooled and gentle enough to be safe for the smaller members of the family, yet has sufficient weight-carrying ability for an adult male. In this case the actual breed is not important, but it is likely that such a horse will have native or cob blood.

RIDING HORSE

In showing terms, riding horses fall into two basic categories: small (between 14.2hh and 15.2hh) and large (over 15.2hh). These types need to be of sensible temperament and good movers – horses suitable for anyone to ride out. The judge rides each horse to assess manners, ride and training, and every competitor must give an individual show.

HACK

Although 'hack' is often used as a general term to cover any horse used for riding out, show hacks have specific requirements. As with the riding horses, for show purposes, hacks are described as either small (between 14.2hh and 15hh) or large (between 15hh and 15.3hh). The small hack must still be capable of carrying an adult and usually has pony or Arab blood. The hack must be more than simply a pleasure to look at. In UK shows, hacks are awarded 40% of marks for conformation, presence, type and action in-hand and 60% for ride, training and manners.

DRIVING

Whilst any horse can be broken to harness, a number of breeds are particularly adept in terms of action and temperament. The Cleveland Bay, Welsh Cob and Hackney are regularly seen between the shafts depending on the type of class.

SPORTS HORSE

Although you will not find a sports horse class at your local show, nonetheless this is a recognised type, particularly on the Continent. It is exactly what you would expect from the name – a horse bred to compete at a high level, possibly from a long line of talented performers. The sports horse may not be pure-bred, but will probably have a high percentage of Thoroughbred blood to suit the requirements of the serious competitor.

IDENTIFYING HORSES

Whilst some pure- and part-bred horses and ponies have official papers and are registered with their relevant breed society, many horses and ponies have no such records. Besides their individual breed or type description, several other methods of identification of horses are used for paperwork such as veterinary certificates, vaccination cards, insurance papers and passports.

SEX

Perhaps the most obvious one, all paperwork should state whether the horse is a filly (female

UK show hunter classifications

Class	Approx. height	Approx. bone measurement below knee	Weight-carrying capacity
Lightweight	16.1hh	8" (20.5cm)	up to 12 stone 7lb (80kg)
Middleweight	16.3hh	9" (23cm)	up to 14 stone (89kg)
Heavyweight	17.0hh	9"+	over 14 stone

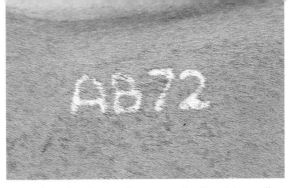

Freeze-branding for security purposes (as shown) is usually done in the saddle area or on the neck. Brands carrying breed or stud information are generally made on the quarters or shoulder.

under three years old), mare (female over three), colt (young male up to three years), stallion or entire (male over three) or gelding (castrated male of any age). A 'rig' is a male horse which has been improperly castrated and, although infertile, still shows stallion-like characteristics (See Chapter Ten).

SIZE

In the UK horses and ponies are still measured in 'hands', although the metric system of metres and centimetres is creeping in and is already well-established in show jumping. Shetland ponies and miniature horses are the only breeds described in units of inches only, rather than hands and inches. A hand is a unit of four inches, the measurement being taken from ground level to the withers. When the precise height of an animal is important for competition purposes, an official height certificate may be issued after measuring by a vet or breed society representative.

The use of the general description 'horse' or 'pony' is not necessarily as straightforward as simply defining a 'pony' as being a horse measuring 14 hands 2 inches or less. Type, general build and body proportions are also significant. Several breeds which measure below the accepted threshold are referred to as horses for this reason, for example the Icelandic, the Caspian and the Falabella (miniature horse).

COLOUR

Coat colouring is generally a secondary consideration for those looking for a pleasure horse. It is worth remembering, however, that for showing purposes some breed societies may specify permitted colours. Other potential owners may actively seek an unusually-coloured or marked horse, such as a piebald, skewbald (collectively known as 'pinto' in the US), palomino or appaloosa, all of which have their own showing and competition classes.

Both the colour of the coat and of the horse's 'points' (i.e. the muzzle, tips of the ears, mane, tail and lower legs) are taken into account when describing a horse as being of a particular colour. The colour is created by the mixture within the coat of red, black and white hairs.

BRANDS

Branding may be carried out either for security purposes (where a code is painlessly frozen onto the horse and grows back as white hair) or to mark a horse with the crest of its particular breed and/or grade within a breed or a herd number, when it is usually done on the shoulder or quarters. Papers

relating to the brand should always change hands with the horse.

SCARS AND OLD INJURIES

These are an indisputable way of recognising a particular animal and will be included on a veterinary certificate even when they are not expected to affect the soundness of the horse. Unless the horse is required for showing purposes, most working animals have taken a knock at some time or another and this is not necessarily a defect.

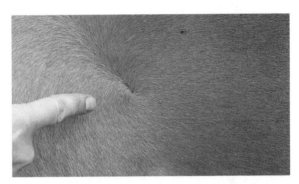

Whorls, where the growth of the coat hair changes direction, are the equine equivalent of the human fingerprint. Every individual has a unique pattern and combination of whorls.

WHORLS

Whorls are points at which the hair changes direction, showing as a specific swirling pattern on the coat. As their number and precise location is unique to each horse, whorls provide another accurate and indisputable means of identifying individual animals in a similar way to human finger-printing. Whorls must be marked on a horse's identification papers.

AGE

The age of a horse or pony is taken from January 1 in the year of its birth. The term 'rising' is used when a horse is approaching its next 'birthday'. Any young animal is described as a 'foal' (colt foal or filly foal depending on the sex) for its first year and 'yearling' for the subsequent year.

Determining the exact age of a horse that does not

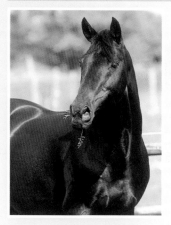

◀ **Black:** *must be totally black all over the body, including the points*

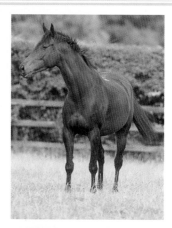

◀ **Brown:** *dark brown (sometimes almost black), but with brown points*

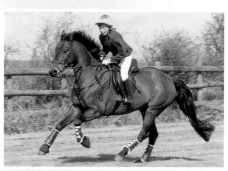

▲ **Bay:** *brown coat varying in shade from tan ('light') to reddish-brown ('bright') or dark brown ('dark'), with black points.*

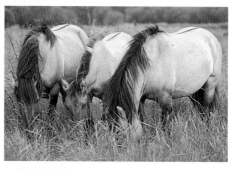

▲ **Dun:** *light-coloured coat with black points, frequently showing eel stripe and possibly, zebra marks on the legs. Body colour varies from 'mouse' (a blueish-grey shade sometimes termed 'blue dun') to shades of golden (often termed 'yellow dun').*

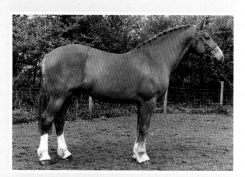

▲ **Chestnut:** *ginger or reddish colour, with mane and tail of the same or slightly darker or lighter shade.*

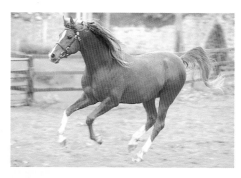

▲ *Variations include 'light', 'dark' and 'liver' (above). Significantly lighter manes and tails are described as 'flaxen'.*

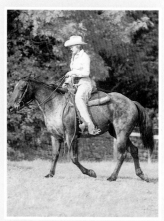

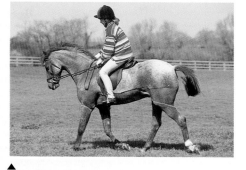

◀ **Roan:** *a coat having an even spread of white hairs within it, described according to the base colour either as 'strawberry' (chestnut base – above), 'red' (bay base – left), or 'blue' (dark brown/bay or black base).*

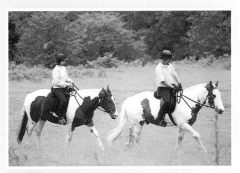

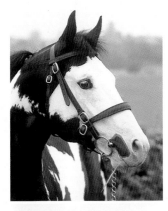

◄ **Piebald:** *large, irregular patches of white and black.*

▲ **Skewbald:** *large, irregular patches of white with any other colour except black.*

In the US, 'broken-coloured' horses, such as the piebald and skewbald, are collectively described as 'pinto'. Here the Pinto has its own breed register and animals are bred for specific characteristics in addition to colour. Coat markings fall into the categories 'overo' (white splashes on a dark base, usually with a white head) and 'tobiano' (regular, solid patterns of dark on a white base).

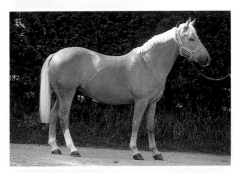

◄ **Palomino:** *golden coat varying in shade from light cream to richer ginger, with flaxen mane and tail. May be registered with its own society in many countries, notably the US where specific breeding criteria also apply.*

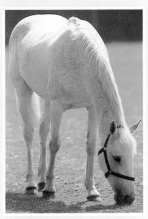

◄ 'Flea-bitten' greys have dark flecks of hair on a light background over the whole body. No horse is ever correctly described as being 'white' – an animal on which white hairs predominate is termed 'light grey'.

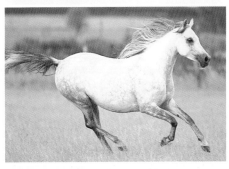

▲ **Grey:** *coat containing mixture of white (unpigmented) and black hairs, the distribution of which determines the exact description. In 'iron grey' black hairs predominate and are evenly spread. A 'dapple grey' (above) has light patches of hair in circles on a darker background.*

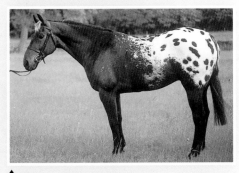

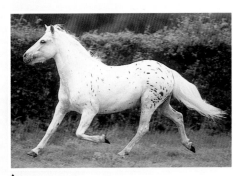

▲
Spotted horses: *a spotted coat can occur within many types, but the spotted 'appaloosa' is officially recognised as a breed in the US. The eight basic spotting patterns are 'snowflake' (dark with white spots all over), 'leopard' (dark spots on a light base); 'frosted hip' (dark with white spots/specks on quarters), 'marble' (mottled roan or bay with darker patches), 'white blanket' (dark forehead with white hindquarters without spotting), 'spotted blanket' (dark forehand, white over quarters with dark spots), 'near leopard' (leopard spotted body with different-coloured head/legs); and 'few-spot leopard' (white with a few scattered roan patches or spots). Skin is always mottled and the eye encircled with white. Hooves are often striped.*

Ahorse may be completely without white markings on either his face or legs. Most animals, however, do have a combination of the following markings.

On the face:

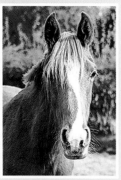

▲ A narrow stripe down the middle of the face and white lip marks, covering all or part of the nostrils.

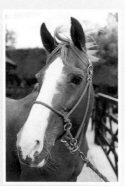

▲ A blaze, which extends over the face from eyes to nostrils.

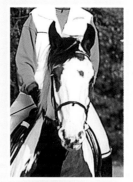

▲ A white face, as above but including the eyes and nostrils.

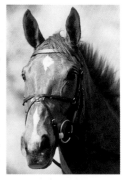

▲ A snip of white between the nostrils and a star between the eyes.

On the legs:

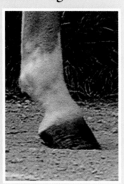

▲ Sock, extending to the fetlock or slightly above.

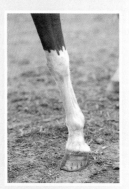

▲ Stocking, extending to the knee or hock.

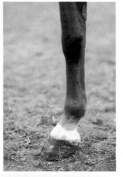

▲ White markings can also be more precisely described by referring to the part of the leg to which they extend, e.g. 'white heel/coronet/pastern', or 'white to half-cannon'.

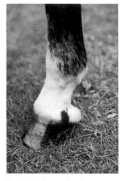

▲ Ermine marks are dark spots or flecks within a white area on the lower legs.

An **eel stripe**, commonly seen on dun-coloured ponies of native origin, is a dark stripe running down the length of the spine from crest to tail (see photo, page 264). **'Zebra' markings**, faint horizontal stripes on the back of the lower legs, are similarly seen on some natives and again indicate primitive breeding.

A **wall eye** is often seen in dun, palomino or cream-coloured horses or those where a white facial marking extends over one or both eyes. It denotes an eye with an unpigmented iris, showing more white than usual around the pupil.

possess official papers is difficult, particularly after the age of five when the full set of adult teeth is established. However, a vet or equine dentist can make an educated guess by looking at the length and shape of the horse's teeth (see panel). Horses are frequently described as simply 'aged' when they pass the age of eight.

PROPHET'S THUMB-MARK
This mark, seen occasionally particularly in horses of oriental breeding, appears as an indentation in the muscle, often on the neck or quarters. It is traditionally said to be a sign of quality, but does not seem to affect the horse in any way.

ASSESSING AGE FROM THE TEETH

Documentary evidence showing the date of birth is the only way to be certain of a particular horse's age. The traditional method of checking teeth to assess the age is now known to be very imprecise, providing only an informed estimate. It is based on changes in the shape, appearance and angle of the incisors as they are gradually worn away through use. However, the link between tooth age and wear is strong only up to around 6 years old, after which it begins to weaken, markedly so beyond the age of 11.

MILK OR PERMANENT?
The temporary milk teeth begin erupting from birth and by the age of two, all are present. These small, white, smooth teeth are upright, with oval surfaces (tables) that carry faint marks. Age determination in young horses is based on when the milk teeth are replaced by the permanent, adult teeth and the point at which these grow to come into contact with the opposite jaw and so begin to be worn (around six months).

At around $2^1/2$ years, the central two milk teeth in the lower jaw are pushed out by the growing permanent teeth. Eruption occurs at $3^1/2$ years for the neighbouring lateral incisors and $4^1/2$ years for the corners, which take until around 6 years of age to come fully into use. The canines appear at around the age of four. The front permanent pre-molars and molars start arriving at around 6 to 9 months and are all present by around 4 years.

WEAR & TEAR?
Once the front teeth are all permanent, by around 5 years, age assessment becomes more difficult. Mouth abnormalities, breeding, stable 'vices', diet and type of grazing can all influence the amount of wear shown by teeth, leading to two horses of the same age appearing to differ widely.

CUP AND STARS
Wear on the patterns on the tables (biting surfaces) of the incisors are the most reliable measurements of age. Young horses have a large, circular, dark depression on the tables, well-defined by a rim of white enamel. This is known as the 'cup mark' or infundibulum. At around 8 years old, a brown streak known as the 'dental star' is also created as the pulp cavity begins to be exposed at the front of the cup. This is less well-defined but becomes wider and more central with age. Both marks are present until around the age of 10 or 12, the cup becoming shallower and smaller, firstly in the central incisors, then the laterals and finally the corners, until by the age of 13, only the dental star is visible.

GROOVES & HOOKS
The back edge of the upper corner tooth sometimes shows a hook at around 7 years old, which tends to wear flat but still overlap the lower corner tooth, by eight. However, this notch can appear at around 11 and 20 years. Inconsistencies like this are common, particularly in the teeth of 6, 7 and 8 year olds. The sides of the upper corner teeth start to show a small, darkly-stained groove at around the age of ten. Known as 'Galvayne's groove', this slowly extends down the tooth until it reaches the whole length at around 20 years. During the next five years it fades from the top half, disappearing completely by 30 years.

INCREASING AGE
An overall impression of advancing age is given by lengthening of the teeth and increased slope, caused by continuing growth and the recession of the gums. Yellowing also occurs, and the tables also take on a more circular and then triangular shape.

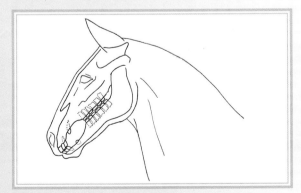

▲ *The arrangement of the teeth in the horse's mouth. In each jaw, an adult horse has six incisors, used for biting and tearing grass, and twelve molars (three pre-molars and three molars) for grinding. Males also have one upper and one lower canine tooth (tushes) which lie between the incisors and molars, at the front of the area of gum known as the 'bars' of the mouth. Small additional pre-molars or 'wolf' teeth are occasionally present in the upper jaw and, rarely, also in the lower jaw.*

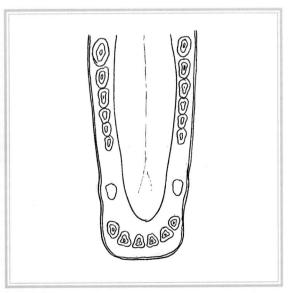

▲ *On both the top jaw and bottom jaw (shown), the middle two incisors are the 'centrals'. The next two are termed the 'laterals' and the next the 'corners'.*

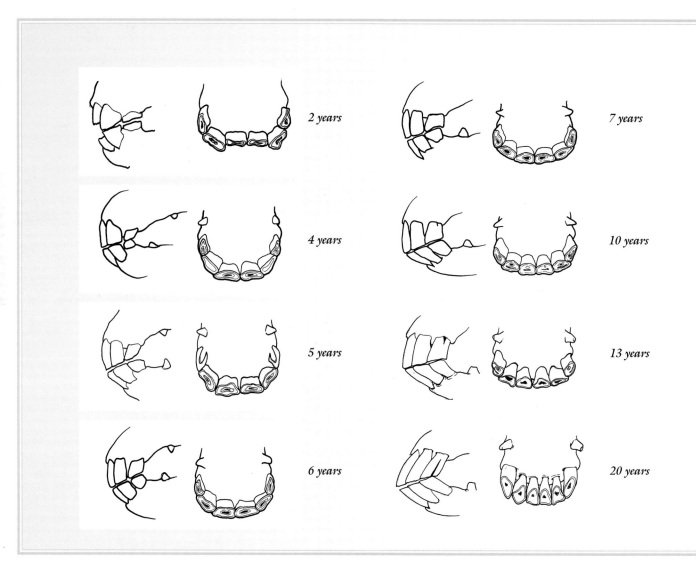

2 years

7 years

4 years

10 years

5 years

13 years

6 years

20 years

POINTS OF THE HORSE

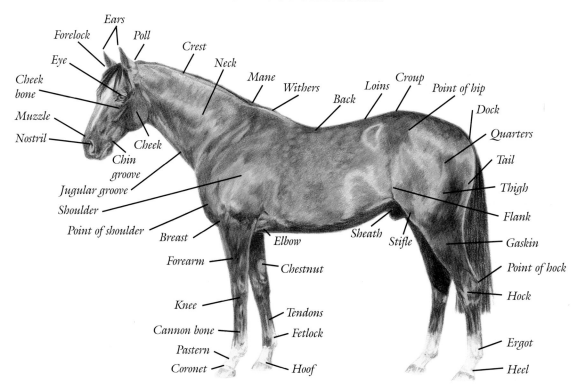

Ears
Forelock
Poll
Eye
Crest
Neck
Cheek bone
Mane
Withers
Back
Loins
Croup
Point of hip
Muzzle
Dock
Nostril
Quarters
Cheek
Tail
Chin groove
Thigh
Jugular groove
Flank
Shoulder
Gaskin
Point of shoulder
Sheath
Stifle
Point of hock
Breast
Elbow
Hock
Forearm
Chestnut
Knee
Tendons
Cannon bone
Fetlock
Ergot
Pastern
Heel
Coronet
Hoof

ASSESSING CONFORMATION

Basic conformation is the foundation framework upon which a horse is made. Good and bad conformation makes for the working capabilities of the animal. A horse with good conformational make-up will stand more work and should stay sound longer than the animal with poor conformation. Although types and, of course, show quality, will vary between different breeds, a horse that is able to withstand the strains and stresses of everyday use must be made up as near to theoretically 'correct' conformation as possible. Fat and muscle on an animal can hide a multitude of faults on the main body mass itself, but the same cannot be said of the feet and limbs.

The business of learning about conformation can be complicated but, if one is willing to watch, look and learn, it is a fascinating subject.

WHAT IS 'IDEAL' CONFORMATION?

It is essential that any horse will, throughout its lifetime, stand up to the kind of work it is expected to do. When assessing conformation, the purpose for which the animal is to be used must be taken into consideration. Event horses, for example, will need correct limbs and feet but can be of the lighter-framed type, or might be a rib 'too long', or have a plain head. Of greater importance is that this horse is a good mover and is hard and tough in his constitution.

Racehorses come in all shapes and sizes, but the one thing trainers insist on is a very well-shaped fore-leg and shoulder, the reason being that at speed, galloping and in jumping, enormous strain is placed on the forehand (the front half of the body).

The conformation of the show horse or pony should be as near correct as possible, but it is the unique overall 'presence' of the horse that gives it that look of something special.

THE BASIC PRINCIPLES OF CONFORMATION

The ground rules of good conformation remain the same for a pony as for a hunter – type should be the only difference between the two. As the animal's make-up and conformation determine its balance, it therefore influences its way of going. This explains why a well put-together animal finds it easier to perform than a poorly-conformed one.

Head A quality animal will have a fine, clean-cut head with good bone structure. For showing, the

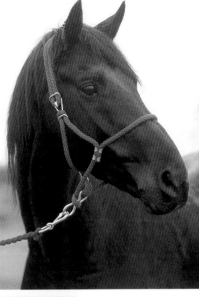

Head shape varies greatly ▶ between breeds and types. The factors common to a good head include clearly-defined bone structure and a kind, bold eye.

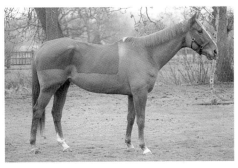

▲ In general terms, a horse or pony with correct conformation forms a balanced whole and an over-all impression that is pleasing to the eye. Each part is in proportion and equally developed.

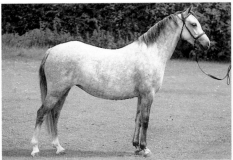

▲ The neck and the way it is set on, must be considered as a unit. The neck should be well-muscled and longer along the 'top-line' than underneath. The 'ewe-necked' horse shown effectively carries his neck 'upside-down' and will find it difficult to flex correctly. His high withers will create problems when fitting the saddle.

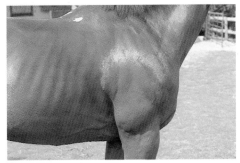

▲ The more upright the shoulder, as shown, the more 'choppy' the horse's action will be. A sloping shoulder allows for free movement and extension of the fore-limbs.

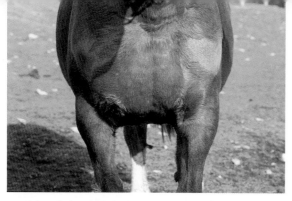

▲ *A broad chest is desirable, although too much width will produce a rolling action.*

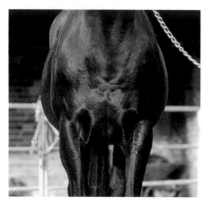

◄ *The narrow-chested horse is likely to knock into himself with his fore-limbs and has little heart-room.*

head should ideally be attractive, but although a quality, chiselled head is desirable, it must always be remembered that a horse will never go lame because he has a plain head!

Neck The neck must be longer on the top-line than underneath, creating an arch from the wither to poll. The top-line should be well-muscled and the general length of the neck should be in balance with the rest of the animal. Avoid the mistake of confusing what is simply a long neck with a 'good front', which is dependent on the neck and shoulders seen together, as a unit. The ideal front consists of a neck that is in proportion to a good, sloping shoulder and well-defined wither. The angle at which the neck leaves the shoulder is significant – too low and the horse will find balancing, and therefore carrying itself, difficult, and being light in front when ridden will not come easily.

Withers These should be pronounced and fine. Withers which sit lower than the top of the quarters give a downhill ride, whereas flat withers cause the saddle to roll about or even to move forwards. Upright shoulders have the same effect, and broad, lumpy shoulders restrict the horse's movement.

Chest The chest should neither be too narrow, nor too broad, when viewed from the front. Too narrow a chest gives the impression of a weak animal and may cause it to move close in front. Too wide creates a 'bosomy' look and a tendency for the horse to roll in its movement.

Body The ideal body is short and deep, enabling the horse to carry condition easily. A long-backed, narrow-bodied horse will have difficulty in carrying condition when in full work. After strenuous work this type will look hollow and empty and may have to wear a breast girth or breast plate to keep the saddle in the correct place. The tall, leggy animal is at a disadvantage in many ways, whereas the compact, deep horse will not only hold its condition but look well. The distance from the last rib to the hip bone should not be too great – a hand's breadth is ideal. A horse that is slack here is weak through the loins and, again, finds holding condition difficult.

Back A hollow back, although comfortable for the rider, is a weakness. The opposite, a roach back, is stronger but less supple makes the horse uncomfortable to ride. The muscles along the side of the back should be higher than the bones of the

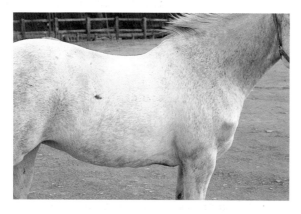

▲ *The hollowed ('dipped' or 'sway') back (above) or over-long back (below) are both prone to muscle and ligament strain and are weak in comparison to a compact, 'short-coupled' horse.* ▼

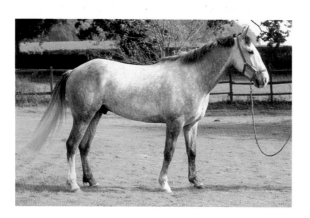

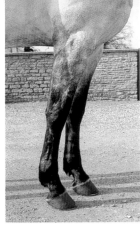
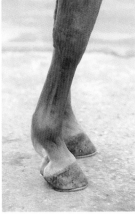

ABOVE LEFT: Forelegs that are 'back at the knee' show a concave, rather than convex profile, and put added strain on the tendons. Frequently they are also 'tied in' below the knee, i.e. the measurement around the cannon at this point is less than that further down.

ABOVE RIGHT: Being 'over at the knee' is not considered a serious fault.

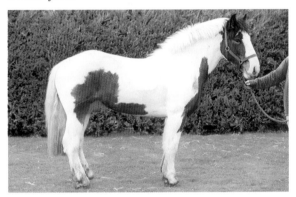

▲ *Hocks should be positioned directly under the centre of gravity of the quarters. Hocks that are too 'bent' or too far forward, as shown, are weak and termed 'sickle hocks'.*

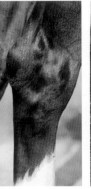
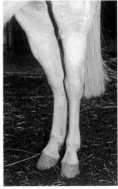
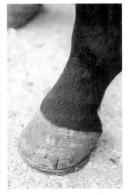

ABOVE LEFT: The hock joint viewed from the side should appear wide above and below, with no lumps or signs of puffiness.

ABOVE MIDDLE: Any deviation in the straightness of the hocks will make them prone to strains. 'Cow hocks' turn inwards, forcing the toes out.

ABOVE RIGHT: An upright pastern (shown) will not absorb concussion well. More length produces a smoother action with greater 'spring'. Over-long pasterns will be weak and force the bodyweight back on to the horse's heels (see Chapter Four) making him susceptible to corns, bruising and other foot problems.

spine. When assessing the back, it should look as if the saddle would sit in position on it without a girth.

Fore-legs The fore-leg should not be light of bone, nor should it have long, weak cannons or small knees. It must have good, flat bone with large knees and fluted tendons. A fore-leg that is 'back at the knee' (see photo, top left) is a fault, as this puts unnecessary strain on the tendons. Being 'over at the knee', however, is not considered a fault. The cannon bone, whether below the knee or the hock, should be the same width all the way down.

Hind legs A good, strong hind leg with a robust second thigh is the ideal. There should not be too much bend in the hock, but neither should the hocks be too straight. They should be placed directly under the centre of gravity and be well let-down, having the appearance of being close to the floor. A hock viewed from the side should look wide above and below, with no signs of puffiness.

The pasterns of the fore and hind legs should be both of average length and angle, able to take the amount of strain given them. Pasterns that are too short and upright lead to jarring and unsoundness, while over-long pasterns are weak and put undue strain on the tendons (see Chapter Four).

Feet The old saying "No foot, no horse" is so true, even today. Animals with bad feet rarely stay sound, they are difficult to keep well-shod and are a groom and a farrier's nightmare. To be correct, the foot should be of average size and of an even, round appearance. Over-large feet often render the animal clumsy and liable to knock its joints. Small feet are undesirable, particularly if of a 'boxy' appearance. Extremes are to be avoided. Big, flat, low-heeled feet often lead to unsoundness and are particularly prone to corns (see Chapter Four). There is often talk of black-coloured hooves being stronger than white ones, although experts will say there cannot be any difference in the hardiness of the horn structure.

Horses with odd feet are often viewed with suspicion, although in some cases this difference is congenital. Foreign-bred horses may be considered cautiously by the British because they often do have small, boxy feet. Nine times out of ten, however, the horse proves everyone wrong by staying extremely sound.

CONFORMATION AND MOVEMENT
A good mover moves from its entire shoulder, with elevation of the knee and extension of the whole

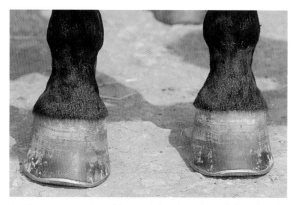

▲ *Foot shape varies with breed, but ideally each foot should create an angle of 45-50 degrees to the ground. Upright, 'boxy' feet (as shown) absorb concussion poorly. Shallow, spread-out feet are generally weak with a flat sole and low heels that give the foot little protection*

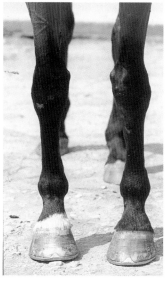

◄ *Straightness is important in all four limbs, with each set of fore and hind limbs making an even pair and pointing straight forwards. Inward-turning ('pigeon') toes, as shown, are unsightly and will put uneven wear on the leg joints. Outward-turning feet make a horse prone to brushing.*

fore-leg. In order to be free-moving, the elbows must be placed well away from the ribs. Take care not to confuse a high knee action with elevation. The elevation that enables the foreleg to move up and out is different to the natural high-stepping action of the Hackney or harness horse (although the best of these do also have elevation). It is the 'up-and-down', choppy action in either a ride or a drive animal that is undesirable.

No horse can be described as a 'good mover' unless it moves equally well behind as in front, a point that is often overlooked. The rear end is the engine that produces impulsion. Hocks brought well underneath the body in turn lighten the forehand, making for a comfortable, well-balanced ride.

The horse or pony should also move dead straight, his hind feet following in the track of the forefeet. A good mover at the walk over-steps with his hind feet the print made by the forefeet. Dishing, or any movement which throws the feet out sideways, is undesirable, as it often causes undue strain of the foreleg, leading to wear on the joints and even to splints. When the two front feet move too closely or even cross over, known as plaiting, the animal will often knock itself, causing repeated injury.

OVERALL IMPRESSIONS

Whilst the overall impression of an animal is very important, it must not be misleading when judging the animal's actual correctness. A pretty animal with a shiny coat and flashy movement should not be allowed to disguise poor limbs and feet. Nevertheless, the initial impression is particularly important for the show horse, which must make a good picture that is pleasing to the eye.

On first walking into a horse's stable, if you do not like the animal then the chances are that you never will. Some animals do 'grow' on you, but this is generally where 'quality' comes in, and quality depends on bone structure. Although apparently having quality, the one horse to avoid is the blood 'weed', a type which oozes 'quality' yet has no substantial 'limb' and will never stand any serious work.

In conclusion, the reasoning behind good conformation is to enable the animal to function correctly. Correct make-up is not a necessity in show animals alone, that must 'look correct'. It is vital to any competition animal to allow it to compete soundly in its chosen sphere. Every small reason behind the rights and wrongs of conformation are factors that enable the animal to stay sound.

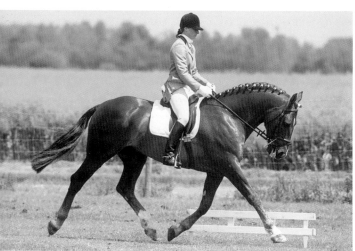

▲ *A horse that moves well uses its whole shoulder to elevate and extend the fore-leg. Hocks brought well forwards under the body create impulsion that lightens the forehand and produces a free, smooth and balanced ride.*